NATIONAL BEST SELLER

Gluten Free

The Definitive Resource Guide

Shelley Case, BSc, RD
Registered Dietitian

July 25/17

Melanie
Nice to meet you on the
Farm to Fork Tour 2017 in
Saskatoon, Saskatchewan!
Blessings,
Shelley

i

Gluten Free – The Definitive Resource Guide

by Shelley Case, BSc, RD (Registered Dietitian)

First Edition (*Gluten-Free Diet: A Comprehensive Resource Guide*) – May 2001
Revised Edition – April 2002
Third Printing – July 2003
Fourth Printing – May 2004
Fifth Printing – January 2005
Expanded Edition – April 2006
Revised-Expanded Edition – October 2008
Eighth Printing – January 2010
Ninth Printing – December 2010
Fifth Edition (*Gluten Free: The Definitive Resource Guide*) – September 2016

Published by:
Case Nutrition Consulting, Inc.
Suite 1403 | 3520 Hillsdale St.
Regina, Saskatchewan
Canada S4S 5Z5

www.shelleycase.com
info@glutenfreediet.ca
Phone/FAX: 306-751-1000

Library and Archives Canada Cataloguing in Publication

Case, Shelley, author
Gluten free : the definitive resource guide / Shelley Case, BSc, RD Registered Dietitian. -- Fifth edition.

Previously published under title: Gluten-free diet : a comprehensive resource guide.
Includes bibliographical references and index.
ISBN 978-0-9937199-0-5 (paperback)

1. Gluten-free diet--Handbooks, manuals, etc. 2. Gluten-free diet--Recipes.
I. Case, Shelley. Gluten-free diet, a comprehensive resource guide. II. Title.

RM237.86.C38 2016   613.2'68311   C2016-905305-9

Cover design by:
Larry Mader, LM Publications, Regina, Saskatchewan

Printed and produced in Canada by:
Friesens Book Division
One Printers Way, Altona, MB, Canada R0G 0B0
204-324-6401
www.friesens.com

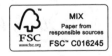

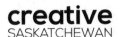

Made possible through Creative Saskatchewan's
Creative Industries Production Grant Program

Dedication

To Jesus Christ

- Who gives meaning and purpose to my life
- For His amazing love, wisdom, strength and answers to prayer
- For His countless blessings, especially my family

To my husband, Blair

- The love of my life for more than 36 years
- For your incredible devotion, patience and support
- Without you I would not be where I am today

To my daughters, Erin and Jennifer

- For your encouragement and unconditional love

To my mother, Helen

- For your wonderful support, generosity and encouragement

To my late father, Gord

- Whose entrepreneurial spirit taught me that anything is possible

Praise for Gluten Free: The Definitive Resource Guide

"Shelley Case has a gift. She takes the complicated issue of gluten intolerance and not only clears the confusion, but shares user-friendly information that consumers can immediately put to use in alleviating symptoms and returning to good health. Her books and website are the first resources I recommend for anyone needing to eliminate gluten and stay well nourished. Shelley is completely immersed in the research and works tirelessly to keep consumers and health professionals accurately informed."
Patricia Chuey, MSc, RD, FDC, The People's Dietitian; Former Chair, Board of Directors, Dietitians of Canada, Vancouver, BC

"Amidst the hype and noise about the gluten-free diet, for those with celiac disease and gluten-sensitivity, it's vitally important to have a reliable source for managing the diet successfully. Shelley's new book is thorough, packed with nutritional information and gives real facts to people who have a medical necessity for a strict gluten-free diet."
Alice Bast, President and CEO, Beyond Celiac

"I give Shelley's book two thumbs up! I recommend this complete, well-researched and useful tool to both patients and health care professionals who need an excellent resource for managing celiac disease and other gluten-related disorders. Thanks Shelley, you make my job easier!"
Pam Cureton, RDN, LDN, Past Chair, Dietitians in Gluten Intolerance Diseases (a subunit of the Medical Nutrition Practice Group, Academy of Nutrition and Dietetics); Dietitian, Center for Celiac Research, Boston, MA

"Shelley's book is the best gluten-free resource and I always recommend it to my patients. I am really looking forward to the new edition, as are my patients. Thank you Shelley, for all you do for patients with celiac disease!"
Dr. Sheila Crowe, MD, Professor of Medicine and Director of Research, Division of Gastroenterology and Director, UCSD Celiac Disease Clinic, Department of Medicine, University of California, San Diego, CA

"I've recommended Shelley Case's book to my patients with gluten-related disorders since the very first edition. I trust the research and respect the dedication and care that she put into writing this educational book. The material is equally useful for those newly diagnosed learning about hidden gluten as for those seeking ways to increase variety in their diets with new products, grains, recipes and meal plans."
Melinda Dennis, MS, RD, LDN, Nutrition Coordinator, Celiac Center at Beth Israel Deaconess Medical Center; Co-Author of *Real Life with Celiac Disease;* Founder/Owner Delete the Wheat, LLC.

"This is the book I have been waiting for, to recommend to ALL my patients with celiac disease. It is a MUST-READ for everyone who needs a gluten-free diet."
Dr. Cynthia Rudert, MD, F.A.C.P., Gastroenterologist, Atlanta, GA

"Shelley has produced a thoughtful, well-researched book. As a leading nutrition expert in celiac disease, she has given the celiac community the foundation for a long, healthy gluten-free lifestyle."
Elaine Monarch, Founder, Celiac Disease Foundation

"The new edition of Shelley Case's book is comprehensive, authoritative and a valuable resource for those currently maintaining or transitioning to a gluten-free diet. Shelley discusses a variety of important topics, from hidden sources of gluten to meal planning and proper nutrition. This book will help you navigate and understand the gluten-free options, stay positive and focused on the foods you can eat and enjoy a healthy, balanced diet."
Marilyn Geller, Chief Executive Office, Celiac Disease Foundation

"This book contains a wealth of information useful for everyone interested in an accurate resource for the gluten-free diet."
Cynthia Kupper, RD, CD, Executive Director, Gluten Intolerance Group of North America, Seattle, WA

"Shelley's book was the first one I read when I started working with gluten-free clients. I believe that all dietitians should have this book in their library. This new edition keeps pace with ever-changing information and research, and it will continue to be my go-to reference for years to come!"
Amy Jones, MS, RDN, LD, Chair, Dietitians in Gluten Intolerance Diseases (a subunit of the Medical Nutrition Practice Group, Academy of Nutrition and Dietetics)

"Shelley Case's *Guide* is an exhaustive and definitive book that will answer all your questions about products, ingredients and the gluten-free diet. It's filled with the most up-to-date information and is a must-have for anyone with celiac disease or gluten sensitivity. I keep a copy at my desk and one in my kitchen. Thanks Shelley. You are a godsend for all of us."
Beth Hillson, Author of *The Complete Guide to Living Well Gluten Free*

"Having been diagnosed with celiac disease and practicing as a Registered Dietitian for over 30 years, I know the importance of professional-looking, detailed and accurate information. Shelley's book accomplishes this and much more! I highly recommend this book to people with celiac disease, as well as dietitians, physicians and other health professionals."
Mark A. Dinga, MEd, RD, LDN, Pittsburgh, PA

"Shelley's book provides solid, evidenced-based information that empowers individuals with celiac disease to lead a happy and healthy gluten-free life. Her contributions to the disease and diet knowledge base, not to mention her insights into the food industry, are fundamental to the quality of life we enjoy today. Sufficient praise cannot be bestowed upon this hard-working, tenacious and ever-optimistic advocate! With this edition, you've done it again, Shelley!"
Ellen Bayens, Founder and President, The Celiac Scene, Victoria, BC, Canada

"Whether you are just starting the gluten-free journey or are a seasoned expert seeking a more healthy diet, Shelley does an outstanding job of researching and presenting all the information you need to know. This resource teaches you how to eat a healthy, nutritionally balanced and safe gluten-free diet. The learning curve is steep, but Shelley makes it feel doable!"
Sheila Horine, Branch Manager, Gluten Intolerance Group of Asheville, NC

"Shelley's book is a wonderful well-researched resource and an indispensable tool for people with celiac disease and for any health professional who is working with the celiac community."
Mary K. Sharrett, MS, RD, LD, CNSC, Nutrition Support Dietitian, Children's Hospital and Founder / Dietitian Advisor of the Gluten-Free Gang, Columbus, OH

"This must-have book is an extremely comprehensive resource for anyone following a gluten-free diet. Well-written and professionally researched, this thorough and invaluable reference helps those who must follow a gluten-free diet regain their quality of life. Highly recommended!"
Kim Koeller, Founder of GlutenFree Passport and Author of *Let's Eat Out Around the World Gluten Free and Allergy Free*

"Shelley Case's book contains an amazing wealth of practical information you can put to immediate use to maintain a healthy gluten-free diet, and keep as a reference for years, as I have. It's like having a wise friend to guide you through the maze of information out there and highlight the best."
Jennifer Iscol, President, Celiac Community Foundation of Northern California

"As cookbook authors, we do not hesitate to recommend the new edition of Shelley's resource guide. We know that it contains the latest information and is well researched, accurate and extremely helpful to a new or seasoned person with celiac disease."
Donna Washburn, PHEc and **Heather Butt, PHEc**, Authors of *Easy Everyday Gluten-Free Cooking*, *Great Gluten-Free Whole-Grain Bread Machine Recipes*, *The Gluten-Free Baking Book*, *125 Best Gluten-Free Bread Machine Recipes*, *250 Gluten-Free Favorites* and *Complete Gluten-Free Cookbook*

"Each edition of Shelley's book keeps getting better. It incorporates the latest information about the gluten-free diet and is full of practical advice."
Dr. Elena F. Verdu, MD, PhD, Associate Professor of Medicine, Division of Gastroenterology, McMaster University, Hamilton, ON, Canada

"As the corporate dietitian for a regional supermarket chain, I know how important it is to guide our customers to science-based, practical resources when they have questions about diseases or special diets. Shelley Case's books have been and will continue to be go-to resources for those who need to follow a gluten-free diet."
Leah McGrath, RD, Corporate Dietitian, Ingles Markets, Asheville, NC

"I needed this book before I accumulated the mountain of computer printouts and handouts that adorn my office. Buy it or spend the next 20 years of your life unnecessarily duplicating this research."
Jacqueline Jones, Humboldt, TN

"Shelley Case is one of the foremost experts on the gluten-free diet. There is a lot of 'bad' information out there about the diet, but Shelley's book can be trusted to be current, accurate, and thoroughly researched."
Danna Korn, Founder of ROCK (Raising Our Celiac Kids) and Author of *Kids with Celiac Disease: A Family Guide to Raising Happy, Healthy, Gluten-Free Children* and *Wheat-Free, Worry-Free: The Art of Happy, Healthy Gluten-Free Living*

"A concise resource with all the key information clinicians AND patients frequently need to get started. I highly recommend this book as the first one to buy to all patients referred to the nutrition clinic here with celiac disease."
Carol Rees Parrish, MS, RD, Nutrition Support Specialist, University of Virginia Health System, Digestive Health Center, Charlottesville, VA

"This is a must-read for anyone living a gluten-free lifestyle. Shelley's tips, tricks and resources are invaluable for those who are new to the gluten-free diet, as well as those who have been living this way for years."
Jen Cafferty, Founder and CEO, The Gluten Free Media Group

"This is a phenomenal book. Shelley has managed to research, compile and organize volumes of valuable information and present it in a logical manner that is easy to understand. It is the most thorough gluten-free reference book on the market today."
Connie Sarros, Author of *Wheat-Free, Gluten-Free* cookbooks

"With all of the confusing and inaccurate information out there today, Shelley does an outstanding job setting the record straight. Her coverage of the gluten-free diet is comprehensive and well-researched. It is an excellent resource for patients and medical professionals alike."
Trisha B. Lyons, RD, LD, Outpatient Dietitian, MetroHealth Medical Center, Cleveland, OH

"I highly recommend this book as a true 'resource' for those who are gluten sensitive."
Ann Whelan, Founder, *Gluten-Free Living* magazine, New York, NY

"Shelley Case should be congratulated for her efforts in contributing such a valuable reference tool to the field of celiac disease."
Mavis Molloy, RDN, Dietitian, Past Member of the Professional Advisory Board, Canadian Celiac Association

"This is a must-have book for dietitians, doctors and patients. It is a critical component to the nutrition education sessions I provide and is an excellent resource for products and recipes."
Jacquelyn Stern, RD, LD, Annapolis Nutrition, Annapolis, MD

"Each edition of Shelley Case's *Resource Guide* gets better and better with more practical information for all people with wheat and gluten sensitivities. A 'must-have' resource for the newly diagnosed person with celiac disease."
Janet Y. Rinehart, Former President, Celiac Support Association

"Shelley Case's book is an excellent guide for anyone following a gluten-free diet. As a researcher and someone living with celiac disease, I am so grateful for this thorough and detailed resource."
Dr. Justine Dowd, PhD, Post-Doctoral Fellow, Health Psychology, University of British Columbia, Okanagan Campus, Kelowna, BC, Canada

"This guide is full of information on what's safe and healthy for people with celiac disease, and is presented in a practical, clearly organized 'no-nonsense' format. It is a must for the celiac bookshelf."
Bev Ruffo, Honorary Life Member, Canadian Celiac Association

"This is more than 5 stars! Without question, this is THE resource to have if you or a family member has celiac disease. It is a book that you will refer to over and over again. And, a great one to share with physicians and teachers."
Andrea S. Levario, JD, Former Executive Director, American Celiac Disease Alliance

"I am tremendously grateful for Shelley's book! This is THE most comprehensive resource on the gluten-free diet. I highly recommend this book to everyone needing accurate and practical information about the gluten-free lifestyle."
Lynn Shadle-Gabriel, Celiac Disease Foundation Minnesota Support Group, Minneapolis, MN

Acknowledgements

When I contemplate the African proverb "It takes a village to raise a child," I think of the wonderful group of people involved in creating this book. I would like to acknowledge them and also the spirit of their contributions. From family and friends, to dietitians, physicians, authors, government departments in Canada and the United States, the food industry and others in the gluten-free community, your generosity in providing information and help has been truly amazing. I am very fortunate to have received such assistance and kindness. The writing of this acknowledgment is a daunting task because there are so very many individuals to whom I owe a great deal.

First and foremost, to my wonderful husband, Blair – words cannot adequately express my heartfelt appreciation for your overwhelming support, patience, understanding, encouragement and love. Thank you for all your help with proofing the manuscript into the wee hours of the morning and all the other "behind-the-scenes" work, not only with this edition but throughout my career. Over the past 17 years of researching and writing each edition and frequently being away from home on speaking engagements, you've always kept the home front running smoothly while also successfully managing your own thriving business. Your incredible sacrifices and selfless devotion to our family and others continues to be one of your very many admirable qualities. I am truly blessed to have such an awesome husband and I love you so much!

Big hugs to my precious daughters, Erin and Jennifer. Thanks for all your fantastic support and love – you're the best!

To my mom, deep gratitude for your support in the production and distribution of my books over the years. Your assistance with editing and proofing is deeply appreciated. Thanks, mom, for *everything*.

I'm forever grateful to Enid Young, former president of the Regina chapter of the Canadian Celiac Association, who believed in my idea for this book from the very beginning. You encouraged and supported me in a variety of ways, including reviewing numerous manuscripts for the first edition of the book.

Wolf Rinke – thank you for inspiring me to "dream big" and change career paths.

My dear friend, mentor and dietitian colleague, Marion Zarkadas – a heartfelt thanks for your excellent advice and editorial assistance with all the editions of my book. Your attention to detail and specific suggestions have been incredibly helpful and I am deeply indebted to you.

Jessica Ethier is an amazing dietitian who has worked tirelessly alongside me for over a year to create this best edition yet. Jessica, your nutrition and gluten-free culinary expertise as well as ability to help me sift through thousands of references and mountains of technical information has been unbelievable. I know you are just as excited as I am to see this book finally published!

Special thanks to dietitian Rhonda Kane for reviewing and editing some of the more challenging sections of the book. Your dedication to sourcing and providing accurate information was outstanding.

Thank you to all the other dietitians, dietetic interns and nutrition students who provided further information, constructive feedback and/or support, especially: Alexandra Anca, Beth Armour, Dina Aronson, Tiffany Banow, Amy Barr, Lisa Chartier, Alex Crerar, Pam Cureton, Jenny Dean, Melinda Dennis, Mark Dinga, Nancy Patin Falini, Kim Faulkner-Hogg, Kelly Fitzpatrick, Jacqueline Gates, Cindy Heroux, Cynthia Kupper, Faith Kwong, Anne Lee, Christine Lionel, Mavis Molloy, Danielle Moore, Carol Rees Parrish, Huda Rashid, Sarah Rohde, Joyce Schnetzler, Jackie See, Mary K. Sharrett, Lauren Swann, Quinci Taylor, Tricia Thompson and Jeannie Zibrida.

I am grateful to the many physicians and scientists who provided technical advice, most notably: Dr. Scott Bean, Dr. Vern Burrows, Dr. Decker Butzner, Dr. Brett Carver, Dr. Carlo Catassi, Dr. Ravi Chibbar, Dr. Pekka Collin, Dr. Sheila Crowe, Dr. Jeff Dahlberg, Dr. Alessio Fasano, Dr. Peter Green, Dr. Don Kasarda, Dr. Ciaran Kelly, Dr. Joseph Murray, Dr. Michelle Pietzak, Dr. Mohsin Rashid, Dr. Lloyd Rooney, Dr. Cynthia Rudert, Dr. Connie Switzer, Dr. Fred Townley-Smith, Dr. Elena Verdu and Dr. Ralph Warren.

Carol Fenster, wonderful friend and colleague, you deserve an enormous Thank You for your expert advice, encouragement and generosity.

My appreciation extends also to all the other gluten-free culinary experts who offered sage advice and practical suggestions, especially Heather Butt, Beth Hillson, Connie Sarros and Donna Washburn.

A special thanks to everyone who contributed recipes: Dina Aronson, Heather Butt, Leslie Cerier, Jessica Ethier, Carol Fenster, Patricia Green, Bruce Gross, Carolyn Hemming, Beth Hillson, Barbara Kliment, Jacqueline Mallorca, Vesanto Melina, Sharon Palmer, Rebecca Reilly, LynnRae Ries, Karen Robertson, Laurie Sadowski, Girma and Ethiopia Sahlu, Rosie Schwartz, Jo Stepaniak, Donna Washburn and Tilly Wiens. Also, thank you to these companies for recipes: Avena Foods, Best Cooking Pulses, The Birkett Mills, Bob's Red Mill, Canadian Lentils, The Flax Council of Canada, Northern Quinoa Corporation, Pulse Canada, Saskatchewan Flax Development Commission, Saskatchewan Pulse Growers, The Teff Company and Wondergrain.

I appreciate all the assistance and academic information from the staff in various agriculture, food and health divisions of government in Canada and the United States.

Thank you to all the food companies and organizations that provided detailed information: Elizabeth Arndt and Don Trouba (Ardent Mills), Steve Rice (Authentic Foods), Margaret Hughes and Trudy Heal (Best Cooking Pulses), Matt Cox, Lindsay Duncan and Cassidy Stockton (Bob's Red Mill), Heather Maskus (Canadian International Grains Institute), Peter Felker (Casa de Mesquite), Raj Sukul and Sylvia Tam (Maplegrove Gluten Free Foods), Josh Deschenes (Nu Life Market), Cynthia Harriman (Oldways / The Whole Grains Council), Elisabeth Carlson (The Teff Company) and Kathleen Apaid (Wondergrain) for their additional support and for digging up hard-to-find information.

Aunt Carolyn – thanks for the many ways in which you helped in the research and reviewing of the book over the years.

Much appreciation goes to Amy Beitel, Donna Poole and Kendra Pottage, my "strong" massage therapists, for helping reduce all those aches and pains resulting from thousands of hours at the computer and on the phone over the past 17 years!

To my editor, Wanda Drury at Green Line Editing – thank you for your amazing attention to detail and ability to shape this book into a polished final version.

I am deeply indebted to Kathryn van der Laan for her incredible proficiency and accuracy in transforming the manuscript into such a professional-looking resource. Kathryn, your willingness to make "a million changes" with such patience and a smile did not go unnoticed!

Thank you to Creative Saskatchewan for supporting this publication through the Creative Industries Production Grant Program.

And to the many other people whose names I have not mentioned but who also contributed to this book, I say a heartfelt Thank You!

Table of Contents

Shelley Case, BSc, RD xii

Preface xiii

Foreword xv

Introduction xvii

Chapter

1   Celiac Disease, Dermatitis Herpetiformis and Non-Celiac Gluten Sensitivity 1
    Celiac Disease 1
    Dermatitis Herpetiformis.. 5
    Non-Celiac Gluten Sensitivity 6
    Medical Nutrition Therapy 8

2   The Gluten-Free Diet 9
    What Is Gluten? 9
    The Gluten-Free Diet Overview 9
    Gluten-Free Diet by Food Groups... 11
    Gluten-Free Additives and Ingredients 25

3   Oats 27
    Overview.. 27
    Reactions to Oats 27
    Gluten-Free Oat Production 28
    Gluten-Free Oat Products 29
    More Information about Gluten-Free Oats 30

4   Alcohol 31
    Distilled Alcohols 32
    Liqueurs 32
    Wines... 32
    Beers.. 33
    Hard Ciders 34
    Specialty Premixed Alcoholic Beverages 34

5   Frequently Questioned Ingredients 35
    Vinegars... 36
    Barley Grass and Wheat Grass 37
    Flavors/Flavorings 37
    Starches 40
    Dextrin 41
    Maltodextrin 41
    Glucose Syrup 41
    Rice Syrup 42

6   Gluten Threshold Levels, Parts Per Million and Testing.............................. 43
    Gluten Threshold Levels.. 43
    Concentration of Gluten in Foods... 44
    Consumption of Gluten-Free Foods 45
    Gluten-Testing Methods.. 46
    Amount of Gluten in Foods 46

7	**Food Labeling**	49
	How to Read a Food Label	49
	Labeling Jurisdictions in North America	51
	Gluten and Food Allergen Labeling	51
	Alcohol Labeling in the United States and Canada	63

8	**Nutrition and the Gluten-Free Diet**	65
	Nutritional Status of Individuals with Celiac Disease	66
	Nutritional Quality of Gluten-Free Specialty Products	66
	Enrichment and Fortification	67
	Specific Nutritional Concerns	67

9	**Gluten-Free Alternatives (Grains, Legumes, Seeds and Starches)**	97
	Grains	97
	Gluten-Free Grains	98
	Legumes	104
	Seeds	108
	Starches	111
	Using Gluten-Free Alternatives	111

10	**Gluten-Free Meal Planning**	115
	Getting Started	115
	A Healthy Gluten-Free Diet	115
	Gluten-Free Meal-Planning Ideas	121

11	**Gluten-Free Shopping**	131
	Shopping Tips	131
	Gluten-Free Shopping List	134

12	**Cross-Contamination: Home and Away from Home**	135
	Preventing Cross-Contamination in the Kitchen	135
	Eating Away from Home	136

13	**Gluten-Free Cooking and Baking**	143
	Gluten-Free Grains	143
	Pulses and Soybeans	145
	Gluten-Free Baking	147
	Thickening Agents in Gluten-Free Cooking	155

| 14 | **Recipes** | 157 |

| 15 | **Gluten-Free Products** | 205 |

| 16 | **Company Directory** | 263 |

| 17 | **Gluten-Free Specialty Retailers** | 287 |

Resources		289
	American Celiac Organizations	289
	Canadian Celiac Organizations	289
	International Celiac Organizations	290
	American Celiac Disease Centers and Programs	291
	Certification of Gluten-Free Products	292
	Websites: Celiac Disease and the Gluten-Free Diet	293
	Books	294

Resources (cont'd)

      Magazines 296

      Cookbooks 297

      Online Cooking Resources 300

      Gluten-Free Product Information 300

      Eating Out and Travel Resources 300

      Gluten-Free Food Service Training and Accreditation Programs 302

      Children's Books 303

      Other Children's Resources 304

      College/University Resources 304

      Medication Resource 304

Appendices 305

  A   Companies with Gluten-Free Oat Products 305

  B   Canadian Celiac Association Professional Advisory Council Position Statement
on Consumption of Oats by Individuals with Celiac Disease 306

  C   American and Canadian Regulations and Guidance Documents 308

  D   Codex Alimentarius Standard for Foods for Special Dietary Use
for Persons Intolerant to Gluten 312

  E   History of Gluten-Free Labeling Regulations:
United States, Canada and the Codex Alimentarius Commission 314

  F   Nutrient Composition of Gluten-Free Grains, Flours, Starches,
Gums, Legumes, Nuts and Seeds 318

  G   Carbohydrate Content of Flours, Starches, Grains, Legumes and Seeds: Highest to Lowest 322

References 324

      Celiac Disease 324

      Dermatitis Herpetiformis 325

      Non-Celiac Gluten Sensitivity 325

      Oats 326

      Foods, Beverages and Ingredients 327

      Gluten Threshold Levels, PPM and Testing 330

      Gluten-Free Labeling Regulations 331

      Codex Alimentarius Commission 336

      Nutrition and the Gluten-Free Diet 336

      Nutrient Composition 338

Index   340

Order Form 349

Shelley Case, BSc, RD

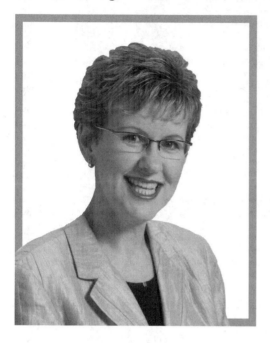

A leading international expert on the gluten-free diet, Shelley is a registered dietitian, author, speaker and consultant with more than 30 years' experience. She is a member of the Medical Advisory Boards of the Celiac Disease Foundation and Gluten Intolerance Group in the United States; Professional Advisory Council of the Canadian Celiac Association; and serves on the Scientific Advisory Board of the Grain Foods Foundation.

Shelley has been featured on radio and television including NBC's *Today* show, CBC, CTV and Global TV, as well as frequently quoted in major print media such as the *Wall Street Journal*, WebMD, *National Post*, *Globe and Mail*, *Food Business News*, *Chatelaine* and *Canadian Living*.

A popular speaker, she delivers presentations at medical, nutrition, celiac and food industry conferences throughout North America. Shelley's best-selling book is highly recommended by health professionals, celiac organizations, consumers and the food industry. Author of many journal articles on celiac disease and the gluten-free diet, she also contributes to a variety of other publications for health professionals and consumers. Her column "Ask the Celiac Expert" is featured in *Allergic Living* magazine.

In recognition of Shelley's major contributions to the field of celiac disease and her dedication to educating health professionals and individuals with celiac disease in North America, she was awarded the Queen Elizabeth Golden Jubilee Medal.

Shelley graduated with a Bachelor of Science Degree in Nutrition and Dietetics from the University of Saskatchewan and completed her Dietetic Internship at the Health Sciences Center in Winnipeg, Manitoba. Over the past 34 years, Shelley has helped thousands of people improve their eating habits and manage a variety of disease conditions through good nutrition. She is founder and president of Case Nutrition Consulting, Inc., a company specializing in celiac disease and the gluten-free diet.

Professionally, Shelley is a member of the Dietitians of Canada, Saskatchewan Dietitians Association and the Academy of Nutrition and Dietetics (U.S.), as well as the Nutrition Entrepreneurs, Dietitians in Business and Communications, Food and Culinary Professionals and the Medical Nutrition Practice Groups of the Academy of Nutrition and Dietetics.

When she is not sharing her nutrition and health expertise, Shelley is very active in her community and church. She is an accomplished musician who enjoys playing piano and keyboard in her church, at special events and for other occasions. She lives with her husband and daughter in Regina, Saskatchewan, Canada.

Preface

In the Beginning

As a new graduate dietitian in 1981, I was excited finally to enter the workforce after five challenging years of university and internship. My passion then, and it continues to this day, was to help people eat nutritiously and thereby to improve their health. In my first job at a large outpatient diabetes and diet education center, I was responsible for counseling children and adults with various conditions including diabetes, heart disease, high blood pressure, obesity, cystic fibrosis, food allergies and gastrointestinal disorders including celiac disease. But while I was well prepared to counsel individuals on many issues stemming from widely varied health concerns, celiac disease definitely was not one of them!

During my internship I had never encountered anyone with the disease, and the relevant information offered in only one nutrition class at university had been minimal, so in that area I clearly was inadequately trained. In preparing to counsel my first client with celiac disease, I remember scrambling to find any useful information whatever about the disease itself, but especially regarding a gluten-free diet. The limited material I did find was out of date and of little use. Realizing I needed help, I contacted the local celiac support group in Regina, Saskatchewan. They welcomed me, taught me a great deal about the disease and diet and provided basic materials for counseling future clients. After attending several meetings, I was asked to be the local celiac chapter dietitian advisor. I accepted the position and, over time, my knowledge of the disease and diet expanded. Ten years later, I was invited to become a member of the Canadian Celiac Association Professional Advisory Board (now called the Professional Advisory Council), a position I have held ever since.

The Birth of an Idea

When I counseled clients with celiac disease, every one of them was seeking very specific and practical information on food labeling and ingredients, names of gluten-free companies/products and where/how to access them, recipes, meal-planning suggestions, tips for eating out, how to prevent cross-contamination and how to locate other gluten-free diet resources. Unfortunately, at that time such information usually was available only from assorted different pamphlets, books, manuals and other sources, which meant that after a counseling session the client went home carrying a loose pile of many papers!

Soon other dietitians in the city and from around the province began to contact me in search of celiac-related information, as they too felt their knowledge of the disease and diet was inadequate. The real and almost urgent need for a more comprehensive resource for both health professionals and clients soon became apparent to me, causing the birth of an idea that eventually evolved into *The Gluten-Free Diet: A Comprehensive Resource Guide*.

Dreams Become a Reality

In 1997 I left a very rewarding career at a hospital to pursue my dream of starting a nutrition consulting business, and a few years later I decided to get serious about turning the gluten-free resource book idea into a reality. I dedicated the next two years to researching and writing that book, which was self-published in May 2001. My next big hurdle was informing health professionals and individuals with celiac disease about this new resource!

Lacking the backing of a large publishing house called for creative promotional strategies on a shoestring budget. As the book became more widely known, I began and continued to receive positive and encouraging feedback both from those with celiac disease and from fellow dietitians. News and enthusiasm about the book continued to spread, and increasingly more of my consulting time became devoted to celiac disease. Through wearing "many hats" – those of marketing representative, shipper and accountant, author and speaker – I gained a new appreciation for the roles of both authors and publishers.

The Continuing Saga

The gluten-free "world" continued to expand. More individuals were being diagnosed with celiac disease, and the number of gluten-free products available in the marketplace was increasing. To reflect the ongoing changes, over the next nine years I published four subsequent editions of my original book. Each edition was updated to include the latest research on the disease itself as well as the current information about products, companies and resources.

In the past five years, there has been an explosion in the type and number of gluten-free products available from both specialty and mainstream food companies, for purchase not only in health food and other retail stores but also online. Further significant changes have occurred in the areas of food labeling and of knowledge about ingredients safety (e.g., oats), as well as an increased awareness about the scope of gluten-related disorders.

In response, I have undertaken a major overhaul of my original book and produced *Gluten Free: The Definitive Resource Guide*. This "labor of love," the result of more than three years of intense effort, unarguably is the best edition yet. The book is jam-packed with new information on frequently questioned ingredients, labeling, gluten testing and meal plan suggestions. It also contains many new shopping, cooking and baking tips; delicious recipes; listings for a host of new products; additional references and much more. And through complete revamping of the layout, the book now is even more highly "user-friendly." I'm thrilled finally to release this new edition that I'm confident will make your gluten-free life easier and healthier!

An Amazing Journey

Thirty-four years ago I never would have dreamed that I would be a dietitian specializing in celiac disease and the gluten-free diet, let alone author of a national best seller or interviewed by Matt Lauer on NBC's *Today* show. Rather ironic for a dietitian from Saskatchewan, the Canadian province known as "the breadbasket of the world!" So, for everyone out there with an idea or dream – pursue it, work hard and never give up. Who knows where your journey will take you?

I'm amazed and truly blessed to have had the opportunity to become involved in the gluten-free world. I have met so many wonderful individuals with the disease, as well as professionals in the fields of health, government, industry and more from around the globe, all working hard to improve the lives of those with gluten-related disorders. The Canadian Celiac Association's motto "Together We're Better" is a worthy ideal. I look forward to working together with you as we continue on this challenging gluten-free journey.

Shelley M. Case, BSc, RD

Foreword

Celiac disease has been part of the medical canon for millennia – since Aretaeus of Cappadocia first described "koiliakos" as "suffering of the bowels" in the second century A.D. For centuries, doctors were puzzled as to what was causing the mainly gastrointestinal and sometimes fatal symptoms (mostly found in children) associated with celiac disease. It was only relatively recently that Dr. Willem-Karel Dicke identified gluten as the food trigger for what is now defined as an autoimmune condition afflicting approximately one percent of the world's population.

In the last 30 years – since I graduated from medical school in Naples, Italy – we have made tremendous strides in treating and diagnosing celiac disease. With new serological markers and genetic tests developed in the late 1990s and beyond, we have highly reliable front line tools to identify individuals most at risk for the disease. In the research arena, we have considerably deepened our understanding of the development and molecular pathways of celiac disease, which provides a model for understanding autoimmunity in general.

Cracking the human genome also has advanced our research efforts. In concert with the genetic pieces of the celiac puzzle, we are now placing an emphasis on the study of the human microbiome. By exploring the microbial colonies in our gut, we are gaining a better understanding of how a person tips from gluten tolerance to full-blown celiac disease. The focus of our research is to lead us to the ultimate goal of preventing this condition, and other autoimmune disorders, before they begin.

Another development during the last three decades, along with a rising rate of celiac disease, is the identification of non-celiac gluten sensitivity or gluten sensitivity. This "new kid on the block" of gluten-related disorders is not an autoimmune condition, although it appears to be connected to mechanisms of the innate immune system. Along with celiac disease, gluten sensitivity also manifests in a variety of extraintestinal symptoms including anemia, "foggy mind," headaches, joint pain and chronic fatigue. Even though many of the symptoms overlap with celiac disease, gluten sensitivity does not result in the intestinal enteropathy that is the hallmark of celiac disease. Unfortunately, at this point in time we have no evidence-based diagnostic biomarker for gluten sensitivity, so it is diagnosed solely by exclusion.

In the meantime, the gluten-free diet, as first implemented by Dicke in 1949, is still the cornerstone treatment for celiac disease, gluten sensitivity and other gluten-related disorders. Trials are underway for alternative treatments to the gluten-free diet, including several promising pharmaceutical treatments and the development of a vaccine. However, the gluten-free diet is still mandatory for all of our patients with celiac disease. Working with a knowledgeable dietitian is key to the successful implementation of the diet to avoid cross-contamination and inadvertent gluten exposure.

The book that you are going to read is similar to having your own personal, highly experienced dietitian guiding you on the gluten-free diet. For more than 30 years, Shelley Case has been a leading figure in the movement to create safe and nutritious eating environments – whether at home or elsewhere – for people with celiac disease and other gluten-related disorders.

First published in 2001, Shelley's book has been used by celiac patients around the world as a guide to safe eating. With a fine eye for detail, Shelley addresses all aspects of the gluten-free diet, from hidden sources of gluten and what foods to avoid to the complex area of food starches and maltodextrin. Her thoroughly researched and accurate information will give readers the confidence they need to shop and eat safely by knowing what to look for, what to avoid and how to read labels.

Once her readers know the basics of the gluten-free diet, Shelley goes on to share all the good things that her patients can eat with meal planning recommendations, healthy recipes and an extensive listing of gluten-free products. As the popularity of the gluten-free diet continues to grow and the number of gluten-free products expands almost daily, it is more important than ever to have a reliable and expert book on the cornerstone treatment for gluten-related disorders. *Gluten Free: The Definitive Resource Guide* is the undisputed leader in teaching individuals the complexities of the gluten-free diet while keeping them safe, well-nourished and healthy.

Alessio Fasano, MD

Director, Center for Celiac Research and Treatment
Massachusetts General Hospital
Boston, Massachusetts, USA

Introduction

In recent years, the term "gluten-free" has become synonymous with good health and been promoted for curing "everything that ails you." It is estimated that today over 30% of the North American population has embraced a gluten-free lifestyle, leading to an explosion in the marketplace of gluten-free foods, beverages, cosmetics, supplements – even pet foods.

This gluten-free boom logically gives rise to the question: Is the diet "necessary or even advantageous" for everyone? The gluten-free diet is a medical necessity for the 1%–2% of the population with the autoimmune condition celiac disease. For these individuals, consuming even small amounts of gluten (found in the grains wheat, rye and barley) unarguably can cause serious health complications. Also, emerging evidence has revealed that others may have non-celiac gluten sensitivity, a condition not yet completely understood and the subject of ongoing debate. However, for the vast majority, the gluten-free diet is not necessary.

For anyone with gastrointestinal problems, a discussion with your physician about testing for celiac disease and other medical disorders is essential before starting a gluten-free diet.

Going gluten free is not a "magic bullet" for optimum health, weight loss, increased energy or many of the other claims made about the diet. Although some may lose weight and/or feel better on a gluten-free diet, this easily could occur due not to the elimination of gluten but rather to other factors. For example, replacing calorie-laden items with more nutritious fruits, vegetables and lean protein foods can lead to weight loss and a feeling of improved well-being. Another reason may be that individuals following this diet begin preparing food "from scratch" at home rather than relying on processed prepackaged foods or eating out, and consequently feel better.

Many believe that gluten-free products are healthy; however, this is not always the case. In fact, many gluten-free items are high in fat and sugar, and as well often are low in key nutrients (e.g., fiber, iron, B vitamins). A reliance on these products thus actually can lead to weight *gain* and poor nutritional status, dispelling the myth that the gluten-free diet is healthier than its gluten-containing counterpart.

For the above reasons and many others, accurate, evidence-based information about the gluten-free diet clearly is needed! *Gluten Free: The Definitive Resource Guide* was written for individuals with celiac disease and dermatitis herpetiformis who must follow a strict gluten-free diet for life, as well as for those who have been diagnosed with non-celiac gluten sensitivity. This book clears up the confusion about which foods and ingredients are "safe," and is packed with information to help individuals successfully adapt to a gluten-free lifestyle.

The guide also is a valuable resource for:

- Family members, friends and caregivers
- Dietitians, nutritionists, physicians, nurses and other health practitioners
- Educators in health science, food service and culinary programs
- Chefs, cooks, servers and other food service staff
- Food manufacturers, including research and development staff and consumer representatives
- Staffs of grocery and specialty food stores

About *Gluten Free: The Definitive Resource Guide*

In an easy-to-read format, this book provides practical information on a wide range of health, food and nutrition topics related to the gluten-free diet. Charts, tables and references are present throughout.

The first chapter offers a brief overview of celiac disease, dermatitis herpetiformis and non-celiac gluten sensitivity including prevalence, symptoms, diagnosis and treatment.

The next four chapters feature comprehensive information about the gluten-free diet. Due to considerable misunderstanding about precisely what constitutes a gluten-free diet, having a good knowledge of which foods and ingredients contain gluten is essential. "The Gluten-Free Diet by Food Groups" chart in chapter 2 organizes foods and ingredients into three categories – Foods Allowed, Foods to Question and Foods to Avoid. In addition, concerns regarding the safety of oats and alcoholic beverages as well as frequently questioned ingredients are addressed.

Many questions arise about parts per million and exactly how much if any ingestion of gluten is safe. Chapter 6 discusses the topics of gluten threshold levels, parts per million, food testing and the amount of gluten in foods.

In order to successfully follow a gluten-free diet, understanding how to read product labels is vital. Detailed information about the labeling of foods, ingredients and alcoholic beverages in the United States and Canada is found in chapter 7.

Chapters 8 outlines the most frequent nutritional complications and deficiencies observed in those with gluten-related disorders, and discusses both how to correct them and how to overcome pitfalls that may arise while following the gluten-free diet.

A wide range of nutritious gluten-free alternatives to wheat, rye and barley increasingly is readily available. Featured in chapter 9 is a broad assortment of "safe" grains, legumes, nuts and seeds, plus many suggestions on how to incorporate them into the diet.

Adapting to a gluten-free diet lifestyle requires some adjustments when it comes to meal planning, shopping, cooking, baking and preventing cross-contamination in the kitchen. A wealth of ideas and tips for these "lifestyle" aspects are offered in chapters 10–13. The culinary properties of many different gluten-free flours and starches as well as substitutions also are covered in chapter 13.

Chapter 14 showcases a variety of delicious recipes from various culinary experts. Each recipe includes a nutritional analysis that will be particularly helpful for individuals who have both celiac disease and type 1 diabetes.

Unique to this guide is the listing in chapter 15 of over 3700 gluten-free products from the following categories: cereals and granolas; baked products; crackers and breadsticks; communion wafers, snacks and snack bars; gluten-free flours, starches and gums; coatings, croutons, crumbs and stuffings; grains, side dishes and entrées; pasta noodles and pasta meals; pizza; broths, bouillons, soups and stocks; sauces (including soy sauce) and gravy mixes; and beers.

Provided in chapters 16 and 17 are contact data for over 220 gluten-free specialty companies, stores and distributors in North America and Europe.

Following chapter 17 is a directory of celiac organizations in the U.S., Canada and other countries around the world, as well as a listing of books, cookbooks, magazines, newsletters and other helpful educational resources. Included in the final section of the book are informative appendices and references.

The information in this guide has been exhaustively researched from a wide variety of sources firmly believed to be reliable and representative of the best current scientific research and opinions on the subject at the time of printing. These sources include health professionals; food scientists; agricultural specialists; medical, nutrition, food and celiac organizations; government and culinary experts; and food manufacturers. Information was obtained through personal communications (telephone and email), the Internet and libraries. Textbooks, manuals, books, position papers, journal articles, professional and trade magazines, newsletters and product labels also were used as references. Inclusion of brand-name products and resources is strictly for information purposes only, and the author does not endorse any of the products or resources listed in this book. Please notify the author of any errors in or recommended changes to this guide.

Celiac Disease, Dermatitis Herpetiformis and Non-Celiac Gluten Sensitivity

A spectrum of conditions are associated with the ingestion of gluten – the collective name given to the storage proteins found in the grains wheat, rye and barley. Celiac disease, dermatitis herpetiformis and non-celiac gluten sensitivity are three major gluten-related disorders discussed in this chapter. Additional information about these conditions can be found in the Resources section (pp. 289–304) and in the References section (pp. 324–339).

Celiac Disease

Celiac disease is a hereditary autoimmune intestinal disorder that affects both children and adults. When an individual with this disorder consumes gluten, an immune reaction is triggered in the small intestine. Tiny finger-like projections or *villi* in the small intestine become inflamed and eventually damaged from continued exposure to gluten. This process, called "villous atrophy," may occur rapidly or gradually over time. As a result, the body is unable to adequately absorb nutrients, especially iron, calcium, vitamin D and folic acid. Also, malabsorption of carbohydrates (e.g., lactose [the carbohydrate in milk]), protein and other nutrients may occur.

Untreated celiac disease can lead to (1) nutrition-related deficiency conditions such as anemia and osteoporosis, (2) neurological complications (e.g., ataxia, seizures and neuropathy), (3) infertility in both women and men, (4) an increased risk of miscarriage or of having a low-birth-weight baby, and (5) an increased risk of certain types of cancers (e.g., gastrointestinal cancers).

Prevalence

Originally thought to be a rare disorder, celiac disease is now recognized as one of the most common inherited diseases. Serological (blood) screening tests have revealed that the global prevalence is approximately 1% of the population, although in some countries (e.g., Finland and Sweden) the rate is as high as 2%–3%. Celiac disease is common in people of North American and European ancestry, as well as in the populations of South America, North Africa, India, Pakistan and the Middle East.

Because it is a genetic condition, all first-degree relatives (parent, sibling, child) of celiac individuals should be screened for the disease. First-degree relatives have a 5%–15% risk of developing celiac disease at any age. However, a negative screening test result does not rule out the possibility that a family member could develop the disease in the future. Therefore, if a family member subsequently experiences celiac-related symptoms in spite of previous negative serology results, repeat testing is recommended.

Causes

The development of celiac disease involves a combination of genetic, environmental and immunological factors. It can present at any age, including in the elderly, and may be triggered by a gastrointestinal or viral infection, severe emotional stress, pregnancy, childbirth or surgery. Researchers also are investigating other factors that may play a role in the development of celiac disease, such as the method of birth (higher rates occur in infants born by Caesarean delivery), breastfeeding, age of gluten introduction and quantity of gluten consumed, as well as changes in the bacterial composition of the gut.

Symptoms

Celiac disease affects not only the gastrointestinal tract but also many other organ systems in the body, causing a wide range of symptoms that can vary in severity from one person to another. Onset of symptoms may appear suddenly or gradually, and may progress slowly or rapidly. Some individuals have "silent celiac disease," displaying no or very subtle symptoms in spite of the presence of villous atrophy. For many adults with undiagnosed celiac disease, one of the most common symptoms is iron-deficiency anemia.

Table 1.1   Symptoms and presentations of celiac disease

• Iron, folic acid and/or vitamin B_{12} deficiencies	• Easy bruising of the skin
• Other vitamin and mineral deficiencies (A, D, E, K, calcium)	• Itchy, blistering rash (dermatitis herpetiformis)
• Chronic fatigue and weakness	• Tingling or numbness in hands and feet (peripheral neuropathy)
• Abdominal pain, bloating and gas	• Swelling (edema) of hands and feet
• Indigestion/reflux ("heartburn")	• Migraine headaches
• Nausea and vomiting	• Mood swings
• Ongoing or intermittent diarrhea and/or constipation	• Depression
• Lactose intolerance	• Mouth ulcers (canker sores)
• Weight loss (note that CD also can occur in overweight or obese individuals)	• Menstrual irregularities
	• Infertility (in both women and men)
• Bone/joint pain	• Recurrent miscarriages
• Muscle cramps	• Elevated liver enzymes

Additional symptoms in children

• Failure to thrive (delayed growth and short stature)	• Delayed puberty
• Irritability and behavioral changes	• Dental enamel abnormalities (discoloration, loss of tooth enamel)
• Concentration and learning difficulties	

Associated Conditions

Celiac disease can occur more frequently when in conjunction with other disorders such as:

- Autoimmune disorders (e.g., type 1 diabetes, autoimmune thyroid disease, autoimmune liver disease, Sjögren syndrome)
- Down syndrome
- Turner syndrome
- William syndrome
- Selective IgA deficiency

The connection between celiac disease and other autoimmune disorders is not completely understood. At present, it is not clear whether there is an increased risk for developing other autoimmune disorders due to continued gluten exposure, or if those disorders occur only by association (due to shared specific genes) or other factors. Individuals with any of the above listed conditions who have celiac-related symptoms should be screened for celiac disease.

Diagnosis

Diagnosis of celiac disease often is very difficult because of its diverse range of symptoms, some of which overlap with other conditions. Many individuals with celiac disease are misdiagnosed as having other disorders such as irritable bowel syndrome (IBS), lactose intolerance, ulcers and/or chronic fatigue syndrome. It has been shown that individuals with celiac disease see multiple physicians over an average of 11 years before receiving a definitive diagnosis, as shown in research studies conducted at Columbia University in New York and by the Canadian Celiac Association. Other countries have reported similar delayed diagnosis rates. In spite of the increased awareness of celiac disease, it continues to be under-diagnosed among all age groups, including the elderly. In Canada and the U.S., estimates indicate that only 5%–20% of those with the disease have been diagnosed.

A gluten-free diet should never be started before the celiac blood and biopsy tests (see following) are completed, as this can interfere with making an accurate diagnosis.

Blood Tests

Various blood tests are used to screen for celiac disease including:

- IgA and IgG tissue transglutaminase (tTG)
- IgA endomysial (EMA)
- IgA and IgG deamidated gliadin peptide (DGP) antibody tests

These tests, particularly IgA tissue transglutaminase (IGA tTG), are very useful as a first step in assessing whether an individual may have celiac disease. It should be noted, however, that 10%–15% of those tested may show negative celiac antibody tests despite having the disease. One reason for this is that some people do not produce sufficient amounts of the antibody IgA (e.g., young children under the age of three, or individuals with selective IgA deficiency which affects about 3%–5% of those with celiac disease) needed for a positive IgA tTG test result. Celiac antibody tests also can be falsely positive even though the person tested does not have celiac disease (e.g., some people with type 1 diabetes, autoimmune thyroid or liver disease may have an elevated IgA tTG).

Small Intestinal Biopsy

The definitive test for diagnosing celiac disease is a small intestinal biopsy, done in a hospital or clinic endoscopy unit. The individual is given sedation and a local anesthetic. A long, thin flexible tube (a scope) with a small camera on the end is passed through the mouth, down the esophagus, through the stomach and into the first part of the small intestine (the duodenum). During this procedure, the camera sends a video image to a monitor so the physician can do a visual assessment, watching for possible inflammation. Then a tiny surgical instrument is inserted through the tube and multiple biopsy samples are taken from various areas of the duodenum and duodenal bulb. A minimum of 4–8 samples is recommended because the disease can cause patchy lesions that can be missed if only 1 or 2 samples are taken. Biopsy samples are sent to a pathologist for microscopic examination to see if the tissue is damaged and presents as villous atrophy.

Genetic Tests

DNA testing from a blood sample or cheek swab can identify specific genetic markers called "Human Leukocyte Antigens" (HLAs) DQ2 and DQ8 that are associated with celiac disease. Genetic testing can be completed regardless of whether an individual is consuming gluten. This test does not confirm celiac disease; however, it is used to determine whether someone with a family history of celiac disease and/or experiencing celiac-related symptoms is at risk for the disease. Celiac antibody and intestinal biopsy tests are required even when the DNA result is positive. If the genetic test is negative, the likelihood of developing celiac disease is rare (although 1%–2% with the disease can have a negative genetic test). A positive test may indicate either that the individual has celiac disease or that s/he could develop it in the future. Nevertheless, approximately 30%–40% of the general population can have positive HLA genetic markers yet only 2%–3% of this group actually will develop celiac disease.

The Gluten Challenge

In order to confirm a diagnosis of celiac disease, the individual needs to be on a gluten-*containing* diet prior to the blood test and/or intestinal biopsy testing. Unfortunately, many people initiate a gluten-free diet before undergoing testing for celiac disease because they have heard that such a diet (1) is "healthier," (2) may alleviate an extensive range of symptoms, and (3) is the treatment for numerous conditions. Another reason why some individuals may undertake a gluten-free diet before undergoing complete testing is because the waiting list for an appointment with a gastroenterologist and/or for an endoscopy often is very long.

For those who have eliminated gluten from their diet, it must be reintroduced prior to testing. At present there is no consensus as to the amount of gluten and length of time on a regular diet necessary for producing positive test results. Some experts recommend between 3–10 grams of gluten per day (e.g., approximately 2–5 slices of bread) for at least two to four weeks, although significantly longer time may be necessary before the serology is positive and evidence of intestinal damage can be detected. Not everyone is able to tolerate a gluten challenge because some individuals may develop severe symptoms, with ingestion of even small amounts of gluten. In this situation, genetic testing may be an option. A negative genetic test would indicate that the symptoms most likely are not a result of celiac disease. It is possible that symptoms in these individuals may be due to non-celiac gluten sensitivity (see pp. 6, 7) or some other condition.

Treatment

Currently, the only treatment for celiac disease is **a strict gluten-free diet for life**. Following the diet will result in improved health and well-being, as well as greatly reduce the risk of celiac-related complications. The time needed for resolution of symptoms and the healing process varies considerably, with children tending to heal more quickly and completely than adults. Individuals with long-standing untreated celiac disease may require several years on the diet before the small intestinal damage is repaired. In some cases complete healing may not occur, especially if the villous atrophy is severe.

In addition to the gluten-free diet, vitamin and mineral supplements may be necessary to correct major nutrient deficiencies. Some individuals may experience temporary lactose intolerance and will need to follow a lactose-restricted diet (see pp. 69, 70).

Alternative Therapies

Researchers are investigating different alternative non-dietary treatments for celiac disease such as enzyme therapies, gluten sequestering polymers, antigen presentation suppressors and modulators of the inflammatory response. These treatments work by either breaking down, binding or blocking gluten. Other potential treatments being examined include a vaccine and modification of wheat. At present these therapies are at various stages of development, with some undergoing clinical trials. It is important to note that commercial enzyme supplements promoted to "digest" gluten, currently sold in stores and online, are **NOT** effective and should **NOT** be used by those with celiac disease.

Dermatitis Herpetiformis

Dermatitis herpetiformis (DH) is another presentation of celiac disease. This chronic skin condition is characterized by an intense itchy and blistering rash. The rash is symmetrically distributed on both sides of the body. Commonly found on the elbows, knees and buttocks, it also can occur on the back of the neck, upper back, scalp and hairline. Initially, groups of small blisters (looking similar to those of chicken pox or herpes) are formed on the skin, and these soon erupt into small erosions. Most people with DH have varying degrees of small intestinal villous atrophy, although some have no gastrointestinal complaints.

Prevalence

Approximately 5%–10% of individuals with celiac disease also have DH. The age of onset is typically between 30–40 years, but DH also can occur in children and in older adults.

Diagnosis

Individuals with DH frequently are misdiagnosed as having other skin conditions such as eczema, contact dermatitis, allergies, hives, herpes or psoriasis. The only way to correctly diagnose DH is with a skin biopsy from unaffected skin adjacent to blisters or erosions. A small intestinal biopsy is not required if the skin biopsy is positive for DH.

Treatment

The treatment for DH is **a strict gluten-free diet for life**. Following the diet allows the gastrointestinal damage to resolve within several months and over time results in an improvement in the skin lesions. Depending on the severity of the rash, between six months to two years on the diet may be necessary in order for the skin to heal completely.

Dapsone, a drug from the sulphone family, may be prescribed to reduce the itching. Response to this medication can be dramatic (usually within 48–72 hours); however, Dapsone has no effect on the ongoing immune response or intestinal atrophy. Thus, it is essential to continue to follow the gluten-free diet both to prevent the rash from recurring and also to prevent other long-term complications associated with celiac disease.

In some cases, symptoms of DH may be exacerbated by ingestion of large quantities of iodine. Seaweed (e.g., kelp and nori, often used in sushi) and shellfish are examples of concentrated sources. DH dermatology experts recommend that these individuals should eliminate high sources of iodine in the diet until lesions are healed; however, a low-iodine diet is not necessary. Consult with a dietitian for more specific advice.

Non-Celiac Gluten Sensitivity

The phenomenon of gluten sensitivity in the absence of celiac disease is not new; it was first described in medical literature in the late 1970s. Since then, clinicians have continued to encounter patients who report adverse reactions to gluten, despite testing negative for celiac disease. This has led to further research and increased publication on the subject.

In 2011, world-renowned scientists and medical experts gathered in London for a meeting on gluten sensitivity for the specific purpose of reviewing the then-current scientific knowledge about gluten-related disorders. At this meeting, the term "gluten sensitivity" was established to distinguish that specific condition as separate from wheat allergy and celiac disease. The following year, the participating experts published an article entitled "Spectrum of gluten-related disorders: Consensus on new nomenclature and classification." A second meeting was convened in December 2012 in Germany, for further exploration of advances in gluten-related disorders. One major highlight of this second gathering was an agreement to change the name of the condition from "gluten sensitivity" to "non-celiac gluten sensitivity." This was done in order to emphasize the importance of ruling out other gluten-related disorders such as celiac disease and wheat allergy before making a diagnosis of non-celiac gluten sensitivity. A further meeting was held in Italy in October 2014 to develop standardized diagnostic criteria for non-celiac gluten sensitivity. Guidelines were established to assist clinicians and to allow for comparisons between research studies.

In spite of these meetings, non-celiac gluten sensitivity continues to be widely debated. Still unclear is whether individuals are reacting to gluten or to some other component in foods such as FODMAP carbohydrates (see pp. 7, 8) or to naturally occurring compounds called amylase trypsin inhibitors (ATIs) in wheat. On the other hand, individuals with so-called non-celiac gluten sensitivity actually may have undiagnosed celiac disease. Several reasons can account for an incorrect diagnosis: (1) the symptoms of non-celiac gluten sensitivity overlap with those of other conditions, especially celiac disease and irritable bowel syndrome, (2) the celiac diagnostic testing was not properly completed, (3) individuals followed a gluten-free diet prior to testing, (4) an inadequate number of intestinal biopsy samples were taken, and/or (5) the biopsy samples were inaccurately interpreted.

Prevalence

The true prevalence of non-celiac gluten sensitivity is unknown at this time, although it is estimated that between 0.5%–13% of the general population may have this condition.

Symptoms

Non-celiac gluten sensitivity is characterized by a wide variety of both intestinal and extra-intestinal symptoms including abdominal pain, bloating, gas, diarrhea or constipation, unexplained anemia, headaches, "foggy mind," depression, chronic fatigue, skin rash, leg numbness and joint pain.

Diagnosis

Due to limited understanding of the pathophysiology, there are no diagnostic markers for non-celiac gluten sensitivity. Unlike those with celiac disease, individuals with suspected non-celiac gluten sensitivity do not develop tissue transglutaminase (tTG) autoantibodies or villous atrophy. Currently, the only way to determine if someone may have non-celiac gluten sensitivity is to first rule out celiac disease and wheat allergy, then observe the response to a gluten-free diet and a gluten challenge. **It is essential that the celiac serology and an intestinal biopsy have been completed before initiating a gluten-free diet.**

Treatment

It is recommended that individuals with non-celiac gluten sensitivity follow a gluten-free diet to alleviate symptoms; however, whether gluten must be strictly avoided for life (as is necessary with celiac disease) is at present unknown.

FODMAP Carbohydrates

Some researchers argue that other components in food such as FODMAP carbohydrates, rather than gluten, may be responsible for digestive symptoms seen in individuals believed to have non-celiac gluten sensitivity. FODMAPs are fermentable, poorly digested, short-chain carbohydrates that can cause bloating, gas and other digestive symptoms. The acronym stands for fermentable oligosaccharides (fructans and galactans), disaccharides (e.g., lactose), monosaccharides (e.g., fructose) and polyols (e.g., mannitol, sorbitol, maltitol, xylitol and some fruits and vegetables). Examples of FODMAP foods and ingredients are found on the following page.

The role of FODMAP carbohydrates in non-celiac gluten sensitivity, as well as in irritable bowel syndrome (IBS), remains controversial. Furthermore, FODMAP intolerance does not explain the extra-intestinal symptoms experienced by those with non-celiac gluten sensitivity. Clearly, the FODMAP dietary approach as treatment for gastrointestinal disorders needs further study.

Table 1.2 Types and sources of FODMAP foods/ingredients

FODMAP Carbohydrates	Examples	
Fructans	Barley* Rye* Wheat* Artichoke Chicory Root Dates	Figs Garlic Inulin Leek Onion Watermelon
Galactans	Black Beans Chickpeas Kidney Beans	Lentils Soybeans
Lactose	Ice Cream Milk	Soft Cheese
Fructose	Agave High-Fructose Corn Syrup Honey	Fruits (Apple, Cherry, Mango, Peach, Pear, Prune, Watermelon) Vegetables (Artichoke, Asparagus, Sugarsnap Peas)
Some Fruits/Vegetables and Sugar Alcohols	Fruits (Apple, Apricot, Blackberry, Nectarine, Peach, Pear, Plum, Prune, Watermelon) Vegetables (Cauliflower, Button Mushroom, Snow Peas, Sweet Corn)	Maltitol Mannitol Sorbitol Xylitol

* Barley, rye and wheat contain fructans (carbohydrates) as well as gluten (protein).

Medical Nutrition Therapy

Due to the complexities of the gluten-free diet, consultation with an expert registered dietitian (RD) is highly recommended. After completing a thorough nutritional assessment, s/he will address any nutritional concerns and will work with the individual to learn how to successfully adapt to the gluten-free lifestyle. Practical information about label reading, meal planning, shopping, budgeting, food preparation, cross-contamination and eating away from home will be provided, as well as suggestions on how to effectively cope with the social and emotional aspects of following the diet. Joining a celiac organization for further information and ongoing support also is beneficial. See pages 289–304 for resources.

The Gluten-Free Diet

2

What Is Gluten?

To a baker, "gluten" is the substance in flour that, when combined with a liquid, is responsible for creating the sticky, elastic texture of raw dough. But what exactly is gluten from a scientific perspective? To answer this question, an explanation of the protein components in grains is necessary.

Grains contain four different protein fractions: prolamins, glutelins, albumins and globulins. Technically speaking, it is the prolamin and glutelin proteins found only in wheat (known respectively as gliadin and glutenin) that correctly define gluten. However, in addition to these wheat proteins, both the glutelins in rye and barley and their specific prolamins (secalin in rye and hordein in barley) must be strictly avoided by those on a gluten-free diet. In general, therefore, the components harmful to those with celiac disease – namely, the prolamin and glutelin proteins found in wheat, rye and barley – are what we refer to as "gluten." And while other grains contain prolamins (e.g., zein in corn, sometimes referred to as "corn gluten"; orzenin in rice), these proteins are not harmful to persons with celiac disease.

Historically, oats were restricted from the gluten-free diet because it was thought that their avenin prolamin caused intestinal damage similar to that caused by the proteins in wheat, rye and barley. However, the main reason for reactions to oats is that they frequently are contaminated with gluten-containing grains during seeding, growing, harvest, storage, transportation and milling. Based on clinical studies over the past 20 years, research has revealed that consumption of pure, uncontaminated oats is safe for the majority of individuals with celiac disease. For more detailed information about oats, see pages 27–30.

The Gluten-Free Diet Overview

The gluten-free diet requires the elimination of all types of wheat including spelt, kamut, einkorn, emmer, farro, durum and triticale, as well as rye and barley (see p. 10). In addition to baked products, cereals and pastas, gluten-containing ingredients often are present in other foods and beverages such as soups, sauces, gravies, salad dressings, burgers, meat substitutes, snack foods, candy and alcoholic beverages. Some medications and nutritional supplements also may contain gluten.

The chart Gluten-Free Diet by Food Groups (see pp. 11–24) provides a comprehensive list of foods, beverages and ingredients, categorized into three groups: (1) allowed, (2) to question and (3) to avoid. Examples of many gluten-free additives and ingredients are found on pages 25 and 26. Frequently questioned ingredients and their gluten-free status are thoroughly discussed on pages 35–42. Also, the Canadian Celiac Association's *Acceptability of Foods and Food Ingredients for the Gluten-Free Diet* pocket dictionary is an excellent resource about the gluten-free status of a wide range of foods and ingredients (see p. 295).

Gluten-Containing Ingredients

Wheat

Atta [1]	Hydrolyzed wheat protein
Bulgur	Kamut [3]
Couscous	Matzoh/Matzo/Matzah
Dextrin [2]	Modified wheat starch
Dinkel (also known as farro, faro or spelt) [3]	Seitan [6]
Durum [3]	Semolina
Einkorn [3]	Spelt (also known as dinkel, farro or faro) [3]
Emmer [3]	Triticale [7]
Farina	Wheat bran
Farro or faro (also known as dinkel or spelt) [3]	Wheat flour
Freekeh [4]	Wheat germ
Fu [5]	Wheat gluten
Graham flour	Wheat starch [8]

[1] A flour usually derived from wheat, although it can be made from another grain or a combination of grains, and is used to make roti or chapatti (Indian flatbreads).

[2] Partially hydrolyzed starch sometimes made from wheat. If derived from wheat, dextrin must be avoided (see p. 41).

[3] Types of wheat.

[4] Young green wheat kernels that have been roasted.

[5] A popular Asian food comprising concentrated wheat gluten and wheat flour, used in vegetarian dishes, soups and desserts.

[6] A meat substitute made from wheat gluten, seasonings and other ingredients. Sometimes referred to as "wheat meat," it is used in many vegetarian dishes.

[7] A cross between wheat and rye.

[8] Derived from wheat flour; therefore contains gluten. However, there are specially processed wheat starches that are used in some gluten-free products (see p. 40).

Barley

Beer (ale, lager, porter, stout) [1]	Malted barley flour
Barley (flakes, flour, pearls)	Malted milk
Brewer's yeast [2]	Malt extract / malt syrup [4]
Malt [3]	Malt flavoring [5]
Malted barley	Malt vinegar [6]

[1] Most beers are made from barley. However, there are gluten-free versions made with buckwheat, corn, rice, millet and/or sorghum (see p. 33).

[2] This dried, inactive yeast is a bitter by-product of the brewing industry and is not gluten free.

[3] Usually derived from sprouted barley, which is not gluten free. However, other cereal grains that are gluten free (e.g., corn, rice) can be malted.

[4] These terms are used interchangeably to denote a concentrated liquid solution of barley malt that is used as a flavoring and browning agent in various foods.

[5] Made from barley malt extract/syrup or from a combination of barley malt extract/syrup and corn syrup.

[6] Made from fermented barley and is not distilled; therefore contains gluten.

Rye

Rye flour

Oats*

Oat bran	Oatmeal
Oat flour	Oats

* Most oats are cross-contaminated with barley, wheat and/or rye so they must be avoided. However, there are gluten-free oats available on the market. For more information about gluten-free oats for those with celiac disease, see pages 27–30. In chapter 15 on pp. 205–262, products that contain gluten-free oats will be identified by an asterisk (*). Appendix A on page 305 is a list of companies with gluten-free oat products.

Gluten-Free Diet by Food Groups

Food Category	Foods Allowed [1]	Foods to Question [2]	Foods to Avoid [3]
Dairy	Milk, buttermilk, cream, sour cream, whipping cream; most ice creams, yogurts, frozen yogurts		Malted milk, packaged granola-topped yogurt, ice cream and frozen yogurt made with not-allowed ingredients (e.g., brownies, cookie dough or crumbs), ice cream cakes
	Cottage cheese, cream cheese (plain), hard cheeses (e.g., cheddar, mozzarella, Parmesan, Swiss), soft cheeses (e.g., brie; blue cheeses: Gorgonzola, roquefort, Stilton), processed cheese, processed cheese foods	Dips with cream cheese or sour cream, cheese sauces, cheese spreads, seasoned/flavored shredded cheese or cheese blends	Specialty cheeses made with barley-based beer
Non-Dairy Alternatives	Most non-dairy beverages (e.g., flax, hemp, potato, quinoa, rice, soy), soy-based cheese and cream cheese, coconut or soy yogurt, ice cream made with non-dairy beverages (e.g., cashew, coconut, rice, soy)		Non-dairy beverages (e.g., flax, hemp, nut, oats*, potato, quinoa, rice, soy) made with barley malt, barley malt flavoring or barley malt extract * Oats used in these beverages are not gluten free.
Grains, Flours and Starches	Amaranth, arrowroot starch, buckwheat, corn bran, corn flour, cornmeal, cornstarch, flax, kañiwa, mesquite flour, millet, nut flours (almond, cashew, chestnut, hazelnut, walnut), gluten-free oats (flour, groats, rolled oats / oatmeal, steel-cut)*, pulse flours (bean, chickpea / garbanzo bean, Garfava™, lentil, pea), potato flour, potato starch, quinoa, rice (black, brown, green, purple, red, white), rice bran, rice flours (brown, glutinous/sweet, white), rice polish, sago, sorghum, soy flour, sweet potato flour, tapioca starch (cassava/manioc), taro (dasheen/eddo), teff, wild rice * See pages 27–30 for information about oats. **Note:** For information on the cross-contamination of all grains, see page 46.	Buckwheat flour Items made with buckwheat flour Oats (oat bran, oat flour, oat groats, rolled oats / oatmeal, steel-cut)* * See pages 27–30 for information about oats.	Atta, barley, bulgur, couscous, graham flour, rye, triticale, wheat (all types including durum, einkorn, emmer, farro, kamut, spelt), freekeh, wheat-based semolina, wheat bran, wheat farina, wheat flour, wheat germ, wheat gluten, wheat starch* * Most wheat starches contain high levels of gluten protein. However, some gluten-free products may contain specially processed wheat starch (see p. 40 for more information).

(1), (2), (3) For further information on Foods Allowed, Foods to Question and Foods to Avoid, see pages 16–24.

Food Category	Foods Allowed [1]	Foods to Question [2]	Foods to Avoid [3]
Grains and Grain-Based Foods	**Hot Cereals*** Amaranth, buckwheat grits (cream of buckwheat), corn grits, cornmeal, cream of rice (brown, white), hominy grits, millet grits, gluten-free rolled oats / oatmeal and steel-cut oats**, quinoa, quinoa flakes, rice flakes, soy flakes, soy grits * For information on the cross-contamination of grains see page 46. ** See pages 27–30 for a discussion about oats.		Hot cereals and infant cereals made with wheat, rye, triticale, barley and/or oats* * See pages 27–30 for a discussion about oats.
	Cold Cereals* Puffed gluten-free grains (e.g., amaranth, buckwheat, corn, millet, rice, sorghum), gluten-free cornflakes, gluten-free crisp rice, gluten-free granola (with or without gluten-free oats)**, rice flakes, soy-based cereals, other cereals with allowed ingredients * For information on the cross-contamination of grains see page 46. ** See pages 27–30 for a discussion about oats.		Cold cereals made with wheat, rye, triticale, barley and/or oats* Cereals made with added barley malt, barley malt extract or barley malt flavoring * See pages 27–30 for a discussion about oats.
	Pastas Macaroni, noodles, spaghetti and other pasta shapes made from: corn; dried beans, lentils and peas; millet; potato; quinoa; rice; soy; wild rice	Buckwheat pasta	Pastas (e.g., chow mein noodles, orzo, udon) made with wheat and/or other not-allowed ingredients
	Rice Plain rice (black, brown, green, purple, red, white), wild rice	Seasoned (flavored) rice mixes, rice pilafs	
	Miscellaneous Gluten-free tortillas/wraps, gluten-free pizza dough/crust	Corn tacos, corn tortillas/wraps, polenta	Wheat flour tacos and tortillas/wraps, pizza dough and crust made with not-allowed ingredients; tabouli/tabbouleh
	Gluten-free communion hosts/wafers, gluten-free matzoh/matzo/matzah	Low-gluten communion hosts/wafers	Regular communion hosts/wafers; matzoh/matzo/matzah made with wheat flour

(1), (2), (3) For further information on Foods Allowed, Foods to Question and Foods to Avoid, see pages 16–24.

Food Category	Foods Allowed [1]	Foods to Question [2]	Foods to Avoid [3]
Meats and Alternatives	**Meat, Poultry, Fish, Seafood** Plain (fresh, frozen, canned) meat, poultry, fish, seafood; gluten-free breaded meat, poultry, fish, seafood	Deli/luncheon meats (e.g., bologna, ham, salami), frankfurters/wieners, sausages; meat and sandwich spreads; pâtés	Meat, poultry, fish and seafood breaded in not-allowed ingredients; frozen chicken breasts injected with chicken broth (containing not-allowed ingredients); frozen turkey basted or injected with hydrolyzed wheat protein; frozen or fresh poultry with bread stuffing
		Burgers (meat, fish, chicken, turkey), meat loaf, ham (ready-to-cook), dried meats (e.g., beef jerky)	
		Imitation bacon bits	
		Imitation crab or lobster (e.g., surimi), seasoned (flavored) fish in pouches	Canned fish in vegetable broth containing hydrolyzed wheat protein
	Eggs Plain whole eggs (fresh, frozen, liquid, powder), plain omelets, scrambled eggs	Seasoned (flavored) egg products (liquid or frozen)	Omelets and scrambled eggs made with gluten-containing ingredients
	Plain egg whites (frozen, liquid, powder)		
	Legumes Beans (black, kidney, navy, pinto, white), chickpeas / garbanzo beans, lentils, peas, soybeans	Canned beans in sauce	
	Nuts and Seeds Plain or salted nuts and seeds (chia, flax, hemp, pumpkin, sesame, sunflower)	Seasoned or dry-roasted nuts, pumpkin seeds and sunflower seeds	
		Nut and seed butters (e.g., almond, hazelnut, peanut, sesame, sunflower)	
	Meat Alternatives Plain tofu	Flavored tofu, tempeh, textured soy protein (TSP) / textured vegetable protein (TVP)	Fu, seitan
		Meat substitutes (e.g., burgers, sausages)	Meat substitutes made with wheat gluten and other not-allowed ingredients

(1), (2), (3) For further information on Foods Allowed, Foods to Question and Foods to Avoid, see pages 16–24.

Food Category	Foods Allowed [1]	Foods to Question [2]	Foods to Avoid [3]
Fruits and Vegetables	**Fruits** Plain fruits and juices (fresh, frozen, canned)	Dates, fruits with sauces, fruit juices and smoothies with barley grass or wheat grass (see p. 37)	
	Vegetables Plain vegetables and juices (fresh, frozen, canned)	French-fried potatoes cooked in oil also used for gluten-containing products, French-fried potatoes or potato wedges with seasonings or "fillers"	Scalloped potatoes containing wheat flour, battered deep-fried vegetables
		Vegetables in sauces	
Soups	Gluten-free bouillon cubes, dried soup bases, prepared broths, cream soups and stocks; homemade broth, soups and stocks made from allowed ingredients	Prepared broths, soups and stocks; dried soup bases, soup mixes, bouillon cubes	Broths, soups and stocks made with not-allowed ingredients; dried soup bases, soup mixes and bouillon cubes containing hydrolyzed wheat protein, wheat starch and/or wheat flour
Snack Foods	Plain crackers made with nuts, rice or other gluten-free grains; plain rice cakes; corn cakes; plain popcorn, potato chips, soy nuts, taco (corn) chips	Seasoned (flavored) crackers, rice cakes, corn cakes, potato chips, soy nuts, taco (corn) chips; wasabi peas	Potato chips made with wheat flour, wheat starch and/or malt vinegar
Desserts	Cakes, cookies, muffins, pies and pastries made with allowed ingredients; gluten-free bread pudding; gluten-free flourless cake; gluten-free ice cream cones, wafers and waffles	Flourless cakes	Bread pudding, cakes, cookies, muffins, pies, pastries, ice cream cones, wafers and waffles made with not-allowed ingredients
	Custard, gelatin desserts, milk puddings, sherbet, sorbet	Crème brûlée	
Sugars, Candies and Other Sweets	Agave nectar/syrup, corn syrup, honey, jam, jelly, marmalade, maple syrup, molasses	Honey powder	
	Brown sugar, coconut sugar, confectioner's/icing sugar, turbinado sugar, white sugar	Icings and frostings, sweet sauces/toppings	
	Chocolates and chocolate bars made from allowed ingredients; gluten-free licorice, marshmallows, whipped toppings	Chocolates, chocolate bars, hard candies, Smarties®	Licorice and other candies made with not-allowed ingredients

(1), (2), (3) For further information on Foods Allowed, Foods to Question and Foods to Avoid, see pages 16–24.

Food Category	Foods Allowed [1]	Foods to Question [2]	Foods to Avoid [3]
Beverages	Cocoa, coffee (instant or ground; regular or decaffeinated), flavored waters, soft drinks, tea	Coffee substitutes, flavored coffees, flavored and herbal teas, hot chocolate mixes	Coffee substitutes made with not-allowed ingredients (e.g., Postum), malt-based beverages (e.g., Ovaltine [chocolate malt and malt flavors])
Alcoholic Beverages	Distilled alcohols (e.g., bourbon, brandy, gin, liqueurs, rum, rye whiskey, scotch whiskey, vodka); gluten-free beer, wine **Note:** For information on alcohol see pages 31–34.	Specialty premixed alcoholic beverages (e.g., Caesar vodka beverage, hard ciders, coolers), sake (rice wine)	Beers derived from barley, wheat and/or rye
Fats	Butter, margarine, lard, shortening, vegetable oils, mayonnaise, salad dressings with allowed ingredients	Baking/cooking spray, salad dressings, suet	Salad dressings made with not-allowed ingredients
Condiments/ Sauces/Dips	Herbs, pepper, salt, spices	Seasonings, seasoning blends/mixes Curry paste	
	Ketchup, mustard (plain prepared), mustard flour (pure), olives, pickles (in clear brine), relish, tomato paste, vinegars (apple cider, balsamic, distilled white/spirit, pure rice, red wine, white wine)	Mustards (specialty prepared), mustard flour (prepared), mustard pickles, rice vinegar	Malt vinegar, miso (made with barley and/or wheat)
	Gluten-free barbecue sauce, gluten-free miso, gluten-free soy sauce, gluten-free tamari soy sauce, gluten-free teriyaki sauce, other sauces and gravies made with allowed ingredients	Barbecue sauces, cooking sauces, Worcestershire sauce	Soy sauce, tamari soy sauce or shoyu soy sauce (made with wheat); teriyaki sauce (made with soy sauce containing wheat); other sauces and gravies made with hydrolyzed wheat protein, wheat flour and/or wheat starch
Miscellaneous	Baking chocolate (pure), carob chips and powder, chocolate chips, cocoa (plain), coconut		
	Baking soda, cream of tartar, monosodium glutamate (MSG), vanilla (pure), vanilla extract (artificial/imitation), vanilla extract (pure), natural vanilla flavor	Baking powder, koji Barley grass and wheat grass (see p. 37)	Tempura
	Guar gum, xanthan gum, psyllium husks		
	Yeast (active dry, baker's, nutritional, torula)	Autolyzed yeast, autolyzed yeast extract / yeast extract	Brewer's yeast

(1), (2), (3) For further information on Foods Allowed, Foods to Question and Foods to Avoid, see pages 16–24.

Notes on Foods Allowed

Food Category	Food Products	Notes
Dairy	Blue Cheese (e.g., Gorgonzola, roquefort, Stilton)	Made from cow, sheep or goat's milk along with starter cultures and mold spores. These spores may be grown on different types of substrates derived from either gluten-free or gluten-containing ingredients (e.g., bread, barley malt extract, wheat-based dextrose). After this fermentation process, the substrate is discarded and the purified spores are added in very small amounts to the milk mixture. Test results by Health Canada found no detectable levels of gluten in various blue cheeses made with gluten-containing substrates.
Grains, Flours and Starches	Amaranth	A broad-leafed plant with thousands of tiny grain-like seeds. The seeds can be eaten whole, popped (like popcorn), puffed (for cereal) or ground and used as a flour.
	Buckwheat	Despite its name, is not wheat or related to wheat. Botanically it is classified as a fruit, not a cereal grain, and is closely related to rhubarb. This plant produces seeds covered by a black shell. The outer shell is removed (hulled) and what remains is known as a groat, which can be either eaten whole or ground into grits or flour.
	Garfava™ Flour	A specialty flour developed by Authentic Foods, made from chickpeas (garbanzo beans) and fava beans.
	Glutinous Rice Flour	Also known as sweet, sticky or sushi rice flour. Made from a sticky type of short-grain rice that is higher in starch than brown or white rice, this flour does not contain any gluten.
	Hominy	Dried whole corn kernels that have been soaked in an alkali liquid and then cooked. This process removes the hull and softens the kernels. Hominy is available as whole kernels as well as coarsely ground into grits or finely ground into masa harina flour.
	Kañiwa	A close relative of quinoa. This seed is about half the size of those of quinoa and often is referred to as "baby quinoa."
	Mesquite Flour	Made from the ground pods of the mesquite tree.
	Millet	Closely related to corn and has very small round seeds that are sold either whole, puffed or ground into grits/meal or flour.
	Gluten-Free Oats (steel-cut)	Whole oat groats that have been cut into smaller pieces to allow for a reduced cooking time.
	Quinoa	The small seed of a South American plant; can be cooked and eaten whole or ground into flour or flakes.
	Rice Polish	Meal comprising bran and germ from the brown rice kernel.
	Sago	An edible starch derived from the pith of the stems of a certain variety of palm tree. Sago usually is ground into a powder then used as a thickener or a flour.
	Sorghum	Also referred to as milo. This major cereal grain either is eaten whole; is flaked, popped or puffed; or is milled into flour.
	Tapioca Starch (Cassava/Manioc)	Often referred to as tapioca flour or tapioca starch flour. This starch is made from the root of the tropical cassava (manioc) plant. It can be used as a thickener, as well as to make baked products and tapioca "pearls."

Notes on Foods Allowed

Food Category	Food Products	Notes
Grains, Flours and Starches (cont'd)	Taro (Dasheen/Eddo)	A tropical plant harvested for its large, starchy tubers, which are consumed as a cooked vegetable or made into breads, puddings or poi (a Polynesian dish).
	Teff	The tiny seed of a grass native to Ethiopia that can be cooked and eaten whole or ground into flour.
	Gluten-Free Communion Hosts/Wafers	Gluten-free hosts/wafers made from soy and rice flour. These hosts are allowed by most major denominations except the Catholic Church.
	Gluten-Free Matzoh/Matzo/Matzah	Made from various flours (e.g., almond, oat, potato) and starches (e.g., corn, potato, tapioca). This unleavened thin cracker-like flatbread is eaten primarily during Passover. It also can be ground and used as an ingredient in a variety of foods.
Meats and Alternatives	Chia	Grown in Central and South America. This flowering plant (belonging to the mint family) produces small seeds that are very high in omega-3 fatty acids, fiber, protein and other nutrients. The seeds can be purchased whole or ground.
	Plain Tofu	Made from the liquid of ground whole soybeans that has been coagulated (changed to a firmer gelled state). Textures of tofu range from soft/silken to extra-firm.
Sugars	Agave Nectar (syrup)	A sweet syrup extracted from the agave cactus.
	Coconut Sugar	Made from a sap produced by flowers of the coconut palm tree.
	Turbinado Sugar	Coarse granules also known as raw or cane sugar, made by pressing sugar cane.
Alcoholic Beverages	Distilled Alcoholic Beverages	Made from a fermented mash of various ingredients including grains, fruits, sugar cane and/or other plants. Some alcoholic beverages are derived from gluten-containing grains; however, the distillation process removes the gluten from the purified final product. Liqueurs (also known as cordials) are made from an infusion of a distilled alcoholic beverage and flavoring agents such as nuts, fruits, seeds or cream (also see p. 32).
	Gluten-Free Beer	Made from fermented amaranth, buckwheat, chestnuts, corn, millet, rice and/or sorghum.
Condiments/Sauces/Dips	Gluten-Free Soy Sauce, Gluten-Free Tamari Soy Sauce	Usually made with fermented soybeans, water and salt; also may contain cornstarch, rice and/or sugar. However, some less expensive brands are made of hydrolyzed soy protein, caramel color and sugar.
	Gluten-Free Miso	An intensely flavored condiment used in Asian cooking to season a variety of foods. It is made from fermented soybeans and rice.
	Mustard (plain prepared)	Made from distilled vinegar, water, mustard seed, salt, spices and flavors.
	Mustard Flour (pure)	A powder made from pure ground mustard seed.

Notes on Foods Allowed

Food Category	Food Products	Notes
Condiments/ Sauces/Dips (cont'd)	Vinegars	Derived from various ingredients as follows: balsamic (grapes), cider (apples), pure rice (fermented rice), distilled white/ spirit (corn and/or wheat), wine (red or white wine). All these vinegars are gluten free (including distilled white/spirit derived from wheat as the distillation process removes the gluten from the final purified product). Malt vinegar is not gluten free (see p. 36).
Miscellaneous	Vanilla (pure), Vanilla Extract (pure)	Derived from the bean pods of the climbing vanilla orchid grown in tropical locations. The vanilla beans are chopped and soaked in alcohol and water then the mixture is aged and filtered. It must contain at least 35% ethyl alcohol by volume. The plain bottled mixture is called pure vanilla; the mixture combined with sugar and a stabilizer and then bottled is called pure vanilla extract.
	Natural Vanilla Flavor	Derived from vanilla beans but contains less than 35% ethyl alcohol. Sugar and a stabilizer may be added.
	Vanilla (artificial/imitation)	Made either from a by-product of the pulp and paper industry or from a coal tar derivative that is chemically treated to mimic the flavor of vanilla. It also contains alcohol, water, color and a stabilizer.
	Baker's Yeast	A type of yeast grown on sugar beet molasses that is available as active dry yeast granules (sold in packets or jars) or compressed yeast (also known as wet yeast, cake yeast or fresh yeast). Compressed yeast must be refrigerated. These active yeasts are used as leavening agents in baked products.
	Nutritional Yeast	A specific strain of baker's yeast grown on molasses that is fermented, washed, pasteurized and then dried at high temperatures. This inactivated yeast contains protein, fiber, vitamins and minerals. Used as a dietary supplement or as a flavoring agent in a variety of foods, it is available in pills, flakes or powder.
	Torula Yeast	Yeast grown on wood sugars (a by-product of waste products from the pulp and paper industry). Used as a flavoring agent, it has a hickory smoke taste.
	Psyllium Husks	The outer coating of the Plantago plant seed, and used primarily as a laxative due to its high soluble fiber content.
	Guar Gum	Extracted from the seed of an East Indian plant. It is used as a thickener and stabilizer, and can be substituted for xanthan gum in gluten-free baked products. Guar gum is high in fiber and may have a laxative effect if consumed in large amounts.
	Xanthan Gum	Produced by fermenting glucose (a naturally occurring simple sugar) with plant-derived bacteria. This fine dry powder is used to thicken sauces and salad dressings, and to improve the structure and texture in gluten-free baked products.

Notes on Foods to Question

Food Category	Food Products	Notes
Dairy	Dips made with Cream Cheese or Sour Cream	May have been thickened with wheat flour or wheat starch. Seasonings may contain hydrolyzed wheat protein, wheat flour, wheat starch and/or autolyzed yeast extract (see p. 37).
	Cheese Sauces, Cheese Spreads, Seasoned/Flavored Shredded Cheese or Cheese Blends	May have been thickened with wheat flour or wheat starch. Seasonings may contain hydrolyzed wheat protein, wheat flour, wheat starch and/or autolyzed yeast extract (see p. 37).
Grains, Flours and Starches	Buckwheat Flour	Gluten free if pure buckwheat flour; however, some brands of "buckwheat flour" also may contain wheat flour.
	Oats (oat bran, oat flour, oat groats, rolled oats / oatmeal, steel-cut)	Most are cross-contaminated with barley, wheat and/or rye so they must be avoided. However, pure, uncontaminated gluten-free oats are available on the market. For more information about gluten-free oats for those with celiac disease, see pages 27–30.
	Buckwheat Pasta	Made from buckwheat flour either alone or in combination with other ingredients such as corn, rice, lentils and/or sorghum. Japanese soba noodles are a type of buckwheat pasta made either from 100% buckwheat flour or from a combination of buckwheat and wheat flours.
	Corn Tortillas/Wraps, Corn Tacos	May contain wheat flour.
	Polenta (precooked and packaged)	Either 100% cornmeal or in a cornmeal/quinoa or cornmeal/potato combination; sometimes made from semolina wheat alone.
	Seasoned (flavored) Rice Mixes and Pilafs	May contain hydrolyzed wheat protein, wheat flour or wheat starch, or added soy sauce that may comprise a combination of soy and wheat.
	Low-Gluten Communion Hosts/Wafers	The Catholic Canon Law, Code 924.2, requires the presence of some wheat in communion hosts/wafers and will not accept the gluten-free hosts/wafers made with other grains. A very low-gluten host/wafer made with a small amount of specially processed wheat starch is available from the Benedictine Sisters of Perpetual Adoration. The level of gluten in these hosts/wafers is extremely small (less than 37 micrograms or 0.037 milligrams per host/wafer). The Italian Celiac Association's scientific committee approved the use of the low-gluten host/wafer, and many health professionals allow the use of it. Some recommend consuming only ¼ of a host/wafer per week. The decision of whether to use this host/wafer should be discussed with your health professional. The hosts/wafers can be purchased by contacting: Benedictine Sisters Altar Bread Department, 31970 State Highway P, Cyde, MO, U.S. 64432 800-223-2772 email: altarbreads@benedictinesisters.org

Notes on Foods to Question

Food Category	Food Products	Notes
Meats and Alternatives	Burgers (meat, poultry, fish), Meat Loaf	May contain fillers (bread crumbs, wheat flour, wheat starch). Seasonings may contain hydrolyzed wheat protein, wheat flour or wheat starch.
	Deli/Luncheon Meats, Frankfurters/Wieners, Sausages, Dried Meats	May contain fillers made from wheat and/or seasonings with hydrolyzed wheat protein, wheat flour or wheat starch.
	Ham (ready-to-cook)	Glaze may contain hydrolyzed wheat protein, wheat flour or wheat starch.
	Imitation Bacon Bits	May contain wheat flour or wheat gluten.
	Imitation Crab or Lobster (e.g., surimi)	May contain fillers such as wheat starch.
	Meat and Sandwich Spreads, Pâtés	May contain wheat flour and/or seasonings with hydrolyzed wheat protein, wheat flour or wheat starch.
	Seasoned (flavored) Fish in Pouches	Seasonings may contain hydrolyzed wheat protein, wheat flour or wheat starch.
	Seasoned (flavored) Egg Products (frozen or liquid)	Seasonings may contain hydrolyzed wheat protein, wheat flour or wheat starch.
	Canned Beans in Sauce	Often thickened with cornstarch which is gluten free; however, some products may be thickened with wheat flour.
	Nut and Seed Butters	Majority of products are gluten free; however, some specialty brands may contain wheat germ or other gluten-based ingredients.
	Seasoned or Dry-Roasted Nuts, Pumpkin Seeds or Sunflower Seeds	May contain hydrolyzed wheat protein, wheat flour or wheat starch.
	Flavored Tofu	May contain soy sauce (made from soy and wheat) and/or other seasonings that may include hydrolyzed wheat protein, wheat flour or wheat starch.
	Meat Substitutes	Often contain hydrolyzed wheat protein, wheat gluten, wheat starch, barley malt and/or soy sauce (made from soy and wheat).
	Tempeh	A cake-like meat substitute made from fermented soybeans and/or grains (e.g., barley, millet, rice, wheat), seeds and other legumes. It may be seasoned with gluten-containing ingredients.
	Textured Soy Protein (TSP) / Textured Vegetable Protein (TVP)	A meat substitute made from defatted soy flour that also may contain hydrolyzed wheat protein.
Fruits and Vegetables	Dates (chopped, diced or extruded)	Packaged with dextrose or with oat or rice flour. Dextrose and oat flour are most commonly used; however, the oat flour is not gluten free.
	Fruit Juices and Smoothies	May contain added barley grass or wheat grass (see p. 37).
	French-Fried Potatoes	Often cooked in the same oil as gluten-containing foods (e.g., breaded fish and chicken fingers), resulting in cross-contamination. Some French fries also may contain wheat or barley flour in the seasonings or as "fillers."

Notes on Foods to Question

Food Category	Food Products	Notes
Soups	Prepared Broths, Soups and Stocks	May contain barley or wheat or wheat-based noodles, macaroni or other types of pasta. Seasonings may contain hydrolyzed wheat protein, wheat flour or wheat starch. Cream soups often are thickened with wheat flour.
	Dried Soup Bases, Soup Mixes, Bouillon Cubes	May contain hydrolyzed wheat protein, wheat flour or wheat starch.
Snack Foods	Multi-Grain Crackers, Rice Cakes, Corn Cakes	May contain barley, oats*, rye and/or wheat. * See pages 27–30 for a discussion about oats.
	Seasoned (flavored) Crackers, Rice Cakes and Corn Cakes; Seasoned (flavored) Potato Chips, Taco (corn) Chips, Soy Nuts	Seasonings may contain hydrolyzed wheat protein, wheat flour, wheat starch, malt vinegar, smoke flavoring (made with malted barley flour), soy sauce (made from soy and wheat).
	Wasabi Peas	Roasted green peas coated in wasabi powder (derived from the wasabi root plant of the same family as horseradish). Some brands of wasabi powder contain wheat flour or wheat starch.
Desserts	Icings and Frostings	May contain wheat flour or wheat starch.
	Crème Brûlée	May contain wheat flour or wheat starch. Some restaurants dust the serving dish with wheat flour before adding the crème brûlée mixture.
	Dessert Sauces/Toppings	May contain barley malt, barley malt extract/syrup, barley malt flavoring, wheat flour and/or wheat starch.
	Flourless Cakes	Traditionally gluten free; however, some may contain wheat flour.
Sugars, Candies and Other Sweets	Chocolates and Hard Candies	May contain barley malt, barley malt extract, barley malt flavoring and/or wheat flour.
	Chocolate Bars	May contain wheat flour, barley malt, barley malt extract/syrup and/or barley malt flavoring.
	Smarties® (Canadian product)	Contain wheat flour.
	Honey Powder	A commercial powder used in glazes, seasoning mixes, dry mixes and sauces; may contain wheat flour or wheat starch.
Beverages	Coffee Substitutes	Gluten-free if made from roasted chicory (the most common coffee substitute). Other coffee substitutes may be derived from wheat, rye, barley and/or malted barley.
	Flavored Coffees	May contain syrups made with barley malt, barley malt extract/syrup or barley malt flavoring and/or toppings made with wheat or barley-based ingredients.
	Flavored or Herbal Teas	May contain barley malt, barley malt extract/syrup or barley malt flavoring.
	Hot Chocolate Mixes	May contain barley malt, barley malt extract/syrup, barley malt flavoring and/or wheat starch.

Notes on Foods to Question

Food Category	Food Products	Notes
Alcoholic Beverages	Flavored Alcoholic Beverages (e.g., coolers and wine coolers, hard ciders, premixed drinks)	May contain barley malt, barley malt extract or barley malt flavoring.
	Sake (rice wine)	Usually made with rice-based koji; however, it can be made with koji derived from barley or wheat (see Koji in "Miscellaneous" at bottom of p. 22).
Fats	Cooking/Baking Sprays	May contain wheat flour or wheat starch.
	Salad Dressings	May contain malt vinegar, soy sauce made from soy and wheat, or wheat flour. Seasonings may contain hydrolyzed wheat protein, wheat flour or wheat starch.
	Suet	The hard fat around the loins and kidneys of beef and sheep. Flour may be added to packaged suet. Suet is used to make mincemeat, steamed Christmas pudding and haggis (a traditional Scottish dish).
Condiments/ Sauces/Dips	Barbecue Sauce	May be made with malt vinegar and/or smoke flavoring (may contain malted barley flour) or contain barley-based beer.
	Cooking Sauces	May contain seasoning blends with hydrolyzed wheat protein, wheat flour or wheat starch; may be thickened with wheat flour or wheat starch.
	Curry Paste	Made from the pulp of the tamarind pod and a variety of spices. Some curry pastes may contain wheat flour or wheat starch.
	Mustard Flour (prepared)	Made from ground mustard seed, sugar, salt and spices, which are gluten free; however, some brands contain wheat flour.
	Mustards (specialty prepared)	May contain wheat flour.
	Mustard Pickles	May contain wheat flour and/or malt vinegar.
	Rice Vinegar	Usually made from fermented rice; however, may also comprise other grains (e.g., barley, millet, sorghum and/or wheat) and/or various seasonings. It may or may not be distilled (see p. 36).
	Seasonings, Seasoning Blends/Mixes	May contain wheat flour, wheat starch or hydrolyzed wheat protein as the carrier agent.
	Worcestershire Sauce	May contain malt vinegar.
Miscellaneous	Autolyzed Yeast / Autolyzed Yeast Extract / Yeast Extract	An ingredient used to flavor a wide variety of foods; can be made from either baker's yeast, brewer's yeast or a combination of both. Brewer's yeast is not gluten free (see pp. 24, 37).
	Baking Powder	Usually is gluten free because most brands are made with cornstarch; however, some brands contain wheat starch.
	Koji	Produced by adding mold spores to steamed grains (rice, barley or wheat) or soybeans. This dried mixture is used as an ingredient in making miso, rice vinegar, sake and soy sauce.

Notes on Foods to Avoid

Food Category	Food Products	Notes
Dairy	Malted Milk	Contains malt powder derived from malted barley.
Grains, Flours and Starches	Atta	A flour that contains bran, germ and endosperm (or just germ and endosperm) usually derived from wheat; however, also may be made from a different grain or from a combination of grains. Atta is used to make roti and chapatti (Indian flatbreads).
	Bulgur	A quick-cooking form of whole wheat used in soups, pilafs, stuffings and salads (e.g., tabouli/tabbouleh). The wheat kernels are parboiled (partially cooked), dried and then cracked before packaging.
	Couscous	Granules of semolina (made from durum wheat), precooked and dried. Cooked couscous is used as a side dish or salad.
	Durum Flour	A type of wheat flour used predominantly for making pasta.
	Einkorn, Emmer, Farro, Kamut, Spelt	Types of wheat used in many "wheat-free" foods. However, remember that "wheat free" does not always mean "gluten free."
	Farina	A coarsely or finely milled cereal, usually made from wheat.
	Freekeh	Young green wheat kernels, roasted, then eaten as a hot breakfast cereal or used in soups and salads.
	Semolina	Derived from the starchy endosperm portion of wheat kernels (usually durum wheat). This coarse meal is used to make porridge and pasta.
	Triticale	A gluten-containing grain crossbred from wheat and rye.
	Wheat Gluten / Vital Wheat Gluten	The protein fraction extracted from wheat flour. Wheat gluten is a fine powder used to improve the texture and volume of breads, and also is an ingredient in meat substitutes.
	Wheat Starch	A starch derived from wheat flour. Depending on the processing method, it can contain varying levels of gluten. Some gluten-free products may contain specially processed wheat starch (see p. 40 for more information).
	Orzo	A type of wheat-based pasta the size and shape of rice grains. Orzo is used in soups and as a substitute for rice.
	Udon	Japanese pasta made from wheat.
	Matzoh/Matzo/Matzah	An unleavened thin cracker-like flatbread eaten primarily during Passover and usually made with wheat and other grains.
	Matzoh/Matzo/Matzah Meal	Finely ground matzoh/matzo/matzah usually derived from wheat and other grains and used in a wide variety of foods during Passover.
	Matzoh/Matzo/Matzah Balls	Dumplings made of matzoh/matzo/matzah meal comprising wheat and other grains.
	Tabouli/Tabbouleh	A salad usually made with bulgur wheat or couscous (therefore not gluten free); however, a gluten-free option can be made with quinoa or sorghum.

Notes on Foods to Avoid

Food Category	Food Products	Notes
Meats and Alternatives	Omelets	In some restaurants may be made with added pancake batter (containing wheat flour) to make the omelet fluffy.
	Fu	A popular Asian food comprising concentrated wheat gluten and wheat flour, and used in vegetarian entrées, soups and desserts.
	Seitan	A meat substitute made from wheat gluten, seasonings and other ingredients. Sometimes referred to as "wheat meat," it is used in many vegetarian dishes.
Snack Foods	Plain Potato Chips	May contain added wheat flour and/or wheat starch.
Candies	Licorice	A candy containing wheat flour; however, some gluten-free versions are available.
Beverages	Coffee Substitutes	May be made with roasted wheat or barley (e.g., Postum).
	Malted Beverage Mix	A powder made with barley malt extract/syrup and other ingredients that is added to hot or cold milk (e.g., Ovaltine).
Alcoholic Beverages	Beer	Made with malted barley, hops (a type of flower), yeast and water. These are only fermented, not distilled; therefore contain gluten.
Condiments/ Sauces/Dips	Malt Vinegar	Made from malted barley. This vinegar is only fermented, not distilled; therefore contains gluten.
	Miso	An intensely flavored condiment used in Asian cooking to season a variety of foods. Miso usually is made from fermented soybeans and grains including barley, wheat and/or rice.
	Soy Sauce Tamari Soy Sauce Shoyu Soy Sauce	Sauces most often made by fermenting a combination of soybeans and wheat.
	Teriyaki Sauce	Contains soy sauce (see Soy Sauce, above).
Miscellaneous	Brewer's Yeast	A dry inactive yeast that is a bitter by-product of the brewing industry. Although not commonly used as a flavoring agent in foods, this yeast is consumed as a nutritional supplement because it is rich in B vitamins and minerals. Current gluten-testing methodologies are unable to accurately determine the amount of gluten in the yeast so it should be avoided.
	Tempura	A Japanese dish of battered then fried foods (e.g., vegetables, meat, poultry, fish, seafood). Tempura batter is made from wheat flour, water and other ingredients.

Gluten-Free Additives and Ingredients

Additives

Acetic Acid	Propionic Acid
Adipic Acid	Propylene Glycol
Benzoic Acid	Rennet
Butylated Hydroxyanisole (BHA)	Silicon Dioxide
Butylated Hydroxytoluene (BHT)	Sodium Benzoate
Calcium Disodium EDTA	Sodium Metabisulphite
Calcium Proprionate	Sodium Nitrate
Fumaric Acid	Sodium Nitrite
Glucono-delta-lactone	Sodium Sulphite
Lactic Acid	Sorbate
Lecithin	Sorbic Acid
Malic Acid	Stearic Acid
Monoglycerides and Diglycerides	Tartaric Acid
Polysorbate 60; 80	Titanium Dioxide

Coloring Agents

Natural colors (e.g., annatto, caramel [see p. 38], carotene, beta carotene, paprika)	Artificial colors (e.g., tartrazine*, sunset yellow FCF, erythrosine, citrus red No. 2, brilliant blue FCF, fast green FCF, titanium dioxide)

Flavoring Agents**

Ethyl Maltol	Vanilla (Pure)
Maltol	Vanilla Extract (Artificial/Imitation)
Monosodium Glutamate (MSG)	Vanilla Extract (Pure)
Natural Vanilla Flavor	

Sugars/Sweeteners

Acesulfame-potassium	Lactose
Agave Nectar/Syrup	Maltitol
Aspartame	Maltitol Syrup
Brown Sugar	Maltose
Cane Sugar	Mannitol
Coconut Sugar	Molasses
Confectioner's/Icing Sugar	Saccharin
Corn Syrup	Sorbitol
Dextrose	Stevia
Fructose	Sucralose
Glucose	Sucrose
Glucose Syrup (see p. 41)	Turbinado Sugar
Honey	White Sugar
Invert Sugar	Xylitol
Isomalt	

* A very small number of individuals may experience an allergic-type reaction to the yellow food color tartrazine; however, this is unrelated to gluten.

** For more information on natural and artificial flavorings, see page 37.

Vegetable Gums

Acacia Gum / Gum Arabic	Guaiac Gum
Agar (Agar-Agar)	Guar Gum
Algin / Alginic Acid	Karaya Gum
Carageenan	Methylcellulose
Carboxymethylcellulose / Cellulose Gum	Tragacanth Gum
Carob/Locust Bean	Xanthan Gum

Miscellaneous

Ascorbic Acid	Maltodextrin (see p. 41)
Baker's Yeast	Nutritional Yeast
Baking Soda	Papain
Beta Carotene	Pectin
Cream of Tartar	Psyllium Husks
Gelatin	Starches (except Wheat Starch; see p. 40)
Inulin	Torula Yeast
Lecithin	

Note: This is not an all-inclusive listing. A more comprehensive listing of gluten-free additives and ingredients can be found in the Canadian Celiac Association's *Acceptability of Foods and Food Ingredients for the Gluten-Free Diet* pocket dictionary (see p. 295).

Oats

3

Overview

Based on the early work of Dutch researcher Dr. W. K. Dicke, oats originally were thought to be toxic for those with celiac disease (CD). A number of studies conducted between 1953 and 1976 appeared to support this conclusion. However, those studies had major limitations, including small size and short duration (less than three months), and the oats consumed were not tested for purity nor the rest of the diet evaluated for hidden sources of gluten. Furthermore, only one of the seven studies used an intestinal biopsy to assess the impact of oats.

In 1995, in Finland, the first large, well-designed research trial concluded that oats did not cause adverse effects in adults with CD. Subsequent research in both Europe and North America confirmed that consumption of moderate amounts of oats was safe for the majority of both children and adults with CD.

Health Canada scientists published a 2007 document entitled *Celiac Disease and the Safety of Oats: Health Canada's Position on the Introduction of Oats to the Diet of Individuals Diagnosed with Celiac Disease* that reviewed the scientific data on oat safety in CD published from 1995–2007. It was concluded that "the majority of people with CD can tolerate limited amounts of pure oats, uncontaminated with other cereal grains such as wheat, barley and rye."

In 2015 Health Canada published an update of its earlier review of the safety of oats, the new document entitled *Celiac Disease and Gluten-Free Claims on Uncontaminated Oats*. It stated: "While recognizing that a few people with CD seem to be clinically intolerant to oats, this review concludes that uncontaminated oats were safely ingested for several years by most patients with CD and that there is no conclusive evidence that the consumption of uncontaminated oats in patients with CD should be limited to a specific daily amount." Another key point from this review was the recommendation to delay the reintroduction of oats until all symptoms of CD were resolved and until the individual had been following a gluten-free diet for at least six months.

Reactions to Oats

In some of the research studies involving oat-containing diets, some individuals with CD experienced gastrointestinal symptoms that were generally mild and gradually resolved over time. The increased fiber intake from oats was thought to be a major contributing factor in the symptoms.

Another reason why participants may have developed clinical reactions could have been due to varying levels of gluten contamination, especially from wheat or barley, in the oat products consumed. Unfortunately, the types, sources and purity of the oats, as well as the gluten test methods and cut-off values used in many of the studies, were not always known or clearly identified. In addition, some investigators used the barley-insensitive omega-gliadin method for evaluating the gluten content or purity of the oats. Thus, it is very possible that the so-called "pure oats" consumed in various studies in reality may have been cross-contaminated with barley, contamination that would not have been detected with this test method.

Over the past few years, scientists also have been examining the avenin protein structure in different cultivars (varieties) of oats and have speculated that certain varieties might be responsible for sensitivity in some individuals with CD. Further research is needed to determine whether specific cultivars or other factors play a role in this oat sensitivity.

Gluten-Free Oat Production

Oats frequently are cross-contaminated with gluten-containing grains because (1) they usually are grown alongside and/or in rotation with wheat, rye and barley, and (2) the equipment used for oat planting, harvesting, storage, transportation and milling often also is used for production of gluten-containing crops.

Several investigators have examined the gluten levels in regular commercial oats available on the market. American dietitian Tricia Thompson tested three brands of commercially available oats (12 samples) and found varying levels of gluten contamination. A 2011 study by Health Canada revealed that 88% of 133 commercial oat samples were contaminated with gluten, ranging from 21–3800 parts per million (ppm). Only one sample tested negative for gluten, and it had a wheat-free claim on the package. Similar results have been reported in other studies.

For the above reasons, consumption of regular commercial oats is not safe for individuals with CD. Fortunately, there are companies around the world that produce gluten-free oats, although the methods used vary among growers and millers.

Purity Protocol

Purity protocol oat production involves a number of steps to prevent cross-contact with gluten-containing grains. Although an industry-wide standard has not been established, most producers have similar protocols that include (1) use of pure oat seed for planting, (2) no wheat, rye or barley grown on the land in the previous two–four years, (3) field inspections, (4) use of dedicated or thoroughly cleaned equipment for planting, harvesting, storing, transportation, milling and processing, (5) analysis by the grower for gluten in the oat seed from the harvested crop before and after cleaning, and (6) frequent testing of oats before, during and after processing at the mill. Due to the complexity and cost of the above processes, the number of purity protocol oat producers is limited.

Mechanically/Optically Sorted Oats

Sophisticated mechanical and optical sorting technologies can separate grains according to their size, shape, density and color, and a growing number of milling companies now are using these technologies to process regular commodity oats for the gluten-free market.

The type and quality of the sorting equipment as well as how it is operated can affect how much gluten-containing grain (i.e., wheat, rye and/or barley) is removed. In spite of the advances in sorting technology, complete elimination of all of the whole and broken kernels of wheat, rye and barley from oats is impossible. This is especially true for barley kernels due to their similarity to oat kernels in size, shape, color and density.

Some millers may choose to source oats from farmers who do not grow any barley in their crop rotations; however, how frequently or if at all this practice occurs is unknown. Another concern is that sorting equipment is unable to remove any gluten-contaminating dust from the oats.

Although this technology is gaining in popularity, currently there is no peer-reviewed published literature on the effectiveness of mechanical and optical sorting for production of gluten-free oats.

Verification and Testing of Gluten-Free Oats

Verification of the purity of oats to ensure they are gluten free is critical, regardless of the production method. This is especially important for commercial oats that have been cleaned with mechanical and optical sorting equipment.

In order to determine the level of gluten contamination in oats, scientifically validated gluten-testing methods must be utilized. Also, an adequate number of test samples needs to be taken to reduce the risk of missing any potential contamination. Gluten contamination is not necessarily evenly distributed throughout a container; there may be "hot spots" within the storage unit. For this reason, multiple samples from different locations in the oat container are required. Each sample should be tested and reported individually, rather than combining all of the samples and testing only the composite sample. (The problem with combining all the samples for testing is that highly contaminated samples can be diluted with lower-value test samples, thus skewing overall results.)

Gluten-Free Oat Products

Many companies sell gluten-free oats (whole groats, steel-cut, rolled, flour and bran) and/or a wide range of products containing oat-based ingredients. Such products include gluten-free cereals, granolas, cookies and snack bars, as well as breads, muffins, baking mixes, entrées, side dishes, veggie burgers, crackers and other foods.

American and Canadian regulatory authorities allow oats in products labeled gluten free. The U.S. Food and Drug Administration (FDA) permits the use of regular commercial oats or gluten-free oats provided the finished product is less than 20 ppm gluten. This applies both to single-ingredient oat products (e.g., bran, flour, groats) and to multi-ingredient products containing oats. Conversely, Health Canada will allow only specially produced or processed oats that do not contain more than 20 ppm gluten in products with a gluten-free claim. More information about gluten-free labeling in the U.S. and Canada can be found on pages 51–58.

Gluten-free products featured in chapter 15 (pp. 205-262) will be denoted by an asterisk (*) if they contain oats. Also, appendix A on page 305 lists the companies in this guide that include oats in some or all of their products. Determining if these oats are processed by mechanical and optical sorting or the purity protocol can be difficult. This is because manufacturers (1) may purchase gluten-free oats from more than one source, (2) may change their supplier(s), and/or (3) will not disclose their sources. Nevertheless, you can contact the manufacturer to ask whether all their gluten-free oats are produced using the purity protocol or by mechanical and optical sorting, or by a combination of both methods.

More Information about Gluten-Free Oats

References about the safety of oats in CD, including Health Canada's documents, are on pages 326 and 327. To read the *Canadian Celiac Association Professional Advisory Council Position Statement on Consumption of Oats by Individuals with Celiac Disease*, see appendix B on pages 306 and 307. Dietitian Tricia Thompson's website (www.glutenfreewatchdog.org) carries an extensive discussion on the controversy surrounding gluten-free oat production and testing protocols (click on "News" and scroll down for the articles).

Oats and Celiac Disease Summary

- Consumption of pure, uncontaminated oats is safe for the majority of individuals with celiac disease.

- Before adding oats to the gluten-free diet, wait until all celiac symptoms have resolved and celiac antibody levels have normalized (may take 6–18 months).

- Always choose oats that are labeled gluten free because regular commercial oats are highly contaminated with wheat, rye and/or barley.

- Oats are high in dietary fiber and may cause gastrointestinal symptoms if initially consumed in large quantities. Therefore, introduce oats in small quantities, for example ¼ cup cooked oats for children and ½ cup for adults, then gradually increase as tolerated.

- Reactions to gluten-free oats are rare. However, if an individual suspects a sensitivity to these oats, it is recommended to stop consumption and contact his/her physician and/or dietitian for further guidance.

Alcohol

4

An extensive selection of distilled alcohols, liqueurs, wines, beers, hard ciders and specialty premixed beverages are available in the marketplace. Depending on the ingredients and/or the production methods used, alcoholic beverages may or may not be gluten free.

This chapter presents information about the production of various alcohols and their gluten-free status. Also, alcohol labeling regulations in the U.S. and Canada are discussed on pages 63 and 64. Pages 327 and 328 of the References section provide further information about alcoholic beverages.

Distilled Alcohols 32

Liqueurs 32

Wines 32

Beers 33
    Gluten-Containing Beers 33
    Gluten-Reduced Beers 33
    Gluten-Free Beers 33

Hard Ciders 34

Specialty Premixed Alcoholic Beverages 34

Distilled Alcohols

Distilled alcoholic beverages are made from various plants including grains, fruits and sugar cane, to name just a few. Examples include:

- Bourbon whiskey (corn and other grains)
- Brandy (wine)
- Gin (malted barley or rye, juniper berries)
- Irish whiskey (barley and other grains)
- Rum (sugar cane)
- Rye whiskey (rye and other grains)
- Scotch whiskey (malted barley and other grains)
- Tequila (agave plant)
- Vodka (e.g., corn, potato, wheat)

Production of distilled alcohol begins with grinding and liquefying the raw base ingredient(s) to form a mash. Next, yeast is added to the mash, causing fermentation and the formation of carbon dioxide and alcohol. This mixture then is heated in large vats for distillation. The alcohol evaporates into special equipment where it cools and forms a pure distilled liquid, while the heavier solid materials remain in the vat. The distilled alcohol is immediately bottled or aged in wooden barrels for specific periods of time to develop distinctive characteristics before bottling.

Even if the alcohol is derived from wheat, rye and/or barley, the gluten proteins do not vaporize; thus, distilled alcohols are free of gluten.

Liqueurs

Liqueurs, also known as cordials, are made from infusing distilled alcohols with flavoring agents (e.g., nuts, fruits, seeds, cream). Examples of the many popular liqueurs include Amaretto, Crème de Cacao, Cointreau, Crème de Menthe, Galliano, Grand Marnier, Kahlua and Irish Cream.

Liqueurs almost always are gluten free, unless a prohibited ingredient is part of the flavoring agent.

Wines

Wines including red, white, port and sparkling (e.g., champagne) are made from different types of grapes, although other fruits and even rice also may be used.

To produce wine, the raw ingredients are crushed or ground and fermented in vats. Select strains of yeast (and sometimes sugar) usually are added to aid in the fermentation process. After fermentation, the wine is filtered and transferred to wooden barrels or stainless steel tanks to age for varying lengths of time. Before bottling, the wine is again filtered to remove any residual sediment.

Previous to the filtration and bottling stages of winemaking, small particles are removed using "fining agents" to improve the clarity. The most common fining agents are egg whites, milk proteins, gelatin and isinglass (a type of fish protein). Occasionally hydrolyzed wheat gluten is used a fining agent, although this is extremely rare.

Expensive red wines usually are aged for longer periods of time in oak barrels, and some vintners may use a very small amount of flour paste to seal the heads of the large barrels. Scientists have tested the wines aged in these barrels using the highly sensitive sandwich and competitive R5 ELISA (Enzyme-Linked Immunosorbent Assay) analytical methods (see p. 46), and no detectable gluten was found in the wines.

Wine is always made with gluten-free ingredients and is considered gluten free.

Beers

Available from large major brewing companies as well as small speciality craft beer companies, this category of alcoholic beverages continues to expand at a rapid pace.

Beers (e.g., ales, lagers, porter, stout) typically are made with malted barley (see p. 37 – barley malt) or wheat, water, specially selected yeast strains and hops (a flowering plant). Some specialty or flavored beers may have other ingredients added (e.g., fruit juice, fruit peels, honey, chocolate, nuts, spices).

To meet the growing demand for gluten-free beer, some brewers are now using various gluten-free grains instead of wheat, rye or barley.

Gluten-Containing Beers

Most beers are made from malted barley and sometimes wheat and/or rye. There are a number of steps involved in the production of these types of alcoholic beverages. First the grain is soaked, germinated (sprouted) then dried. This malted grain is then combined with hot water to create a "mash" that results in a sticky, sweet liquid called "wort." Yeast and other ingredients are added over the course of several steps causing the mixture to ferment over time. The final end product is filtered and bottled.

Since beer is only fermented and does not undergo a distillation process (see p. 32), it contains gluten and must be avoided.

Gluten-Reduced Beers

Special gluten-reduced beers made with gluten-containing grains are being marketed as "gluten free." Manufacturers are not required to disclose how these beverages actually are processed, although some brewers claim that they use a specific enzyme preparation to break down the gluten. Unfortunately, this enzyme affects the ability of the competitive R5 ELISA test to accurately detect gluten in the finished product.

In addition, Health Canada has stated that "there is uncertainty around the complete removal of gluten from beer or beer-like products made using barley, wheat or their hybridized strains." Therefore, individuals with celiac disease should avoid gluten-reduced beers.

Gluten-Free Beers

The process to make gluten-free beer is similar to that of making beer with gluten-containing grains. However, gluten-free beers are made with gluten-free grains (e.g., amaranth, buckwheat, chestnuts, corn, millet, quinoa, rice and/or sorghum) and NOT barley, rye and/or wheat as the starter ingredients.

It is important not to confuse "gluten-free beers" with the "gluten-reduced barley-based beers" which are **NOT** gluten free. Be aware that some establishments (e.g., restaurants, bars, pubs) may offer so-called "gluten-free beer" that actually may be a gluten-*reduced* beer. If unable to confirm whether the beer is made with non-gluten-containing ingredients, do not consume.

For a select list of the more widely available gluten-free beers, see page 262.

Hard Ciders

Hard ciders are fermented beverages usually made from apples although other fruits (e.g., apricots, peaches, pears) or a combination of fruits may be used as the base ingredients. These beverages also may contain flavoring agents (e.g., spices and fruit juice), including barley malt.

Most ciders are gluten free, but those made with barley malt must be avoided.

Specialty Premixed Alcoholic Beverages

Specialty premixed alcoholic beverages such as hard lemonades, coolers and wine coolers are made from distilled alcohol or wine in combination with other ingredients (e.g., barley malt, fruit juices, seasonings). If barley malt or hydrolyzed wheat protein is added, the beverage is not gluten free.

Alcohol Summary

- All distilled alcohols and liqueurs are gluten free, unless a gluten-containing ingredient has been added after distillation.

- Wine is gluten free.

- Regular beer and gluten-reduced beers made from barley, rye and/ or wheat are NOT gluten free.

- Hard ciders are gluten free, unless they contain barley malt.

- Premixed alcoholic beverages are gluten free, unless they contain barley malt or hydrolyzed wheat protein.

Frequently Questioned Ingredients

5

Individuals following a gluten-free diet often are confused about the safety of various ingredients, especially those derived from gluten-containing grains. In this chapter, some of the more frequently questioned ingredients, including the ways they are produced and their gluten-free status, are discussed. Because this chapter refers to gluten testing, parts per million (ppm) gluten and ingredient-labeling regulations, reading pages 43–64 will provide useful background. In addition, more in-depth information about ingredients can be found in the References section on pages 327–330.

Vinegars 36
    Balsamic Vinegars 36
    Distilled White Vinegar 36
    Malt Vinegar 36
    Rice Vinegars 36
    Blended Vinegars 36

Barley Grass and Wheat Grass 37

Flavors/Flavorings 37
    Autolyzed Yeast and Autolyzed Yeast Extract / Yeast Extract 37
    Barley Malt 37
    Barley Malt Extract / Barley Malt Syrup 38
    Barley Malt Flavoring 38
    Caramel 38
    Hydrolyzed Plant/Vegetable Proteins 39
    Smoke Flavoring 39
    Spices, Herbs and Seasonings 39

Starches 40
    Wheat Starch 40
    Modified Food Starch 40

Dextrin 41

Maltodextrin 41

Glucose Syrup 41

Rice Syrup 42

Vinegars

Different vinegars result from the type of starter ingredient(s) used: balsamic (grapes), cider (apples), distilled white/spirit (corn and/or wheat), malt (barley), wine (red or white wine), sugar (honey, molasses, sugar cane) or rice. When yeast is added to the starter ingredient, fermentation begins and produces alcohol and carbon dioxide. Next, a specific bacteria called *Acetobacter* is combined with the alcohol, converting it to acetic acid and other compounds. This acid mixture then is diluted with water and the end result is vinegar. In some vinegars (e.g., distilled white/spirit), the alcohol is distilled before the bacteria is added.

Balsamic Vinegars

Traditional Italian balsamic vinegar is produced from the liquid extracted from pressed grapes, which is boiled and simmered in order to reduce the water content by up to 50%. It next is mixed with an aged balsamic vinegar "starter" containing yeast and bacteria that initiate fermentation. The liquid then is placed in wooden barrels to age for many years. North American commercial balsamic vinegars are considerably less expensive because they are made from fermented wine vinegar combined with other ingredients (e.g., caramel) to simulate the traditional balsamic vinegar taste. Balsamic vinegar is gluten free.

Distilled White Vinegar

This vinegar, also known as "spirit" or "grain" vinegar, is derived from corn and/or wheat-based alcohol. The protein component of the grain is removed in the distillation process; therefore, distilled white vinegar is gluten free.

Malt Vinegar

This vinegar is made from malted barley. Because it is fermented and not distilled, malt vinegar contains gluten and must be avoided.

Rice Vinegars

These vinegars usually are produced from fermented rice although the starter material also may comprise other grains (e.g., wheat, barley). Most are distilled; however, it is difficult to determine whether rice vinegars from Asia are made with gluten-containing ingredients and/or have been distilled. Rice vinegar is gluten free, but if made with wheat or barley and not distilled, it must be avoided.

Blended Vinegars

Blended vinegars usually are a combination of two or more vinegars such as malt and distilled white; rice and balsamic; distilled white and wine. Other ingredients also may be added. Seasoned/flavored vinegars may be infused with fruits (e.g., raspberries, lemon, oranges), herbs and spices, and may have added sugar and salt. Check the ingredient list to make sure blended and seasoned vinegars do not contain malt vinegar.

Barley Grass and Wheat Grass

These young green grasses are used as nutritional supplements and may be added to beverages and smoothies. Barley and wheat grasses are available either as an intact grass, a powder or a liquid.

After the wheat or barley grain seed is planted in soil it germinates, takes root then sprouts a stem with grassy leaves. As the leaves continue to grow, a "head" filled with grain kernels begins to develop. The grass portion of the grain does not contain gluten, but the kernels do. Barley grass or wheat grass easily can be contaminated with the kernels during harvesting and processing, resulting in varying levels of gluten. Therefore, products containing barley grass or wheat grass should be avoided unless there is a "gluten-free" claim on the label and the product has been tested to be less than 20 ppm gluten.

Flavors/Flavorings

The several thousand substances used to flavor foods are derived both from natural sources (e.g., fruits, vegetables and other plant materials; spices, meats, fish, poultry, eggs, dairy products and yeast) and from artificial sources (i.e., obtained by chemical synthesis).

Flavoring agents that must be avoided due to their gluten content include barley malt, barley malt extract/syrup, barley malt flavoring, hydrolyzed wheat protein, autolyzed yeast and autolyzed yeast extract / yeast extract (if derived from barley), seasonings containing wheat flour, wheat starch or hydrolyzed wheat protein as the carrier agent and smoke flavoring (if barley flour is the carrier agent). More details about these flavorings are discussed below.

Autolyzed Yeast and Autolyzed Yeast Extract / Yeast Extract

Yeasts are single-celled micro-organisms belonging to the fungi family. There are numerous species and strains of yeast, with *Saccharomyces cerevisiae* the most commonly used in foods and beverages due to their unique fermentation, leavening and flavoring properties. Selected strains of *Saccharomyces cerevisiae* are grown on various substrates resulting in different types of yeast: baker's yeast and nutritional yeast (on molasses), torula yeast (on wood pulp) and brewer's yeast (on barley).

Derived from baker's or brewer's yeasts, autolyzed yeast and autolyzed yeast / yeast extracts are flavoring agents found in many foods. Autolyzed yeast is partially broken down yeast containing all its components. Autolyzed yeast extract / yeast extract is a separated portion of the autolyzed yeast.

Most autolyzed yeasts and autolyzed yeast extracts / yeast extracts are made from baker's yeast, and thus are gluten free. However, if they are made from brewer's yeast, they are not gluten free.

Barley Malt

Barley malt is used in the production of malted beverages (e.g., beer, malted milk), distilled alcoholic beverages and malt vinegar. It also may be added to different types of dough to increase the fermentation rate and improve baking properties.

It is derived from whole-grain barley that has been soaked, germinated (sprouted) then dried. Barley malt can be further processed into various extracts/syrups (see p. 38).

Altering the length of time and the temperature of the drying process produces an extensive variety of malts of many different flavors and colors. Brewer's malts contain high levels of active enzymes, starches and sugars that are necessary in the fermentation process. Other types of barley malts have lower levels of enzymes and sugars available for fermentation so therefore are more often used as flavoring agents.

Barley malt contains varying levels of gluten; therefore, should be avoided.

Barley Malt Extract / Barley Malt Syrup

The names "barley malt extract" and "barley malt syrup" are interchangeable. This ingredient is used by both the brewing and the food industries for its unique flavoring and coloring properties. In addition to its use in fermented beverages, barley malt extract/syrup is found in many foods such as cold cereals and granola, baked products including crackers and cookies, and beverages.

Several steps are involved in the production of barley malt extract/syrup. A mixture of malted barley and water is steeped, mashed then filtered. Next, through evaporation excess water is removed and a sweet, viscous liquid comprising approximately 75%–80% solids remains. Because malt extract/syrup is made from whole-grain malted barley, it contains proteins, free amino acids, nutritive carbohydrates, phytochemicals, vitamins and minerals. These constituents increase the nutritional value of malt extract compared to that of starch-based glucose syrups (e.g., corn, wheat) that are highly processed and void of these nutritional components. It is these nutritional constituents in barley malt extract/syrup that account for its fermentation and browning properties.

Barley malt extract/syrup contains varying levels of gluten; therefore, should be avoided.

Barley Malt Flavoring

Malt flavoring can be made from barley malt extract/syrup or from a combination of barley malt extract/syrup and corn syrup. Most companies use a combination of barley malt extract/syrup and corn syrup.

This flavoring must be avoided as it contains varying levels of gluten. For example, recently tested corn and rice cereals with barley malt flavoring recently were found to contain over 200 ppm gluten.

Caramel

Caramel is used as a coloring agent and flavor enhancer in a wide variety of foods and beverages. Examples include baked products and mixes, cereals, snack foods, soups, sauces, gravies, spice blends, processed meat products, soft drinks and alcoholic beverages.

There are many types of caramel on the market ranging from tan-yellow to reddish-brown to nearly black. It has an odor of burnt sugar and a pleasant but slightly bitter taste.

Caramel is produced by carefully controlled heat treatment of food-grade sweeteners and starches including fructose, dextrose (glucose), invert sugar, lactose, molasses, barley malt extract/syrup, sucrose and/or starch hydrolysates, in the presence of food-grade acids, alkalis and/or salts.

Although gluten-containing ingredients (e.g., barley malt extract/syrup, starch hydrolysates from barley or wheat) can be used in the production of caramel, North American companies use starch hydrolysates from corn as they have a longer shelf life and result in a superior product. European companies use glucose syrup derived from wheat or barley starch hydrolysates; however, because caramel is highly processed the European product contains little or no gluten. Furthermore, it is added to foods in small amounts; thus caramel is gluten free.

Hydrolyzed Plant/Vegetable Proteins

Hydrolyzed plant/vegetable proteins are used as flavoring agents in many different foods (e.g., soups, sauces, gravies and seasoning mixtures). Most are made from corn, soy or wheat (or a combination of those) but they also can be derived from other sources such as peanut.

Hydrolysis involves breaking down the protein component using acids or enzymes. Depending on the type and degree of hydrolysis, the protein is not always completely broken down, resulting in residual protein levels in the final product. For this reason, hydrolyzed wheat protein should be avoided.

Smoke Flavoring

This potent flavoring agent is found in a range of food products, especially processed meat, poultry, fish, cheese, snack foods, sauces and seasoning blends. It also can be purchased as a liquid labeled as liquid smoke or as a dried powder labeled as smoke flavoring, smoke seasoning or smoke powder.

Smoke flavoring production begins with burning wood chips (e.g., mesquite, hickory). The smoke produced is collected and chilled in specialized equipment that liquefies it, then that liquid is filtered to remove impurities. Sometimes the liquid smoke is aged in wooden barrels for varying lengths of time before bottling. As well, other ingredients may be added to the liquid smoke (e.g., caramel color, molasses, vinegar).

Powdered smoke flavoring is a mixture of dried liquid smoke and a carrier agent (e.g., maltodextrin, malted barley flour or dextrose). Silicon dioxide (an anti-caking agent), sugar, salt and/or other spices may be added. Smoke powder containing malted barley flour is not gluten free.

Spices, Herbs and Seasonings

The main culinary role of spices, herbs and seasonings is for flavoring foods, although some spices (e.g. paprika, turmeric) are used as coloring agents.

Spices, herbs and seeds (e.g., celery seed, fennel seed) do not contain gluten. An anti-caking agent may be added to spices, but often it is a gluten-free ingredient such as silicon dioxide, calcium silicate or sodium aluminum silica (NOT wheat flour or wheat starch). Some ground black peppers contain other ingredients such as buckwheat hulls or ground rice in addition to black pepper.

In general terms, "seasonings" are blends of flavoring agents (e.g., spices, herbs, hydrolyzed wheat protein, smoke flavoring) and sometimes an anti-caking agent (e.g., calcium silicate), which then often are combined with a carrier agent such as salt, sugar, lactose, whey powder, starch or flour. Wheat starch, wheat flour and malted barley flour are common carrier agents in seasoning blends/mixes, especially in snack foods, gravy mixes and sauces. If the seasoning blend contains wheat flour, malted barley flour, wheat starch or hydrolyzed wheat protein, it must be avoided.

Starches

Starches act as thickeners, binders, stabilizers or carrier agents (especially in seasonings) in a wide variety of foods. The most commonly used starches are derived from corn, waxy maize (a type of corn), potato, tapioca, arrowroot, rice and wheat.

All starches are gluten free, except for barley starch and the majority of wheat starches. There are some specially processed wheat starches that may be included in gluten-free products (see below and p. 58).

Wheat Starch

There are different types of wheat starch: unmodified, modified and specially processed.

Wheat flour contains fiber, protein and starch fractions. The extracted starch fraction, in its original unmodified state, is used in some food products. However, it usually is further treated (modified) using acid, enzymes or heat to change its functionality, thus making it more suitable in a larger range of food products.

Depending on the production processing method, wheat starches contain varying levels of gluten protein, ranging from less than 5 ppm to over 10,000 ppm. Regular wheat starch and modified wheat starch contain high levels of gluten, so therefore must be avoided.

Regular unmodified wheat starch may be specially processed by repeatedly washing the starch to reduce or remove a significant portion of the gluten proteins. The resulting specially processed wheat starch is used to improve the texture and taste of gluten-free baked products. Although controversial, it has been used for many years in European gluten-free products and recently has been introduced into North American gluten-free products.

In the past, the safety of gluten-free products containing specially formulated wheat starch for individuals with celiac disease was widely debated, especially when the international Codex Standard for gluten-free foods was higher at 200 ppm. Because the Codex Standard was changed to less than 20 ppm, manufacturers have responded by creating wheat starches with lower levels of gluten.

Researchers now have concluded that the consumption of gluten-free products containing wheat starch with less than 20 ppm gluten is safe for the majority of those with celiac disease. The U.S. Food and Drug Administration allows the use of wheat starch in foods labeled "gluten-free," provided the final product contains less than 20 ppm gluten. Health Canada permits the use of this ingredient, but only if it is specially processed and does not exceed the 20 ppm gluten threshold. In addition, the final product must not exceed 20 ppm gluten.

Modified Food Starch

Starches can be modified by acid, enzymes or heat to alter their physical properties and thereby make them useful/appropriate in different types of foods. They are commonly used as texture-stabilizing agents, thickeners, binding agents and anti-caking agents.

Modified food starch can be produced from corn, waxy maize, tapioca, potato, wheat and other starches. In North America, modified corn, waxy maize and potato are the most common sources, with tapioca and wheat used occasionally. Modified wheat starch is NOT gluten free because it is treated differently than specially processed wheat starch; it contains significantly higher levels of gluten and must be avoided.

Dextrin

Dextrin is a type of starch that is used as a thickener, as a stabilizer and as a binder or surface finishing agent in cosmetics, medications and industrial applications. It is not commonly used in foods.

This starch has been partially hydrolyzed by heat alone or by heating in the presence of food-grade acids and buffers from any of several grain- or root-based unmodified starches (e.g., corn, waxy maize, milo, waxy milo, potato, arrowroot, wheat, rice, tapioca, sago). Usually made from corn or tapioca, dextrin occasionally is derived from wheat.

As dextrin is only partially hydrolyzed, varying levels of protein remain in the final product. Wheat-based dextrin, when used in foods, must be avoided due to residual gluten levels.

Maltodextrin

Maltodextrin is used as an anti-caking and free-flowing agent, a formulation and processing aid, a carrier agent for flavors, a bulking agent, a stabilizer, a thickener and a surface-finishing agent in many foods.

It is a purified, concentrated, non-sweet nutritive mixture of saccharide polymers obtained by hydrolysis (breaking down) of edible starch. Maltodextrin can be derived from a variety of starches including corn, waxy maize, potato, rice or wheat. In North America, the most common sources of maltodextrin are corn, waxy maize and potato, although wheat-based maltodextrin is now used more frequently.

Maltodextrin derived from wheat is highly processed and purified significantly more than are modified food starches. North American and European scientists, using the most sensitive R5 ELISA (Enzyme-Linked Immunosorbent Assay) test, have found very low or no gluten levels in wheat-based maltodextrin. As this ingredient is added to food products in only small quantities, the final product contains insignificant levels of gluten and is allowed on a gluten-free diet. In 2007, the European Food Safety Authority (EFSA) permanently exempted wheat-based maltodextrin (as well as glucose syrup) from allergen labeling.

Glucose Syrup

Glucose syrup is added to foods for sweetening, browning, texture modification, bulking and moisture control, as well as for extending shelf life.

It is derived from various highly purified starches including corn, tapioca, potato, wheat, sorghum, barley or rice. In North America cornstarch is the most common source of glucose syrup, whereas in Europe wheat starch is the more frequent source.

The starch is highly processed and purified (significantly more than that used for modified food starch) and combined with enzymes, causing the starch to break down and create glucose syrup.

Scientists and research centers in Europe, Australia and other countries applying the highly sensitive R5 ELISA tests have found very low levels or no gluten in glucose syrups derived from wheat or barley starch. As glucose syrup is added to food products in only small quantities, the final product contains insignificant levels of gluten. In 2007, the EFSA permanently exempted wheat-based and barley-based glucose syrups from allergen labeling. Regardless of the source of starch, glucose syrup is gluten free.

Rice Syrup

Rice syrup (one type of glucose syrup) is a common ingredient in rice beverages, snack bars, cereals, baked goods and other foods. Consumers and the food industry use it as a substitute for sugar, honey and other refined sweeteners. Like most starch-based syrups, rice syrups have other functions in addition to sweetening such as browning, texture modification, bulking, controlling moisture and enhancing shelf life.

Rice syrup, sometimes referred to as "rice malt," does not result from the process of germination/sprouting undergone by malted barley. It is made from brown or white rice in combination with laboratory-produced enzymes (bacterial or fungal), koji enzymes (derived from rice, barley, wheat or soybeans) or barley malt enzymes. The mixture of rice, water and enzymes is gently heated and cooked, causing the starch, protein and fat to be broken down and eventually producing thick, sweet syrup.

Unlike other glucose syrups, which are derived from only the starch component of grains and are highly processed, rice syrup is made from the whole grain (brown rice syrup is from the whole grain including the fiber) and is less processed. As a result, rice syrups (especially brown rice syrup) contain a small amount of protein, vitamins and minerals.

Most rice syrups in North America are gluten free because they are made using bacterial or fungal enzymes. Occasionally, the syrup is made with koji (from barley or wheat) or barley malt enzymes so therefore may contain very low levels of residual gluten.

Frequently Questioned Ingredients Summary

- Balsamic, cider, distilled white, sugar and wine vinegars are gluten free. Malt vinegar is NOT gluten free. Rice vinegar is gluten free unless made with wheat or barley. Blended vinegars are gluten free unless malt vinegar has been added.

- Barley grass and wheat grass may be contaminated with gluten and should be avoided unless labeled gluten free.

- Autolyzed yeast and autolyzed yeast extract / yeast extract are gluten free, unless derived from brewer's yeast.

- Barley malt, barley malt extract / barley malt syrup and barley malt flavoring are NOT gluten free.

- Caramel is gluten free.

- Hydrolyzed plant/vegetable proteins are gluten free, except hydrolyzed wheat protein.

- Smoke flavoring is gluten free, unless malted barley flour is used as the carrier agent.

- Spices and herbs are gluten free.

- Seasonings are gluten free, unless the blend includes a gluten-containing ingredient.

- Starches and modified starches are gluten free, except for regular wheat starch and modified wheat starch. However, specially formulated wheat starch is approved for use in gluten-free products.

- Dextrin is gluten free; wheat-based dextrin is not gluten free.

- Maltodextrin is gluten free.

- Glucose syrup and rice syrup are gluten free.

Gluten Threshold Levels, Parts Per Million and Testing

6

The gluten-free diet requires the complete elimination of wheat, barley and rye. Although obvious sources of gluten are relatively easy to avoid, eliminating all traces of gluten from the diet can be difficult. For people with celiac disease even small amounts of gluten may trigger symptoms and cause damage to the small intestinal villi, as well as lead to other complications as explained in chapter 1 on pages 1 and 2. For those with non-celiac gluten sensitivity, the level of gluten exposure that results in symptoms varies considerably and at present it is not clear whether gluten consumption among this group can lead to long-term health-related problems.

This chapter highlights four areas of research on gluten in celiac disease, namely (1) gluten threshold levels, (2) concentration of gluten in foods, (3) studies examining the consumption of gluten-free foods and quantifying the amount of gluten in foods, and (4) gluten testing. Key references for this chapter are found on pages 330 and 331.

Gluten Threshold Levels

Investigations by medical experts have focused on determining the levels of gluten exposure that can lead to symptoms and complications in celiac disease. Early studies (1985–1993) of both children and adults introduced varying levels of gluten over different lengths of time. The results indicated that the extent of inflammation and/or intestinal damage correlated directly with the amount of gluten ingested.

A landmark Italian study in 2007 by Catassi measured the impact of ingesting 0, 10 and 50 mg of gluten per day for three months by 49 adults with celiac disease who had been following a strict gluten-free diet. One patient developed clinical symptoms (vomiting, bloating and diarrhea) at the 10 mg per day intake. However, because this patient refused to undergo a repeat intestinal biopsy, it is unknown what degree of intestinal damage, if any, occurred. Surprisingly, none of the patients consuming 50 mg experienced any symptoms, yet the majority demonstrated negative histological changes in the intestinal mucosa (inflammation and/or villous atrophy). The researchers concluded that the amount of gluten ingested should be less than 50 mg per day to prevent villous atrophy and other complications.

In 2008, Akobeng and Thomas conducted a systematic review of 13 studies that evaluated the effects of gluten in subjects with celiac disease. Comparing the results of these studies was challenging due to considerable variations in study designs, the amount of gluten consumed, the duration of the gluten challenge and how adverse effects were measured. Nevertheless, Akobeng and Thomas stated the following: "The amount of tolerable gluten varies among people with coeliac disease.

Whilst some patients tolerated an average of 34–36 mg of gluten per day, other patients who consumed about 10 mg of gluten per day developed mucosal abnormalities. Although there is no evidence to suggest a single definitive threshold, a daily gluten intake of <10 mg is unlikely to cause significant histological abnormalities."

The above studies were instrumental in helping regulatory authorities worldwide to establish recommendations for threshold levels for consumption of gluten by individuals with celiac disease. Most experts now agree that a safe threshold level should be less than 10 mg of gluten per day (approximately 1/250th of a slice of wheat bread). Therefore, because of this very low gluten threshold in celiac disease, a gluten-free diet must be followed strictly and all possible steps must be taken to reduce the risk of gluten contamination in foods. To learn more about cross-contamination, see pages 135–142.

These studies also enabled the development of standards for the labeling of gluten-free foods. Both the U.S. and Canada have established a 20 parts per million (ppm) maximum of gluten in a food labeled as "gluten free." These standards also take into consideration gluten that may occur as a result of contamination or from the processing methods used to remove gluten from specific ingredients derived from wheat, rye and barley. Gluten-free labeling standards are discussed in depth on pages 51–58.

Concentration of Gluten in Foods

The amount of gluten in foods is defined as a concentration in parts per million. A 20 ppm gluten threshold level means there is a maximum of 20 parts of gluten in one million parts of the food. To understand how small the 20 ppm ratio is, think of 20 pennies in $10,000.

Table 6.1 below shows how ppm is equivalent to milligrams per kilogram (mg/kg) or milligrams per 100 grams (mg/100 g). For example, if a food contains exactly 20 ppm of gluten, this is the same as 20 mg of gluten in one kg or 2 mg of gluten in 100 g of the food.

Table 6.1   Gluten equivalents

ppm	mg/kg	mg/100 g
5	5	0.5
10	10	1
20	20	2
100	100	10
200	200	20
1 kg = 2.2 lbs 100 g = 3.5 oz		

To put this in perspective, if a slice of gluten-free bread (weighing approximately 30 grams) contains 20 ppm of gluten, this is equivalent to 0.6 mg of gluten. Keep in mind that this calculation assumes that the bread contains *exactly* 20 ppm. When the manufacturer states that a product has less than 20 ppm, it may actually contain either no gluten or up to 2 mg per 100 grams.

Table 6.2 on the following page provides an example illustrating what the maximum daily gluten intake would be based on different amounts of consumed gluten-free products containing varying levels of gluten contamination.

Table 6.2   Daily gluten intake based on varying concentrations of gluten (in ppm) in different quantities (in grams) of gluten-free products*

Gluten content in product (in ppm)	Gluten-free products consumed per day					
	50 grams	100 grams	200 grams	300 grams	400 grams	500 grams
20 ppm	1 mg	2 mg	4 mg	6 mg	8 mg	10 mg
50 ppm	2.5 mg	5 mg	10 mg	15 mg	20 mg	25 mg
100 ppm	5 mg	10 mg	20 mg	30 mg	40 mg	50 mg
200 ppm	10 mg	20 mg	40 mg	60 mg	80 mg	100 mg

* Adapted from: Collin P, Thorell L, Kaukinen K, et al. "The safe threshold for gluten contamination in gluten-free products: Can trace amounts be accepted in the treatment of coeliac disease?" *Aliment Pharmacol* Ther 2004; 19:1277–83.

Consumption of Gluten-Free Foods

A limited number of studies have been conducted to assess the quantity and range of gluten-free products (e.g., breads, cereals, pastas, etc.) consumed by those following a gluten-free diet and to estimate their risk of gluten exposure.

In a 2006 study by Gibert, more than 1900 individuals with celiac disease from Italy, Spain, Norway and Germany completed a ten-day diet diary that included recording the type and weight of gluten-free products consumed per day. For each country, the results were compiled on the basis of grouping these foods into seven different categories, namely breads, breakfast cereals, biscuits, pastries, pasta, pizza and bread crumb-coated foods. The total amounts consumed were listed by percentiles (10th, 30th, 50th, 70th and 90th) for every category and for the total daily intake. The median (50th percentile) for the total daily intake of gluten-free products was as follows: Italy 265 g, Spain 173 g, Norway 226 g and Germany 268 g.

Gibert's subsequent 2013 study (see table 6.3) analyzed 205 gluten-free products from six of the seven categories in their 2006 study (above). Based on the gluten-free product consumption intake from that study and the fact that 99.5% of the 205 products tested less than 20 ppm, the estimated number of people consuming more than 10 mg gluten per day would be extremely low.

Unlike Gibert's 2006 study that reported the actual amounts of gluten-free food consumed, a 2014 Canadian study by La Vielle estimated the food intakes and potential gluten exposure of individuals following a gluten-free diet. As there was no Canadian food consumption data for those with celiac disease, La Vielle used the dietary intake data from the 2004 Canadian Community Health Survey (CCHS 2.2). The CCHS 2.2 survey combined 24-hour dietary recall of food intake with the individual's stated usual daily intake.

Using this data, La Vielle estimated the consumption of grain-containing foods per day for the 50th percentile ("average eaters") and the 97th percentile ("heavy eaters"). The information was applied to six exposure scenarios based on different combinations of gluten-free store-purchased products and homemade items using grains, flours and starches with or without a gluten-free claim.

For two of the six scenarios, it was assumed that all foods would contain 20 ppm gluten. In the other four scenarios, the gluten content of ingredients in home-prepared foods that contained gluten-free grains, flours and starches was calculated from testing conducted by Health Canada (see Koerner, 2013 in table 6.3 on p. 48) and a 20 ppm gluten level was assigned to all the purchased products. Analysis of these six scenarios revealed that as long as the packaged gluten-free grain-containing foods and ingredients did not exceed 20 ppm, the daily gluten intake was less than 10 mg per day.

Gluten-Testing Methods

A wide range of laboratory tests using different analytical methods have been developed to measure the gluten content of ingredients and finished products, and to verify the effectiveness of a company's quality control programs. The detection and measurement of gluten levels in food and beverages is complicated. Many factors can affect the accuracy of the results, such as (1) how a product is processed (e.g., heated, hydrolyzed [broken down], fermented), (2) other components present in the food, (3) how the sample is extracted and prepared for testing and (4) the type of analytical method chosen.

The most sensitive methodologies require expensive equipment and highly trained technicians, so therefore tests usually are conducted in specialized laboratories and research facilities. Manufacturers most commonly use ELISA (Enzyme-Linked Immunosorbent Assay) analytical methods, particularly the R5 ELISA. The *Codex Alimentarius Standard for Foods for Special Dietary Use for Persons Intolerant to Gluten* (see pp. 312, 313) developed by the international Codex Alimentarius Commission (see p. 55) has identified the R5 ELISA as "the method for determination of gluten."

Depending on the type of product, different R5 ELISA kits are used for the detection of gluten. The "R5 sandwich ELISA" must be used for products containing intact gluten protein, whereas the "R5 competitive ELISA" tests those items that have been hydrolyzed or fermented (e.g., malt extract, glucose syrup, soy sauce, beer).

The lowest level at which gluten can be quantified in a food or beverage is 5 ppm using the R5 sandwich ELISA and 10 ppm using the R5 competitive ELISA. It should be noted that if a product contains no gluten, the test result will be reported as less than 5 ppm for the R5 sandwich ELISA and less than 10 ppm for the R5 competitive ELISA. However, if a product contains more than 5 ppm of gluten, using R5 sandwich ELISA the specific amount will be reported (e.g., 8 ppm). Similarly, if a product contains more than 10 ppm of gluten, using the R5 competitive ELISA, again the specific amount will be reported (e.g., 14 ppm).

Amount of Gluten in Foods

The presence of gluten in naturally gluten-free foods and in gluten-free specialty products has been investigated by scientists in the U.S., Canada and Europe. Varying amounts of gluten have been found in products labeled "gluten free." While some samples contained more than 20 ppm gluten, the vast majority tested under 20 ppm (see table 6.3). A significant percentage of products that tested over 20 ppm lacked a "gluten-free" claim or included a gluten precautionary warning statement (e.g., "May contain wheat" or "Made in a facility that processes wheat") on the label.

Of all categories of naturally gluten-free foods and specialty products tested, grains and flours on average tended to have higher levels of gluten contamination, and especially if there was no "gluten-free" claim on the product package. The main reason for this is because inherently gluten-free grains (and thus flours made from them) are easily contaminated with wheat, barley or rye during seeding, harvest, transport, milling, processing and/or packaging. This is why it is essential to purchase grains and flours that have a "gluten-free" claim on the package label.

Table 6.3   Studies from different countries examining the gluten content of foods

Author, date	Country	Categories of foods tested	Number of products tested	Gluten content < 5 ppm	Gluten content 5 to < 20 ppm	Gluten content > 20 ppm	Notes
Sharma et al. 2015	U.S.	Gluten-free and non-gluten-free labeled foods (baked products, cereals, grains, pasta, snack foods, soups and miscellaneous)	461 *	19/461 (4.1%)	403/461 (87.4%)	39/461 (8.5%) ** †	* Labeling claims for all products: - 275/461 (59.7%) "gluten-free" claim - 186/461 (40.3%) no "gluten-free" claim ** Labeling claims for 39 products over 20 ppm: - 3/275 (1%) "gluten-free" claim - 36/186 (19.4%) no "gluten-free" claim † 1/29 (3.5%) products with both a "gluten-free" claim AND a gluten precautionary warning was over 20 ppm.
Thompson, Simpson 2014	U.S.	Labeled gluten-free foods (same as Thompson 2013 study with additional products in each category as well as more miscellaneous items)	158 * †	137/158 (86.7%)	13/158 (8.2%)	8/158 (5.1%) **	* 112/158 products were previously reported in Thompson 2013 study. Forty-six additional products were added to this study. † 46/158 (29.1%) certified; 112/158 (70.9%) not certified. ** Labeling claims for products over 20 ppm: - 2/46 (4.3%) certified "gluten free" - 6/112 (5.4%) not certified
Thompson et al. 2013	U.S.	Labeled gluten-free foods (baking mixes, breads, cereals, cookies, flours, grains, pasta, tortillas, snack foods, soups and miscellaneous)	112 * †	609/672 (90.6%)	46/672 (6.8%)	17/672 (2.5%) **	* 3 different packages from 112 separate products for a total of 336 samples; these 336 samples were each tested in duplicate for a total of 672 extractions. † 36/112 (32.1%) certified "gluten free," 76/112 (67.9%) not certified. ** 4/112 products were from only 3 manufacturers.

Author, date	Country	Categories of foods tested	Number of products tested	Gluten content < 5 ppm	Gluten content 5 to < 20 ppm	Gluten content > 20 ppm	Notes
Thompson et al. 2010	U.S.	Naturally gluten-free grains, seeds and flours (no gluten-free claim on package)	22	13/22 (59%) *	2/22 (9%) **	7/22 (32%) **	* 3/13 had a wheat precautionary statement. ** 9/22 had a wheat precautionary statement.
Koerner et al. 2013	Canada	Naturally gluten-free flours and starches; gluten-free flour mixes	640 * †	This category was not included in article	579/640 (90.5%) 20 ppm or less	61/640 (9.5%) **	* Labeling claims for all products: - 268/640 (41.9%) "gluten-free" claim - 298/640 (46.6%) no "gluten-free" claim - 74/640 (11.5%) gluten precautionary warning statement † Gluten level range 5–7995 ppm. ** Labeling claims for products over 20 ppm: - 3/268 (1.1%) "gluten-free" claim - 30/290 (10.1%) no "gluten-free" claim - 28/74 (37.8%) gluten precautionary warning statement
Gibert et al. 2013	Spain	Gluten-free specialty products (breads, breakfast cereals, biscuits, pastries, pasta and pizza)	205 *	191/205 (93.2%) **	13/205 (6.3%) **	1/205 *** (0.5%)	* Analyzed the gluten concentration of foods from each of the four countries (Spain, Norway, Italy and Germany). Results in this chart are the total number of food products from all four countries. ** Study reported % for <5 ppm as 94% although the actual is 93.2%. *** Product had 27.8 ppm gluten.

Food Labeling

7

How to Read a Food Label

Product labels provide valuable information to help the consumer choose safe gluten-free options. The most important areas to focus on are the "ingredient" list (and "Contains" statement, if present); any "gluten-free" claims, symbols or certifications; and the manufacturer's contact information. Remember, reading the label every time is essential because at any point, manufacturers may change ingredient formulations and thus a product's gluten-free status may be altered.

This chapter includes practical information on (1) how to read a label and determine if a product is gluten free, (2) understanding the difference between the "Contains," the "May Contain" and other precautionary statements, (3) the various "gluten-free" claims and certification programs, (4) American and Canadian food and beverage allergen and gluten-labeling regulations, and (5) the international Codex Standard for gluten free.

Ingredient List and Contains Statement

In the U.S. and Canada, an ingredient list is required on most prepackaged food products that contain two or more ingredients. The ingredients are listed in descending order of predominance by weight by their common or usual names. Major/priority food allergens (8 in the U.S. and 11 in Canada) must be declared by their food source names either in the ingredient list or in a separate Contains statement immediately following the list of ingredients. When a Contains statement is used, all the major/priority food allergens present must be declared. It should be noted that the U.S. and Canada have different regulations regarding how allergen and gluten sources must be declared on a product label. To learn more about these regulations, see pages 51–58.

When reading a label for gluten content, look for any of the following words: **wheat, rye, barley, oats*, malt and/or brewer's yeast** in the ingredient list. The following example shows three different ways in which the presence of wheat might be declared on the label for a multi-ingredient food product:

INGREDIENTS: Canola oil, water, distilled vinegar, sugar, salt, garlic, wheat flour, xanthan gum, potassium sorbate.

OR

INGREDIENTS: Canola oil, water, distilled vinegar, sugar, salt, garlic, flour (wheat), xanthan gum, potassium sorbate.

OR

INGREDIENTS: Canola oil, water, distilled vinegar, sugar, salt, garlic, flour, xanthan gum, potassium sorbate.
        Contains: Wheat.

---

* More information about the gluten-free status of oats is found on pages 27–30.

Precautionary Advisory Statements

Precautionary advisory statements such as "May contain wheat," "May contain traces of wheat or gluten" or "Made in a facility that also processes wheat or barley" are strictly voluntary and are undefined. These warning statements usually appear near the ingredient list or the Contains statement and are intended to alert consumers to the possible unintentional presence of an allergen or gluten source in a product. Some manufacturers choose to use these types of statements while others may not include any such precautionary statements on their product labels.

Both the U.S. Food and Drug Administration (FDA) and Health Canada (HC) state that the use of precautionary statements on food labels should be truthful and not misleading, and should not be used as a substitute for "Good Manufacturing Practices" (GMPs). Manufacturers are required to have GMPs that include strict quality control policies and procedures to prevent the risk of cross-contamination from allergens and gluten sources.

Gluten-Free Claims, Symbols and Certification Programs

In addition to checking for the absence of gluten-containing ingredients, look for any "gluten-free" claims, certification logos and/or symbols on the product label. These indicators commonly are found on the front of the package, but can appear elsewhere. However, also note that even if a label does not include a symbol or wording to indicate the package contents to be "gluten free," the product could still be free of gluten.

Gluten-Free Claims and Symbols

Manufacturers are permitted to use a gluten-free claim on a product provided the claim is in compliance with the gluten-free labeling regulations in the country where the item is to be sold (not the country where it is produced/manufactured/packaged). For products to be sold in the U.S., one of four terms can be used: "gluten free," "no gluten," "free of gluten" or "without gluten"; whereas in Canada, only "gluten free" is allowed. Further details about these gluten-free regulations are discussed on pages 51–58.

Regardless of whether a product exhibits a gluten-free symbol, the words "gluten free" and/or another similar term, you should always check the list of ingredients and the Contains statement. If in doubt about the safety of a product with or without a gluten-free claim or symbol, contact the manufacturer to determine if it is gluten free.

Gluten-Free Certification Programs

American and Canadian celiac associations, as well as various certification organizations, have developed gluten-free certification programs. These voluntary programs have specific criteria that manufacturers are required to meet in order to receive a license for the use of the certifying agency's logo on their product labels. The four major North American programs are listed below. Refer to page 292 for contact information for these programs.

- Gluten Free Certification Program (GFCP) – Canadian Celiac Association
- Gluten Free Certification Program (GFCP) – Beyond Celiac (formerly known as the National Foundation for Celiac Awareness)
- Gluten Free Certification Organization (GFCO) – Gluten Intolerance Group
- Recognition Seal Program – Celiac Support Association

Labeling Jurisdictions in North America

The U.S. and Canada both have specific regulations and policy guidelines for the labeling of foods, beverages and supplements. The development, revisions and enforcement of labeling regulations fall under different jurisdictions within various government departments in the U.S. and Canada (see below). American and Canadian gluten-free regulations can be found on pages 53, 54 and 56–58.

United States

There are three departments involved in the labeling of foods and beverages:

- Food and Drug Administration (FDA) of the U.S. Department of Health and Human Services
- Food Safety and Inspection Service (FSIS) of the U.S. Department of Agriculture (USDA)
- Alcohol and Tobacco Tax and Trade Bureau (TTB) of the U.S. Department of the Treasury

The FDA regulates the vast majority of food products and some alcoholic beverages while the USDA regulates most meat, poultry and egg products. The TTB regulates the labeling of wines that contain 7% or more alcohol by volume, malt beverages (made with both malted barley and hops) and all distilled spirits, regardless of their alcohol content.

The regulations for these three government departments are found in the publication called *Code of Federal Regulations (CFR)*. All of the regulations developed by the FDA are found in Title 21 of the *CFR*. The USDA regulations are in Title 9 and the TTB regulations are located in Title 27. These agencies also have various compliance policy guidance documents and rules that provide further regulatory information. The links to these regulatory documents can be found in appendix C (pp. 308–311) and gluten-free labeling regulation references on pages 331–333.

Canada

In Canada, the regulation of foods and alcoholic beverages as well as drugs, cosmetics and medical devices falls under the *Food and Drugs Act*. Health Canada and the Canadian Food Inspection Agency (CFIA) share the administration of the *Food and Drugs Act*, including the labeling of all prepackaged foods, meat, poultry, egg products and alcoholic beverages. Health Canada is responsible for establishing policies and regulations relating to the health, safety and nutritional quality of foods sold in Canada, whereas the CFIA is involved in the development of regulations and policies relating to non-health and -safety requirements for food labeling (e.g., common name, country of origin, list of ingredients). The CFIA also is responsible for all food inspection, compliance and enforcement activities as designated in the *Food and Drugs Act*, as well as for numerous agricultural-related acts. The regulations for foods, alcoholic beverages and drugs are found in the Food and Drug Regulations (FDR). The links to these regulatory documents can be found in appendix C (pp. 308–311) and labeling regulation references on pages 334 and 335.

Gluten and Food Allergen Labeling

Globally, some (but not all) countries have regulations governing "gluten-free" claims, the labeling of foods and ingredients, what terminology and symbols can be used on the product label, and the gluten threshold level allowed in products. However, there is no single worldwide uniform definition for the term "gluten free."

Both similarities and significant differences exist between the gluten-free labeling and food allergen regulations of the U.S. and those of Canada. The following section is an overview of the various regulations in each of those two countries. Also included is a summary of the gluten-free standards of the World Health Organization (WHO) and the Food and Agriculture Organization (FAO) international Codex Alimentarius Commission.

United States

Food Allergen Labeling and Consumer Protection Act of 2004 (FALCPA)

This legislation requires that all ingredients containing **protein** from any of the eight major food allergens (i.e., milk, eggs, soy, peanuts, tree nuts, fish, shellfish and **wheat**) must be declared by their specific food source names (e.g., milk, eggs, soy, peanuts, walnut, tuna, crab and wheat) on the labels of all prepackaged foods under the FDA's purview. All species of wheat belonging to the genus *Triticum* (e.g., spelt, einkorn, emmer and kamut) and triticale (a cross between wheat and rye) are subject to food allergen labeling requirements established by this law. *FALCPA* labeling requirements DO NOT apply to the other gluten-containing grains (barley and rye). However, with growing consumer demand for information about the presence of gluten in products, many manufacturers voluntarily declare the presence of barley and rye on their package labels.

When a product contains **protein** from any of the eight major food allergens, the allergen's specific food source name must be declared either in the ingredient list or in a separate Contains statement at the end of the ingredient list. Major food allergens present as ingredients in flavorings, colorings, seasoning mixtures and incidental additives also must be listed in accordance with these requirements. For example, if a snack food has seasonings containing whey powder and flour, the terms "milk" and "wheat" must be identified either in the ingredient list or in a Contains statement. It could be labeled in the ingredient list as "whey powder (milk)" and "flour (wheat)" or alternatively, "Contains: Milk, Wheat" immediately after the ingredient list. However, in the case of an ingredient such as distilled vinegar derived from wheat, the word "wheat" would not have to be declared on the food label. The reason for this exception to allergen labeling is because the distillation process removes the wheat protein so it therefore is not found in the final product.

FALCPA requirements apply both to products manufactured in the U.S. and to items imported from abroad to be sold in the U.S. These include all conventional foods (including eggs in shells), dietary supplements, infant formulas and medical foods regulated by the FDA, but exclude meat, poultry and certain egg products in liquid, frozen or dried forms (e.g., egg whites, yolks), which are regulated by the USDA.

The USDA does not have mandatory allergen labeling regulations. Nevertheless, the FSIS developed guidance documents on allergen labeling that the agency strongly encourages the food industry to follow. The FSIS indicates that the majority (80%–90%) of manufacturers voluntarily list the specific food source names of the major food allergens on the product label either in the ingredient list or in a separate Contains statement, consistent with FDA allergen labeling requirements. In addition, alcoholic beverages regulated by the TTB are not subject to *FALCPA* food allergen labeling requirements. However, a report by the House of Representative Committee on Energy and Commerce that accompanied the *FALCPA* bill (S. 741) that was enacted into law stated that the Committee expected TTB to determine how to apply allergen labeling requirements to alcoholic beverages under TTB's purview. The report also indicated an expectation that TTB and FDA would work together in the development of allergen labeling regulations for such products. For more information about products regulated by USDA, see pages 59–62 and TTB see pages 63 and 64.

Gluten-Free Labeling of Food

A directive in the *FALCPA* required the Secretary of Health and Human Services to issue a final rule to define the food-labeling term "gluten-free." The Secretary delegated the responsibility for this rule-making to the FDA, one of the major federal agencies overseen by the U.S. Department of Health and Human Services. On August 5, 2013, the FDA published the final rule, called "Gluten-free labeling of food," that established requirements for food labeled "gluten free." These requirements are found in Title 21 of the *Code of Federal Regulations*, Part 101, Section 101.91 (21 CFR 101.91) (see p. 332). The following is an excerpt from the final rule that was adopted in the *CFR*:

(a) Definitions

(1) The term "gluten-containing grain" means any one of the following grains or their crossbred hybrids (e.g., triticale, which is a cross between wheat and rye):

    (i)   Wheat, including any species belonging to the genus *Triticum*;

    (ii) Rye, including any species belonging to the genus *Secale*; or

    (iii) Barley, including any species belonging to the genus *Hordeum*.

(2) The term "gluten" means the proteins that naturally occur in a gluten-containing grain and that may cause adverse health effects in persons with celiac disease (e.g., prolamins and glutelins).

(3) The labeling claim "gluten-free" means:

    (i)   That the food bearing the claim in its labeling:

        (A) Does not contain any one of the following:

            (1) An ingredient that is a gluten-containing grain (e.g., spelt wheat);

            (2) An ingredient that is derived from a gluten-containing grain and that has not been processed to remove gluten (e.g., wheat flour); or

            (3) An ingredient that is derived from a gluten-containing grain and that has been processed to remove gluten (e.g., wheat starch), if the use of that ingredient results in the presence of 20 parts per million (ppm) or more gluten in the food (i.e., 20 milligrams (mg) or more gluten per kilogram (kg) of food); or

        (B) Inherently does not contain gluten; and

    (ii) Any unavoidable presence of gluten in the food bearing the claim in its labeling is below 20 ppm gluten (i.e., below 20 mg gluten per kg of food).

Canada

1220 – Enhanced Labelling for Food Allergen and Gluten Sources and Added Sulphites

Canada's *Food and Drug Regulations* require the labeling of all ingredients that contain **protein** from any of the priority allergens, including milk, eggs, soy, peanuts, tree nuts (almonds, Brazil nuts, cashews, hazelnuts, macadamia nuts, pecans, pine nuts, pistachios and walnuts), crustaceans, shellfish, fish, sesame seeds, mustard seeds, **wheat** or **triticale** and **gluten sources (wheat, rye, barley, triticale and oats)** and added sulphites (over 10 ppm). These allergens, gluten sources and sulphites must be declared on the label in the list of ingredients or in a Contains statement.

Although oats are included in the list of gluten sources, Health Canada differentiates between regular oats and specially processed gluten-free oats (see following page).

The Gluten-Free Regulation

The *Food and Drug Regulations* regulate "Foods for Special Dietary Use" that have been specially processed or formulated to meet the particular needs of individuals for whom a physical or physiological condition exists. Section **B.01.010.1(1)** defines the term **"gluten"** and **B.24.018** defines the terms for food labeled as **"gluten free,"** as follows:

B.01.010.1(1)

gluten means

(a)   any gluten protein from the grain of any of the following cereals or from the grain of a hybridized strain that is created from at least one of the following cereals: (i) barley, (ii) oats, (iii) rye, (iv) triticale, or (v) wheat; or

(b)   any modified gluten protein, including any gluten protein fraction, that is derived from the grain of any of the cereals referred to in paragraph (a) or from the grain of a hybridized strain referred to in that paragraph (gluten).

B.24.018

It is prohibited to label, package, sell, or advertise a food in a manner likely to create an impression that it is a gluten-free food if the food contains any gluten protein or modified gluten protein, including any gluten protein fraction, referred to in the definition *gluten* in subsection B.01.010.1(1).

In addition to the above regulations (see first link under Gluten-Free Labeling on p. 334), *Health Canada's Position on Gluten-Free Claims* states: "Based on the available scientific evidence, Health Canada considers that gluten-free foods, prepared under good manufacturing practices, which contain levels of gluten not exceeding 20 ppm as a result of cross-contamination, meet the health and safety intent of B.24.018 when a gluten-free claim is made." The link for this document is found on page 334 under Gluten-Free Labeling.

Oats and Gluten-Free Labeling in Canada

Health Canada published a position paper in 2007 entitled *Celiac Disease and the Safety of Oats: Health Canada's Position on the Introduction of Oats to the Diet of Individuals Diagnosed with Celiac Disease (CD)* (see pp. 27, 335). The scientists from Health Canada concluded that most people with celiac disease could consume moderate amounts of pure, uncontaminated oats. However, although pure, uncontaminated oats had been available in Canada for a number of years, manufacturers were not allowed to include a gluten-free claim on the label because the then-existing gluten-free regulations included oats in the list of prohibited grains.

Due to subsequent advances in the understanding of celiac disease and the gluten-free diet (including the safety of pure, uncontaminated oats), Health Canada acknowledged the gluten-free regulations needed revising. In 2011, the gluten-free regulation was revised after an extensive consultation with stakeholders. Four years later, on November 14, 2015, Health Canada published a "Notice of Intent" to permit gluten-free claims on specially produced oats, provided the oats did not contain more than 20 ppm of gluten. On May 19, 2015, the Minister of Health issued a "Food Marketing Authorization" allowing the use of "gluten-free" claims for specially produced oats and foods containing these gluten-free oats (see p. 335).

That same month, Health Canada also published an updated document called *Celiac Disease and Gluten-Free Claims on Uncontaminated Oats* that incorporated the latest scientific research about the safety of oats for those with celiac disease (see pp. 27, 335). Based on the new evidence, Health Canada confirmed its 2007 conclusions that consumption of uncontaminated oats was safe for the majority of people with celiac disease. Furthermore, the research revealed there was no evidence of a need to limit the amount of oats consumed per day.

International Codex Alimentarius Gluten-Free Labeling

As mentioned earlier, another standard for gluten-free labeling is that developed by the Codex Alimentarius Commission. The World Health Organization and the Food and Agriculture Organization formed the Codex Alimentarius Commission in 1963 with a mandate to develop internationally agreed-upon food standards. This organization includes representatives from around the world including the U.S., Canada and most European countries as well as countries from Africa, Asia and Latin America, although not all participating countries adopt the standards developed by the Commission and many have their own standards and specific regulations.

The *Codex Standard for Foods for Special Dietary Use for Persons Intolerant to Gluten* allows two levels of gluten for foods making gluten-related claims. One is for naturally gluten-free foods and the other is for gluten-reduced specially processed foods. The following excerpts are key sections from this standard which was last amended in 2015. To read the entire standard, see appendix D on page 312.

Codex Standard for Foods for Special Dietary Use for Persons Intolerant to Gluten
(Codex Stan 118-1979; Adopted in 1979. Amendment: 1983 and 2015. Revision: 2008.)

2.1.1   Gluten-free foods

Gluten-free foods are dietary foods

a) consisting of or made only from one or more ingredients which do not contain wheat (i.e., all *Triticum* species, such as durum wheat, spelt, and khorasan wheat, which is also marketed under different trademarks such as KAMUT), rye, barley, oats[1] or their crossbred varieties, and the gluten level does not exceed 20 mg/kg in total, based on the food as sold or distributed to the consumer, and/or

b) consisting of one or more ingredients from wheat (i.e., all *Triticum* species, such as durum wheat, spelt, and khorasan wheat, which is also marketed under different trademarks such as KAMUT), rye, barley, oats[1] or their crossbred varieties, which have been specially processed to remove gluten, and the gluten level does not exceed 20 mg/kg in total, based on the food as sold or distributed to the consumer.

2.1.2   Foods specially processed to reduce gluten content to a level above 20 up to 100 mg/kg

These foods consist of one or more ingredients from wheat (i.e., all *Triticum* species, such as durum wheat, spelt, and khorasan wheat, which is also marketed under different trademarks such as KAMUT), rye, barley, oats[1] or their crossbred varieties, which have been specially processed to reduce the gluten content to a level above 20 up to 100 mg/kg in total, based on the food as sold or distributed to the consumer. Decisions on the marketing of products described in this section may be determined at the national level.

[1] Oats can be tolerated by most but not all people who are intolerant to gluten. Therefore, the allowance of oats that are not contaminated with wheat, rye or barley in foods covered by this standard may be determined at the national level.

Comparison of Current Gluten-Free Labeling Regulations in the United States and Canada

Both the FDA and Health Canada have gluten-free labeling regulations that permit manufacturers to include a gluten-free claim on products on a voluntary basis. Regardless of where a product is manufactured, the label must meet the gluten-free requirements of the country where the item is sold. Table 7.1 provides a comparative summary of the gluten-free labeling regulations in the U.S. and Canada. To learn more about these labeling regulations for each country, see pages 331–335 in the References section.

Table 7.1   Gluten-free labeling regulations in the United States and Canada

	United States	Canada
	FDA	**Health Canada**
Name of Regulation	Title 21 of the *Code of Federal Regulations*, Part 101, Section 101.91 (21 CFR 101.91) "Gluten-Free Labeling of Food"	*Food and Drug Regulations* B.24.018
Publication Date	August 5, 2013	Officially enacted in 1995 and revised February 16, 2011
Compliance Date	August 5, 2014	August 4, 2012
Mandatory or Voluntary Use of Gluten-Free Claim	Voluntary	Voluntary
Categories of Products Covered	Packaged foods, dietary supplements, infant formulas, medical foods FDA-regulated alcoholic beverages (see p. 64)	Prepackaged foods, alcoholic beverages
Categories of Products Not Covered	USDA-regulated products (meat, poultry, egg products) TTB-regulated alcoholic beverages (see pp. 63, 64) Cosmetics, prescription and non-prescription drugs	Vitamin and mineral supplements, herbal and plant-based remedies, probiotic supplements, prescription and non-prescription drugs
Foods Eligible to Make a "Gluten-Free" Claim	Any foods, including naturally gluten-free foods (e.g., packaged raw carrots, grapefruit juice), **not made** with a prohibited ingredient (e.g., a gluten-containing grain) and that do not contain 20 ppm or more gluten	Foods that have been specially processed or formulated to be gluten free provided they do not exceed the 20 ppm gluten threshold level

	United States	Canada
	FDA	**Health Canada**
Allowed Gluten-Free Labeling Terminology	"Gluten-free" "No gluten" "Free of gluten" "Without gluten" However, statements such as "Made with no gluten-containing ingredients" or "Not made with gluten-containing ingredients" that may appear on a food label are NOT equivalent to a "gluten-free" claim. If these statements are present **without** the inclusion of a "gluten-free" claim, there is no guarantee the product was manufactured to comply with FDA requirements for gluten-free foods.	"Gluten-free"
Low Gluten or Reduced Gluten Claims	FDA discourages the use of such claims.	Not allowed
Maximum Gluten Level in the Packaged Food	Less than 20 ppm	Cannot exceed 20 ppm
Quantitative Statements (e.g., "Contains less than 5 ppm gluten")	Allowed but must be truthful and not misleading	Allowed but must be truthful and not misleading
Prohibited Grains as Ingredients	All types of wheat, barley, and rye and their crossbred hybrids (e.g., triticale, which is a cross between wheat and rye)	All types of wheat, barley, rye, triticale, spelt, kamut, oats* *Oats are a prohibited grain unless specially produced and meet the gluten-free regulation B.24.018 (see p. 54).
Other Prohibited Ingredients	Barley-based ingredients: malt, malt syrup (also known as malt extract) and malt vinegar	Barley-based ingredients: malt, malt syrup (also known as malt extract) and malt vinegar
Oats as Ingredients	Oats sold as a single ingredient labeled "gluten free" must contain less than 20 ppm gluten. When oats are used in a multi-ingredient food, the final product must be less than 20 ppm gluten. Oats do not have to be specially produced to be used as ingredients in foods labeled "gluten free."	Specially produced "gluten-free" oats sold as a single ingredient must not exceed 20 ppm gluten. In a multi-ingredient product, only specially produced "gluten-free" oats can be used and the final product also must not exceed 20 ppm gluten.

	United States	Canada
	FDA	Health Canada
Ingredients Derived from Gluten-Containing Grains	Not allowed unless ingredients are processed to remove gluten (e.g., wheat starch [and other ingredients derived from wheat starch such as glucose syrup, maltodextrin, caramel]). When these ingredients are used in a food, the final product must be less than 20 ppm gluten. If a product labeled "gluten free" is made with an ingredient derived from wheat that was processed to remove gluten, but that ingredient still contains ANY wheat protein residue, the word "wheat" must be declared in the ingredient list or in a separate Contains statement immediately after the ingredient list with an asterisk carrying this wording: "The wheat has been processed to allow this food to meet the Food and Drug Administration requirements for gluten-free foods."	Not allowed unless ingredients are processed to remove gluten (e.g.,wheat starch [and other ingredients derived from wheat starch such as glucose syrup, maltodextrin, caramel]). When used in a food product, wheat starch and wheat starch derivatives must not contain 20 ppm or more gluten. If a product labeled "gluten free" is made with an ingredient derived from wheat that was processed to remove gluten, but that ingredient still contains ANY wheat protein residue, the word "wheat" must be declared in the ingredient list or in a separate Contains statement immediately after the ingredient.
Gluten Cross-Contamination	Final food product as packaged must be less than 20 ppm gluten.	Health Canada states "cross-contamination should be as low as reasonably achievable." Final product must not exceed 20 ppm gluten.
Precautionary Statements and "Gluten-Free" Claims	Precautionary statements such as "Made in a facility that also processes wheat products" and a gluten-free claim are allowed, provided the food meets all requirements for gluten-free labeling.	Precautionary statements such as "Made in a facility that also processes wheat products" and a gluten-free claim are allowed, provided the food meets all requirements for gluten-free labelling.
Gluten Testing of Ingredients or Final Products	Not specifically mandated, but manufacturers are responsible for ensuring that their foods bearing a gluten-free claim meet all requirements, including not containing 20 ppm or more gluten; otherwise, the food is misbranded.	Not specifically mandated, but manufacturers are responsible for ensuring that their foods bearing a gluten-free claim meet all requirements, including not containing 20 ppm or more gluten; otherwise, the food is misbranded.
Gluten-Testing Methodology Requirements	No regulatory requirements established for manufacturers, but FDA "recommends the use of scientifically valid methods in order for the gluten test results obtained to be reliable and consistent." Method of analysis used to determine the amount of gluten in a food must be appropriate for the type of product (e.g., R5 sandwich Enzyme-Linked Immunosorbent Assay [ELISA] is not appropriate for hydrolyzed, fermented or enzymatic processed food products).	Does not specify the test to be used. Health Canada's "Position on Gluten-Free Claims" (see p. 334) discusses the importance of using scientifically validated methods. Method of analysis used to determine the amount of gluten in a food must be appropriate for the type of product (e.g., R5 sandwich Enzyme-Linked Immunosorbent Assay [ELISA] is not appropriate for hydrolyzed, fermented or enzymatic processed food products).
Third Party Gluten-Free Certification	Allowed but not required.	Allowed but not required.

Labeling of Frequently Questioned Ingredients in the United States and Canada

Certain ingredients derived from wheat, rye and barley may be labeled differently between the U.S. and Canada. The processing methods and the quantities of the ingredient used in a product also can impact the allergenicity and gluten-free status of foods (see chapter 5 on pp. 35–42). Table 7.2 below highlights the main differences in how these ingredients are listed on the package label between the U.S. and Canada.

Table 7.2 Labeling requirements in the U.S. and Canada for foods made with ingredients derived from possible gluten sources

	United States		Canada
	FDA	**USDA**	**Health Canada**
Labeling of Allergens and Gluten Sources	FDA regulations require, in most cases, all ingredients to be listed by their specific "common or usual names." When an ingredient contains **protein** from a **major food allergen** (see p. 52), the name of the allergen **must** appear on the label in the ingredient list or in a Contains statement. For example – flour (wheat) or Contains: Wheat.	USDA regulations require, in most cases, ingredients to be listed by their specific "common or usual names." When an ingredient contains **protein** from a **major food allergen**, USDA encourages manufacturers to **voluntarily** follow the FDA's food allergen labeling requirements. However, the USDA does not have mandatory allergen labeling regulations.	Canadian regulations require, in most cases, ingredients to be listed by their specific "common or usual names." When an ingredient contains **protein** from a **priority food allergen** or **gluten** source (see p. 53), the protein name **must** appear in the ingredient list or in a Contains statement. For example – malt vinegar (barley) or Contains: Barley.
Starch See page 40	The terms "starch" and "cornstarch" are interchangeable common or usual names for the food starch made from corn. All other starches must include their source (e.g., wheat starch, potato starch, tapioca starch) when declared in an ingredient list.	The single word "starch" refers to cornstarch or wheat starch; therefore, wheat may not always be declared on the label.	The common name of the plant plus starch must be declared in the ingredient list (e.g., corn starch, potato starch, wheat starch).
Modified Food Starch See page 40	If this modified starch is derived from wheat, the term "wheat" must be declared in the ingredient list or in a Contains statement. For example – modified food starch (wheat) or Contains: Wheat.	The source of the modified starch is not required to be declared. When wheat is the source, the label may read "modified food starch" or "modified wheat starch."	The common name modified plus the name of the plant starch must be declared in the ingredient list (e.g., modified wheat starch, modified tapioca starch).
Dextrin See page 41	Dextrin derived from wheat must declare the word "wheat" in the ingredient list or in a Contains statement.	The source of the dextrin is not required to be identified on the label. When wheat is the source, the label will read either "wheat dextrin" or "dextrin."	Dextrin derived from wheat must declare the word "wheat" in the ingredient list or in a Contains statement.

	United States		Canada
	FDA	**USDA**	**Health Canada**
Maltodextrin Maltodextrin is considered gluten free, even if derived from a gluten source. See page 41	If wheat-based maltodextrin contains any residual wheat protein, then "wheat" must be declared either in the ingredient list or in a Contains statement.	If maltodextrin is derived from wheat, then "wheat" may or may not be declared in the ingredient list or in a Contains statement.	If wheat-based maltodextrin contains any residual wheat protein, then "wheat" must be declared either in the ingredient list or in a Contains statement.
Glucose Syrup Glucose syrup is considered gluten free, even if derived from a gluten source. See page 41	If wheat-based glucose syrup contains any residual wheat protein, then "wheat" must be declared in the ingredient list or in a Contains statement. There is no requirement that "barley" be declared on the food label when barley-based glucose syrup is used as an ingredient.	Wheat or barley-based glucose syrup may or may not identify wheat or barley in the ingredient list or in a Contains statement.	If wheat-based glucose syrup contains any residual wheat protein, then "wheat" must be declared in the ingredient list or in a Contains statement. If barley-based glucose syrup contains any residual barley protein, then "barley" must be declared in the ingredient list or in a Contains statement.
Caramel Caramel is considered gluten free, even if derived from a gluten source. See page 38	If wheat-based caramel contains any residual wheat protein, then "wheat" must be declared in the ingredient list or in a Contains statement. There is no requirement that "barley" be declared on the label when barley-based caramel is used as an ingredient.	The source of caramel is not required to be identified on the label. If wheat or barley was used in the production of caramel, these sources may or may not be declared in the ingredient list or Contains statement.	If wheat-based caramel contains any residual wheat protein, then "wheat" must be declared in the ingredient list or in a Contains statement. If barley-based caramel contains any residual barley protein, then "barley" must be declared in the ingredient list or in a Contains statement.
Malt See page 37	The term "malt" is the common or usual name for this ingredient that is made from barley. There is no requirement that the word "barley" be declared on the food label when malt is used as an ingredient.	The term "malt" is the common or usual name for this ingredient made from barley. There is no requirement that the word "barley" be declared on the food label when malt is used as an ingredient.	The term "malt" is the common or usual name for this ingredient made from barley. Malt from barley must be listed as "barley malt" or "malt (barley)," or "Contains: Barley."
Malt Extract / Malt Syrup See page 38	"Malt extract" and "malt syrup" are interchangeable common or usual names for this ingredient made from barley. There is no requirement that the word "barley" be declared on the food label when malt extract or malt syrup is used as an ingredient.	"Malt extract" and "malt syrup" are interchangeable common or usual names for this ingredient made from barley. When used to flavor a meat or poultry product, the name "malt extract" or "malt syrup" must be declared in the ingredient list. There is no requirement that the word "barley" be declared on the food label when malt extract or malt syrup is used as an ingredient.	"Malt extract" and "malt syrup" are interchangeable common or usual names for this ingredient made from barley. The word "barley" must appear in the list of ingredients or in a Contains statement.

	United States		Canada
	FDA	**USDA**	**Health Canada**
Malt Flavoring See page 38	Malt flavoring is made from barley. There is no requirement that the word "barley" be declared on the food label when malt flavoring is used as an ingredient.	Malt flavoring is made from barley. There is no requirement that the word "barley" be declared on the food label when malt flavoring is used as an ingredient.	Malt flavoring is made from barley. The word "barley" must appear in the list of ingredients or in a Contains statement.
Hydrolyzed Proteins See page 39	Hydrolyzed protein cannot be declared in the list of ingredients as "flavor" or "natural flavor." A hydrolyzed protein's common or usual name must include the identity of the food source from which it was derived (e.g., hydrolyzed wheat protein, hydrolyzed soy protein).	Hydrolyzed protein cannot be declared in the list of ingredients as "flavor" or "natural flavor." A hydrolyzed protein's common or usual name must include the identity of the food source from which it was derived (e.g., hydrolyzed wheat gluten, hydrolyzed soy protein).	Hydrolyzed protein cannot be declared in the list of ingredients as "flavour" or "natural flavour." The word hydrolyzed plus the name of the plant plus protein (e.g., hydrolyzed wheat protein, hydrolyzed soy protein) must be declared in the ingredient list.
Autolyzed Yeast and Autolyzed Yeast Extract / Yeast Extract See page 37	Must be declared in the list of ingredients and not as "natural flavor." If derived from brewer's yeast, there is no requirement that the word "barley" must appear on the food label.	Must be declared in the list of ingredients and not as "natural flavor." If derived from brewer's yeast, there is no requirement that the word "barley" must appear on the food label.	Must be declared in the ingredient list and not as "natural flavour." If derived from brewer's yeast, the word "barley" must appear in the ingredients list or in a Contains statement.
Natural Flavors See page 37	If a natural flavor contains any protein derived from a major food allergen, including wheat, the allergen must be declared in the ingredient list or Contains statement. For example – natural flavor (wheat) or Contains: Wheat.	If a natural flavor contains any protein derived from a major food allergen or gluten source, it must be identified in the ingredient list by its common or usual name (e.g., hydrolyzed wheat protein, malt flavoring).	If a natural flavour contains any protein derived from a priority food allergen or gluten source, the allergen or gluten source must be declared in the ingredient list or in a Contains statement. For example – natural flavour (wheat) or Contains: Wheat. Another example – natural flavour (barley) or Contains: Barley.
Seasonings See page 39	Each ingredient in a seasoning blend must be declared in the ingredient list by its common or usual name, with the exception of a few spices, natural flavors, artificial flavors and some coloring agents. If any ingredient contains wheat protein, the term "wheat" must appear in the ingredient list or in a Contains statement. There is no requirement that the word "barley" be declared on the food label.	Most ingredients in a seasoning blend must be declared by their common or usual name in a sub-list after the term "seasonings" in the ingredient list. For example, "seasonings (spices, hydrolyzed soy protein, corn starch, monosodium glutamate)." "Barley" or "wheat" may or may not be declared on the label.	If an ingredient in a seasoning blend contains any protein derived from a priority food allergen or gluten source, the allergen or gluten source must be declared in the ingredient list or in a Contains statement.

	United States		Canada
	FDA	**USDA**	**Health Canada**
Smoke Flavoring See page 39	Smoke flavoring may be declared on the label as "smoke flavoring," "natural flavoring," "artificial flavoring" or "artificial smoke flavoring." Malted barley flour, if used as the carrier agent in the smoke flavoring, may or may not be declared in the list of ingredients by its common or usual name – i.e., "malted barley flour."	Natural smoke flavoring must be declared on the label as "natural smoke flavoring" or "smoke flavoring" and cannot be listed as "natural flavor" or "artificial flavor." Artificial smoke flavoring must be declared on the label as "artificial smoke flavoring." Malted barley flour, if used as the carrier agent in the smoke flavoring, must appear on the label by its common or usual name – i.e., "malted barley flour."	Natural smoke flavour must be declared on the label as "natural smoke flavour" or "smoke flavour" and cannot be listed as "natural flavour" or "artificial flavour." "Artificial smoke flavour" must be declared on the label as "artificial smoke flavour." Malted barley flour, if used as the carrier agent in the smoke flavouring, must be declared as "barley" in the ingredient list or in a Contains statement.
Vinegar See page 36	The single word "vinegar" refers to vinegar made from apples and is also called "cider vinegar" or "apple vinegar." "Malt vinegar" is derived from barley. This must be declared as "malt vinegar" and not simply as "vinegar." There is no requirement that the word "barley" be declared on the food label when malt vinegar is used as an ingredient.	The single word "vinegar" refers to vinegar made from apples and is also called "cider vinegar" or "apple vinegar." Distilled vinegar also can be labeled as "vinegar." "Malt vinegar" is derived from barley. This must be declared as "malt vinegar" and not simply as "vinegar." There is no requirement that the word "barley" be declared on the food label when malt vinegar is used as an ingredient.	The single word "vinegar" refers to wine vinegar, spirit vinegar, alcohol vinegar, white vinegar, grain vinegar, malt vinegar, cider vinegar or apple vinegar, singly or in combination. If the vinegar (after processing) contains any protein from the priority food allergens or gluten sources, the protein must be declared in the list of ingredients or in a Contains statement. For example – vinegar (barley), malt vinegar (barley) or Contains: Barley.

Alcohol Labeling in the United States and Canada

Between the U.S. and Canada, labeling regulations for alcoholic beverages differ. In the U.S., the labeling of alcoholic beverages is regulated by both the Alcohol and Tobacco Tax and Trade Bureau (TTB) and the Food and Drug Administration (FDA), with jurisdiction depending on the type of alcohol. Health Canada regulates all foods and beverages, including alcohol. The following summarizes the jurisdictions, as well as ingredient and gluten-free regulations for alcoholic beverages in both countries.

For more information about alcoholic beverages, see pages 31–34 and pages 327 and 328 in the References section.

United States

Alcohol and Tobacco Tax and Trade Bureau

The U.S. Alcohol and Tobacco Tax and Trade Bureau regulates the majority of alcoholic beverages including distilled alcohols, wines (more than 7% alcohol by volume), beer (made <u>with both</u> malted barley and hops), hard ciders (more than 7% alcohol by volume) and malt beverages (containing barley).

Allergen Labeling

Labels for alcoholic beverages under the jurisdiction of the TTB currently are not required to list ingredients or allergen sources. The exceptions to this rule are the mandatory declarations of sulphites, aspartame and certain coloring agents. However, the TTB published both an interim rule and a proposed rule on July 26, 2006, that addressed the issue of allergen labeling for alcoholic beverages (*Major Food Allergen Labeling for Wines, Distilled Spirits, and Malt Beverages*). The interim rule stated that manufacturers are permitted to declare the presence of major food allergens in the product on a voluntary basis; whereas, the proposed rule recommends mandatory declaration of all allergens. Currently, allergen labeling for TTB-regulated alcoholic beverages is still voluntary.

Gluten-Free Labeling

The TTB issued an interim policy entitled *Gluten Content Statements in the Labeling and Advertising of Wines, Distilled Spirits and Malt Beverages* on May 24, 2012. "Gluten-free" claims are permitted for wines, ciders and distilled alcohols not derived from wheat, rye or barley provided no cross-contamination has occurred during manufacturing. A "gluten-free" claim is NOT permitted for fermented barley-based beverages (e.g., beer) and distilled alcohols made from wheat, rye or barley (e.g., whiskey). When alcoholic beverages are made from these gluten-containing grains that have been "[processed or treated or crafted] to remove gluten," one of the following statements is permissible on the product label and in advertisements:

1. **"Product fermented from grains containing gluten and [processed or treated or crafted] to remove gluten. The gluten content of this product cannot be verified, and this product may contain gluten."**

   This statement would apply to barley-based gluten-reduced beers (see discussion about these types of beers on p. 33). There may be situations where a gluten-reduced beer may still include a "gluten-free" claim. Alcoholic beverages sold in the U.S. must have prior approval of the product label by the TTB before entering the market. However, if a product is brewed and sold only in the same state and does not cross the state line, the company is not required to receive label approval from the TTB.

2. **"This product was distilled from grains containing gluten, which removed some or all of the gluten. The gluten content of this product cannot be verified, and this product may contain gluten."**

    Even though the distillation process (if done correctly following "Good Manufacturing Practices") would completely remove all proteins from the final purified alcohol, the TTB will not allow a "gluten-free" claim on distilled alcoholic beverages made from gluten-containing grains.

Food and Drug Administration

Beers (made <u>without both</u> barley and hops), hard ciders (less than 7% alcohol by volume) and wines (less than 7% alcohol by volume) are under the jurisdiction of the FDA.

Alcoholic beverages under the jurisdiction of the FDA must follow *FALCPA* labeling requirements and may bear a "gluten-free" claim provided they meet all FDA's requirements for gluten-free labeling (e.g., not made with a gluten-containing grain). See pages 52 and 332 about *FALCPA* and pages 56–58 about gluten-free claims.

Canada

Ingredient Declarations

Standardized alcoholic beverages such as distilled alcohols (e.g., rum, whiskey, vodka), wines and beer are not required to list ingredients on the label; however, any priority food allergens, gluten sources or added sulphites (at 10 ppm or more) must be declared in an ingredient list or Contains statement. Exceptions to this rule are that wines produced before 2012 and all standardized beers are not required to list allergens, gluten sources or added sulphites on the label.

Non-standardized alcohols (e.g., coolers, ciders and beers not made with barley) must identify the ingredients and any allergens on the product label. If a "fining agent" used to clarify wine contains protein from allergens (e.g., milk, egg, fish, wheat) and is present in the final product, it must be declared on the label in a Contains statement.

Gluten-Free Claims

Health Canada permits the use of a "gluten-free" claim on distilled alcohols provided they meet the requirements of the gluten-free regulation B.24.018. Because the distillation process removes the gluten protein from the final product, a distilled alcohol made with wheat, rye or barley is rendered gluten free (see p. 32). If a gluten-containing ingredient is added after the distillation process (e.g., malt flavoring), the alcohol is no longer gluten free and thus would not qualify for a gluten-free claim.

Wines inherently are gluten free, as they are made from grapes or other fruits and do not undergo a distillation process (see p. 32). For these reasons, Health Canada does not permit a gluten-free claim on wine.

Beer made from non-gluten-containing grain(s) is allowed to make a gluten-free claim as long as it meets the gluten-free labeling regulations. "Gluten-reduced beer" derived from barley, wheat or rye is prohibited from making a "gluten-free" claim. However, Health Canada has stated that if a manufacturer can provide "evidence to substantiate their claim, including a detailed description of the method used to remove gluten from the product, appropriate gluten assay results for the finished product, and the name and the manufacturer of the assay," the wording below can appear on the product label:

> **"This product is fermented from grains containing gluten and [processed or treated or crafted] to remove gluten. The gluten content of this product cannot be verified, and this product may contain gluten."**

Nutrition and the Gluten-Free Diet

8

Learning about a nutritious and balanced gluten-free diet is equally important as knowing about the foods that are gluten free. Unfortunately, the nutritional quality of the gluten-free diet often is overlooked. This chapter covers (1) the nutritional issues affecting those with celiac disease, (2) practical strategies and tips for improving the nutritional quality of the gluten-free diet, and (3) the nutrient composition of various gluten-free foods and ingredients. Also, appendix F on page 318 includes the nutritional composition of numerous gluten-free grains, flours, starches, gums, legumes, nuts and seeds. References for this chapter are found on pages 336–339. The chapter is organized as follows:

Nutritional Status of Individuals with Celiac Disease 66

Nutritional Quality of Gluten-Free Specialty Products 66

Enrichment and Fortification 67

Specific Nutritional Concerns 67
    Weight Management 68
    Lactose Intolerance 68
    Calcium 70
    Vitamin D 74
    Bone Disease 77
    Iron 79
    Folate 84
    Vitamin B_{12} 89
    Dietary Fiber 91

Nutritional Status of Individuals with Celiac Disease

The nutritional status of people with celiac disease varies considerably between individuals and is influenced by several key factors. The length of time the disease is active prior to diagnosis; the degrees of inflammation, intestinal damage and malabsorption; and nutritional adequacy of the diet before eliminating gluten all can impact overall nutritional health.

Researchers have investigated nutritional deficiencies and associated conditions at diagnosis in both children and adults with celiac disease. In these studies many were deficient in a number of nutrients, especially iron, folate, calcium, vitamin D and/or zinc. Most of these nutrients are absorbed in the upper portions of the small intestine (duodenum and jejunum) that are damaged in celiac disease. A deficiency in some of these nutrients can lead to nutrition-related complications such as anemia and osteoporosis, two (among other) conditions frequently observed in this population. Also, in many individuals, damage to the intestinal villi causes lactose intolerance.

Studies of both children and adults have shown that in spite of the malabsorption, most individuals were not underweight at diagnosis. In fact, many actually were overweight or obese, particularly the adults. Because damage in the small intestine often is patchy, healthy areas still remain and have the capacity to absorb some nutrients including proteins, carbohydrates, fats, vitamins and minerals.

Following a strict gluten-free diet is essential for healing of the damaged small intestinal villi and more effective absorption of the nutrients in foods. While a gluten-free diet currently is the sole treatment for celiac disease, in some cases this may not be nutritionally adequate. Research from various countries has demonstrated that intakes of fiber, iron, folate, calcium, vitamin D, magnesium and zinc in a gluten-free diet frequently were low, while calories, fat, sugar and other refined carbohydrates tended to be high. Some of the reasons why a gluten-free diet may be nutritionally unbalanced are:

- Nutrient-poor gluten-free substitutes are chosen as replacements for wheat-based products
- Intake of gluten-free whole grains is inadequate
- Dairy products are eliminated or restricted due to lactose intolerance

It is important, therefore, to make wise food choices to ensure an adequate intake of nutrients. However, vitamin and mineral supplementation also may be needed to correct any nutritional deficiencies.

Due to the nutritional issues associated with celiac disease, the complexity of the gluten-free diet and the challenges of learning how to adapt to this new lifestyle, consultation with a registered dietitian (RD) having expertise in celiac disease is highly recommended in order to (1) assess the nutritional adequacy of the gluten-free diet, (2) review the results of laboratory tests and (3) address any challenges encountered while on the diet.

Nutritional Quality of Gluten-Free Specialty Products

Just because a food is gluten free, it is not necessarily a healthy option. Studies from Australia, Italy, Spain, Austria, Canada and the U.S. examined the nutritional quality of many individual gluten-free products. A common theme was that many of those products were lower than their gluten-containing counterparts in fiber, protein, iron, folate and other B vitamins. The most significant differences were found in the pasta, bread, cereal and flour categories. Typically, the gluten-free versions of those foods are made with refined flours and starches that often are not enriched or fortified with vitamins and/or minerals. Furthermore, the baked products tend to be higher in calories because more sugar and fat are added to improve their flavor, texture and shelf life. Therefore, the focus should be on selecting products made with more nutritious whole grains (e.g., brown rice, millet, oats, quinoa, sorghum, teff) and/or enriched with iron and B vitamins. To learn more about healthy alternative grains, see pages 97–104.

Enrichment and Fortification

Enrichment refers to the process whereby vitamins and minerals lost during processing subsequently are added back into the food product. For instance, during the milling of a grain, if the bran and germ are removed, the resulting "refined" grain contains substantially lower levels of fiber, B vitamins, iron and other nutrients. When the removed nutrients then are added back to that refined grain, it is labeled "enriched." In contrast, fortification is the addition of nutrients (e.g., vitamins, minerals, omega-3 fatty acids) to a product that originally were not present in the food or were present only in very insignificant amounts. The additions of vitamin D to fluid milk or calcium to orange juice are examples of fortification.

Unlike wheat-based baked products, cereals and pastas, the majority of gluten-free items in these categories usually are not enriched with iron and B vitamins. To illustrate this point, the percent daily value of iron in a particular brand of enriched wheat-based pasta contains 10% of the daily value for iron versus 2% for the non-enriched gluten-free pasta. Fortunately, some gluten-free specialty products are enriched/fortified. Following is a select list of companies that enrich/fortify some of their gluten-free products:

• All But Gluten	• gfJules	• Kinnikinnick
• Barbara's	• Gluten Free Café	• 1-2-3 Gluten Free
• Cooksimple	• Glutino	• Pastato
• DeBoles	• Kellogg Company	• President's Choice
• Duinkerken	• KIND	• Schär
• Ener-G	• King Arthur Flour	• Udi's Gluten Free
• Enjoy Life		

Specific Nutritional Concerns

In this section, the most common nutrition-related issues in celiac disease are discussed, beginning with information about weight management and lactose intolerance and followed by a discussion of key nutrients of particular concern. The main function of each nutrient is described, followed by the consequences of a deficiency, recommendations for daily intake,* dietary sources (listed from highest to lowest in value) and practical tips to increase intake.

* The "**Dietary Reference Intakes**" (DRIs) are reference values for the daily intake of over 40 nutrients specific for age, gender and life stage. They were developed in 1997 by the National Academy of Science's Food and Nutrition Board, Institute of Medicine of the National Academies.

Weight Management

As the symptoms of celiac disease resolve – especially bloating, abdominal pain and gas – there tends to be an improved sense of well-being and as a result, appetite often increases. Regardless of whether an individual was underweight, overweight or at healthy weight at the time of diagnosis, excess weight gain on the gluten-free diet frequently occurs because food now is being more completely absorbed. Therefore, making careful food choices and controlling serving sizes are essential. Many gluten-free products are low in fiber and protein and tend to digest quickly, thus increasing a craving for more food. Also, these foods often contain more calories than their gluten-containing counterparts. Following are some healthy strategies for successful weight management:

- Limit nutrient-poor, high-fat and/or high-sugar items such as gluten-free cookies, cakes, pastries, chips, candy and soft drinks.

- Incorporate more fiber-rich foods (e.g., fruits, vegetables, whole grains, nuts, seeds and legumes) into meals and snacks.

- Choose whole grains such as amaranth, buckwheat, brown rice, millet, oats, quinoa, sorghum and teff instead of white rice and other refined grain-based foods.

- Eat smaller meals and snacks throughout the day to prevent cravings.

- Include a protein-rich food with each meal to slow down the digestion process and increase satiety (the feeling of "fullness"). Good sources of protein include lean meats, fish, seafood, poultry, legumes, nuts, seeds and low-fat dairy products.

- Choose low-fat milk, yogurt and cheese.

- Use smaller amounts of butter, margarine, oils and salad dressings.

- Drink plenty of water.

- Stay active and exercise regularly.

Lactose Intolerance

Lactose is a naturally occurring sugar found in milk and milk products. Individuals who are lactose intolerant lack enough of the enzyme lactase, located in the tips of the small intestinal villi, to completely digest the lactose into two simple sugars (glucose and galactose). If lactose is not digested it passes through the intestinal tract, drawing fluid along with it. When it reaches the large intestine, naturally occurring bacteria ferment the lactose and produce fatty acids and gas. Symptoms of lactose intolerance can include abdominal cramping, bloating, gas, nausea, diarrhea and/or headache. These symptoms can appear within 15–30 minutes or as long as several hours after consumption of lactose.

Causes of Lactose Intolerance

Primary lactase deficiency
In some people, the level of lactase enzyme activity may gradually decrease with age to the point where they no longer are able to tolerate as much lactose as they once did. This type of intolerance affects approximately 70% of the world's population and is more prevalent among Asians, Africans, Hispanics, African Americans and North American Aboriginals.

Secondary lactase deficiency
This usually is a temporary condition in which the level of lactase has decreased as a result of injury to the gastrointestinal tract because of conditions such as celiac disease, inflammatory bowel disease, surgery, infection or the use of certain medications.

Lactose Intolerance in Celiac Disease

Individuals with celiac disease may or may not present with lactose intolerance at diagnosis. The extent of intestinal damage and the level of lactase in the villi affect lactose digestion. If significant gastrointestinal symptoms persist in spite of following a strict gluten-free diet, lactose may need to be reduced or eliminated until the villi are healed and the lactase enzyme levels are restored. Most individuals can digest small amounts of lactose; therefore, it usually is not necessary to completely eliminate lactose from the diet. Because tolerance to lactose varies greatly, an individualized approach needs to be taken with respect to the type and amount of lactose-containing foods consumed.

Dairy products are an excellent source of many nutrients, especially calcium and vitamin D. Although they contain differing amounts of lactose (e.g., one cup of milk has 11 grams compared to 1 gram of lactose in an ounce of cheddar cheese), it nonetheless is possible to consume these nutritious foods with some adaptations. The following information and practical tips can help in the management of lactose intolerance:

Milk

- Avoid drinking large quantities of milk at one time. Small amounts (e.g., ¼–½ cup), spaced throughout the day, often are better tolerated.

- Consume milk or milk products with meals or snacks rather than on an empty stomach.

- Try lactose-reduced or lactose-free milk. Lactase enzymes have been added to the milk, converting the naturally occurring lactose to simple, easily digested sugars. These types of milk are slightly sweeter than regular milk but have the same nutritional value. They also can be used in cooking and baking.

- Dried milk powder and non-fat milk solids are very high in lactose.

Yogurt

- Yogurt generally is better tolerated than milk. Live and active bacteria cultures that are added to milk during the production of yogurt have the ability to break down some of the lactose and create lactic acid in the process, contributing to yogurt's taste and texture.

Cheese

- Aged hard cheeses (e.g., cheddar, Swiss, Parmesan, mozzarella) are low in lactose. The majority of the lactose is removed with the whey and the small amount remaining is broken down during the aging process.

- Soft cheeses such as creamed cottage cheese, feta, quark and ricotta contain varying amounts of lactose. Limit consumption to small amounts with meals.

Miscellaneous Foods

- Avoid or limit the quantity of ice cream, ice milk, cream, whipping cream and sour cream.

- Soups, salad dressings and sauces also may contain lactose from milk, cream and/or added milk solids.

- Non-dairy beverages, cheeses, yogurts and frozen desserts made from ingredients such as coconut, nuts (e.g., almond, cashew), rice, soy or other ingredients (e.g., pea protein) do not contain lactose. When choosing such beverages look for those enriched with calcium, vitamin D and other nutrients. Check the label to make sure they do not contain barley malt flavoring.

Lactase Products

- Lactase enzyme products are available in different strengths and forms (tablets, caplets and drops). These enzyme preparations break down the naturally occurring lactose found in milk and milk products. Tablets or caplets should be taken just before consuming a food that contains lactose. Lactase drops must be added to the milk at least 24 hours in advance of consumption in order for the lactose to be broken down.

Calcium

This most-abundant mineral in the body is found in the skeleton, teeth, blood, muscles and fluid between cells. The majority of calcium (99%) is located in the bones and teeth. Calcium is involved in building and maintaining strong bones and teeth, blood clotting, contraction and relaxation of muscles, nerve transmission, regulation of the heartbeat, and the secretion of enzymes and hormones.

During childhood and adolescence, bones increase in size, density and strength. This process continues until peak bone mass (maximum amount of calcium deposited in the bones) is achieved, usually before age 30. However, because approximately 90% is acquired by age 18–20, consuming enough calcium and vitamin D during this crucial growth and development period is essential.

The body has a tightly regulated system that ensures a constant level of calcium is within the fluids and tissues at all times. It does this in several ways, by (1) absorbing calcium from foods, (2) slowing down the amount of calcium lost through the urine and (3) if necessary, pulling calcium out of the bones when there is an insufficient dietary intake. To prevent this loss of calcium from bones that can lead to osteoporosis, adequate amounts of calcium need to be consumed on a daily basis throughout life.

Table 8.1 Dietary Reference Intake for calcium

	Age	Calcium (mg/day)
Infants	0–6 mo	200*
	7–12 mo	260*
Children	1–3 y	700
	4–8 y	1000
Males	9–18 y	1300
	19–50 y	1000
	51–70 y	1000
	>70 y	1200
Females	9–18 y	1300
	19–50 y	1000
	51–70 y	1200
	>70 y	1200
Pregnancy	≤18 y	1300
	19–30 y	1000
	31–50 y	1000
Lactation	≤18 y	1300
	19–30 y	1000
	31–50 y	1000

* Adequate Intake (AI)

Food Sources of Calcium

Milk and milk products are major sources of calcium and many other nutrients. In the North American diet, dairy products provide more than 75% of the total calcium intake. Other foods also supply calcium (e.g., broccoli, spinach, almonds, dried beans), but generally in smaller amounts or in a form that the body absorbs less efficiently. (Nevertheless, these foods still provide a diverse range of nutrients and should be included in the diet.) Note that an adequate vitamin D intake is needed for the absorption of calcium (see p. 74). Practical tips for getting enough calcium are as follows:

- Choose foods high in calcium (see pp. 72–74).

- For those who do not like drinking plain milk, use it in cream soups, sauces, tea, coffee, smoothies or baking. Try drinking chocolate milk.

- If restricting dairy products, choose orange juice, non-dairy beverages and cereals that have been fortified with calcium.

- A calcium supplement also may be necessary if dietary intake is not sufficient. Discuss supplementation with a dietitian, pharmacist or physician. In addition, here are some key points to keep in mind when selecting a supplement:

  – Calcium is available in different forms such as calcium carbonate, calcium citrate, calcium lactate, calcium gluconate, calcium phosphate and calcium citrate. The most commonly available forms of calcium in supplements are carbonate or citrate.

  – Check the label to determine the amount of total "elemental" calcium in the supplement. This is the amount of calcium that can be absorbed by the body. On average, calcium supplements contain 300–600 mg of elemental calcium, whereas most multivitamin/mineral supplements contain lower amounts (e.g., 100–200 mg).

  – Calcium is absorbed more effectively when taken in divided doses throughout the day, e.g., a maximum of 500 mg at one time twice daily, rather than 1000 mg in a single daily dose.

  – For maximum absorption, calcium carbonate should be consumed with food or immediately after eating. Conversely, calcium citrate can be taken at any time as it does not depend on stomach acid for its absorption.

  – Some individuals may experience gas and/or constipation when taking calcium supplements. Strategies to alleviate the gastrointestinal symptoms include (1) starting with a smaller dose (e.g., 200–300 mg elemental calcium) for 1–2 weeks, then gradually increasing the amount, (2) spreading the dose throughout the day, (3) increasing fluid intake and/or (4) trying a different brand or form of calcium (calcium carbonate tends to cause more side effects than does calcium citrate).

Table 8.2   Calcium content of dairy products (highest to lowest)

Milk	Amount	Calcium (mg)
Milk – Calcium Fortified (non-fat/skim)	1 cup	504
Milk (reduced-fat/2%)	1 cup	350
Chocolate Milk (low-fat/1%)	1 cup	322
Milk (non-fat/skim)	1 cup	316
Milk (low-fat/1%)	1 cup	314
Milk Powder – Dry Instant (non-fat/skim)	1/3 cup	283
Buttermilk – Whole	1 cup	282
Milk – Whole (3.25%)	1 cup	276
Milk – Evaporated (non-fat) (canned)	1/4 cup	186

Cheese	Amount	Calcium (mg)
Swiss Cheese	2 oz.	498
Mozzarella Cheese (partly skimmed)	2 oz.	443
Cheddar Cheese	2 oz.	403
Mozzarella Cheese	2 oz.	286
Feta Cheese	2 oz.	280
Camembert Cheese	2 oz.	220
Processed Cheese Slices	1 slice	219
Parmesan Cheese (grated)	4 Tbsp.	171
Ricotta Cheese (partly skimmed)	1/4 cup	169
Ricotta Cheese	1/4 cup	128
Processed Cheese Spread	2 Tbsp.	118
Brie Cheese	2 oz.	104
Cottage Cheese (low-fat/1%)	1/2 cup	69

Yogurt and Ice Cream	Amount	Calcium (mg)
Yogurt – Plain (low-fat)	6 oz.	311
Yogurt Beverage	1 cup	264
Yogurt – Fruit (low-fat)	6 oz.	258
Yogurt – Greek, Plain (non-fat)	6 oz.	187
Yogurt – Greek, Strawberry (low-fat)	6 oz.	150
Frozen Yogurt	1/2 cup	108
Ice Cream – Vanilla	1/2 cup	84

Table 8.3 Calcium content of flours and starches (highest to lowest)

Flours and Starches	1 cup (weight in grams)	Calcium (mg)
Flaxseed Meal / Ground Flax	112	286
Almond Meal (natural with skins)	100	269
Almond Flour (blanched)	112	264
Teff Flour	160	254
Soy Flour (defatted)	105	253
Navy Bean Flour (whole)	149	238
Amaranth Flour	120	203
Mesquite Flour	146	196
Black Bean Flour (whole)	129	181
Soy Flour (full-fat)	84	173
Corn Flour – Yellow (masa, enriched)	114	157
Pea Flour – Yellow (whole)	166	134
Hazelnut Flour	112	128
Garfava™ Flour	157	104
Potato Flour	160	104
Lentil Flour (whole)	180	99
Pinto Bean Flour (whole)	130	96
Chickpea / Garbanzo Bean Flour (whole)	111	85
Chestnut Flour	102	73
Rice Bran (crude)	118	67
Oat Flour	120	66
Oat Bran (raw)	94	55
Quinoa Flour	112	52
Arrowroot Starch/Flour	128	51
Buckwheat Flour (whole groat)	120	49
Corn Bran (crude)	76	32
Tapioca Starch/Flour	120	28
Potato Starch	192	19
Millet Flour	119	17
Rice Flour – Brown	158	17
Rice Flour – White	158	16
Sorghum Flour – White (whole grain)	121	15
Sorghum Flour – White (refined, unenriched)	161	10
Corn Flour – Yellow (whole grain)	117	8
Cornmeal – Yellow (whole grain)	122	7
Rice Flour – Sweet	160	6
Cornmeal – Yellow (degermed, enriched and unenriched)	157	5
Corn Flour – Yellow (degermed, unenriched)	126	3
Cornstarch	128	3

Table 8.4 Calcium content of various foods (highest to lowest)

Various Foods	Amount	Calcium (mg)
Almond Beverage – Fortified, Sweetened, Vanilla Flavor	1 cup	451
Tofu – Regular (processed with calcium sulfate)*	½ cup	434
Almonds (whole, natural with skins)	1 cup	385
Sardines (canned, with bones)	8 small	367
Orange Juice – Calcium Fortified	1 cup	349
Almonds (whole, blanched)	1 cup	342
Soy Beverage – Fortified, Plain	1 cup	299
Salmon – Pink (canned, drained, solids with bones)	3.5 oz.	281
Salmon – Sockeye (canned, drained, solids with bones)	3.5 oz.	230
White Beans (cooked)	1 cup	161
Collards (cooked)	½ cup	134
Brazil Nuts	½ cup	107
Shrimp (canned)	½ cup	93
Baked Beans	1 cup	86
Peanuts (dry, roasted)	1 cup	85
Chickpeas / Garbanzo Beans (cooked)	1 cup	80
Chili Con Carne	1 cup	80
Bok Choy (cooked)	½ cup	79
Broccoli (cooked)	1 cup	62
Crab – Blue (canned)	½ cup	61
Orange – Navel	1 medium	60
Red Kidney Beans (cooked)	1 cup	50
Kale (cooked)	½ cup	47
Sesame Seeds (kernels, dried, decorticated)	½ cup	45
Figs (dried)	3	41
Salmon – Sockeye (cooked)	3.5 oz.	11

* The calcium content for tofu is an approximation based on products available on the market. Calcium content varies greatly from one brand to the other and can be quite low. Tofu processed with magnesium chloride contains less calcium.

Vitamin D

The chief function of this vitamin is to enhance the absorption of calcium and phosphorus in the small intestine, thereby making a significant contribution to bone health. It also is required by the immune system, muscles, heart, lungs and brain. Medical experts have been investigating the relationship between vitamin D and a wide range of diseases such as autoimmune disorders, diabetes, heart disease, stroke, cancer and neurocognitive disorders. However, while there is increasing evidence indicating that vitamin D is associated with such diseases, further research is needed to determine whether it can reduce the *risk* of specific disorders.

Vitamin D is unique because it can be produced naturally by the body when the skin is exposed to sunlight. Although it can be obtained from a limited number of foods as well as from supplements, sun exposure is the major source for most people. Nevertheless, several factors can impair or limit the body's ability to synthesize vitamin D from sunlight:

- In the sunlight of northern latitudes during the winter months, specific wavelengths required for the conversion of the inactive form of vitamin D in the skin are blocked by the atmosphere due to the angle of the sun.

- The use of sunscreen with a sun protection factor (SPF) of 8 or greater can interfere with vitamin D synthesis. While regular use of sunscreen is essential for prevention of skin cancer, sun exposure of the hands, arms and legs without sunscreen for only 10–15 minutes at least two to three times per week can help meet vitamin D requirements. After 10–15 minutes of such exposure, sunscreen should be applied.

- Heavy cloud cover or significant air pollution (smog) can block certain wavelengths of the sun needed to convert vitamin D in the skin to its active form.

- Sunlight through a window cannot stimulate the skin synthesis of vitamin D.

- Dark-skinned individuals with greater amounts of the pigment melanin require longer sun exposure time to produce vitamin D.

- Housebound individuals (e.g., the elderly) or those who wear robes / head coverings / all-covering clothing are less likely to get an adequate amount of vitamin D from sunlight.

- Vitamin D synthesis declines with age.

Dietary Reference Intake for Vitamin D

Vitamin D levels are expressed as micrograms (mcg) or International Units (IU). The biological activity of 1 mcg of vitamin D is equivalent to 40 IU. The daily requirement for vitamin D is listed in the table below. When these DRIs were revised in 2011, the Institute of Medicine's panel of experts focused primarily on vitamin D's effect on bone health. Other organizations recommend higher levels of vitamin D due to emerging research concerning its role in a wide variety of other conditions.

Table 8.5 Dietary Reference Intake for vitamin D

	Age	Vitamin D (mcg/day)*
Infants	0–6 mo	10
	7–12 mo	10
Children	1–3 y	15
	4–8 y	15
Males	9–13 y	15
	14–18 y	15
	19–50 y	15
	51–70 y	15
	>70 y	20
Females	9–13 y	15
	14–18 y	15
	19–50 y	15
	51–70 y	15
	>70 y	20
Pregnancy	≤18 y	15
	19–30 y	15
	31–50 y	15
Lactation	≤18 y	15
	19–30 y	15
	31–50 y	15

* Expressed as cholecalciferol. 1 microgram (mcg) of cholecalciferol = 40 IU vitamin D.
  Recommended amounts in the absence of adequate exposure to sunlight.

Food Sources of Vitamin D

This fat-soluble vitamin, also known as the "sunshine vitamin," is found in a small number of foods such as fatty fish (e.g., mackerel, salmon, tuna, sardines), fish liver oils, beef liver, egg yolks and in some types of mushrooms that have been exposed to ultraviolet light. In North America, fortified foods are the major dietary sources of vitamin D. The fortification regulations and policies in the U.S. and Canada differ (see table 8.7 on p. 77). In the U.S., although a range of foods are permitted to be fortified with vitamin D on a voluntary basis (e.g., milk, yogurt, cheese, margarine, cereals, rice, cornmeal, pasta, plant-based beverages, fruit drinks and juices), fluid milk and ready-to-eat cereals are the most common fortified sources. In Canada, vitamin D fortification of milk (fluid, evaporated and dry) and margarine is mandatory. While other foods could be fortified, this is done less extensively than in the U.S.

Vitamin D Supplements

Vitamin D is available in various supplements. Most multivitamin and mineral supplements contain at least 10 mcg (400 IU) and some calcium supplements have added vitamin D. It also is available as a single-dose supplement ranging from 5–25 mcg (200–1000 IU). Cod liver oil is rich in naturally occurring vitamin D, while other fish oil supplements may contain varying levels, if any. Omega-3 fatty acids from fish oils usually do not contain any vitamin D; however, some companies may add it to these supplements.

Supplementation often is required because achieving an adequate vitamin D status can be difficult for a significant percentage of the population. This is especially important for individuals with celiac disease, due not only to the small intestinal inflammation and malabsorption but also to the fact that many individuals already have some degree of bone loss at diagnosis.

Table 8.6   Vitamin D content in foods (highest to lowest)

Foods	Amount	Vitamin D (IU)
Cod Liver Oil	1 Tbsp.	1360
Salmon – Sockeye (canned, drained, solids with bones)	3.5 oz.	834
Salmon – Sockeye (cooked)	3.5 oz.	664
Salmon – Pink (canned, drained, solids with bones)	3.5 oz.	575
Mackerel (cooked)	3.5 oz.	453
Mushrooms – White (exposed to ultraviolet light, raw)*	4 small	418
Sardines (canned in oil, drained)	8 small	185
Soy Beverage – Plain (fortified with vitamin D)	1 cup	119
Milk (low-fat/1%) (fortified with vitamin D)	1 cup	117
Orange Juice (fortified with vitamin D)	1 cup	100
Yogurt – Fruit (non-fat) (fortified with vitamin D)	6 oz.	88
Margarine**	1 Tbsp.	60
Beef Liver (cooked)	3.5 oz.	49
Tuna (canned in water, drained)	3.5 oz.	47
Pudding (made with fortified milk)	½ cup	45
Egg (whole, cooked)	1 large	44
Ready-To-Eat Cereal (fortified with vitamin D)	1 cup	40
Mushrooms – White (raw)	4 small	3
Yogurt – Fruit (non-fat)	6 oz.	0

*   Mushrooms naturally produce vitamin D, when growers expose them to UV light.
** Margarine in Canada must be fortified with vitamin D.

Table 8.7 American and Canadian vitamin D fortification regulations/policies for select food and beverages

Food or Beverage	Vitamin D Fortification	
	United States	Canada
Fluid Milk	Optional*	Mandatory
Milk Powder – Dry (non-fat)	Optional	Mandatory
Milk Powder – Dry (whole)	Optional	Mandatory
Evaporated Milk	Mandatory	Mandatory
Margarine	Optional	Mandatory
Yogurt and Yogurt-Based Beverages	Optional	Optional; however, vitamin D cannot be added directly to the yogurt; it must come from vitamin D-fortified fluid milk
Cheese	Optional	Optional; however, vitamin D cannot be added directly to the cheese; it must come from vitamin D-fortified fluid milk
Non-Dairy Plant-Based Beverages (e.g., nut, rice, soy)	Optional	Optional
Calcium-Fortified Orange Juice	Optional	Optional
Calcium-Fortified Fruit Drink	Optional	Not permitted
Meal Replacements (e.g., in beverage form)	Optional	Optional
Ready-To-Eat Cereals	Optional	Permitted, but needs prior approval from Health Canada
Enriched Rice	Optional	Not permitted

* Nearly all milk sold in the U.S. is fortified with vitamin D.

Bone Disease

A range of nutrients is necessary for the formation and maintenance of healthy bones and teeth throughout the life cycle. Deficiencies or alterations in the metabolism of nutrients, especially calcium and vitamin D, are common in untreated celiac disease and can lead to osteomalacia, osteopenia and osteoporosis.

Table 8.8 Types of bone diseases

Condition	Description
Osteomalacia	Is failure to deposit calcium into newly formed bones, causing them to become soft, flexible and weak.
	Is caused by a deficiency of vitamin D, calcium and/or phosphorous.
	Can occur in children and adults.
	In children, is called rickets. Symptoms can include bone pain, skeletal deformities (e.g., bow legs, curved spine), dental deformities (e.g., delayed formation of teeth, holes in the enamel, cavities), bone fractures and short stature.
	In adults causes symptoms including bone pain, muscle weakness and fractures.

Condition	Description
Osteopenia	Although not as severe as osteoporosis, causes mild thinning of the outer bone tissue and loss of bone mineral density.
	Is caused by a deficiency of calcium and/or vitamin D.
	Is a risk for the development of osteoporosis.
	Is indicated by a bone density reading between 1 and 2.5 standard deviations below the normal.
Osteoporosis	Is significant thinning of the outer bone tissue and loss of bone mineral density.
	Is caused by a variety of factors such as: – failure to obtain maximum bone mineral density in childhood and adolescence. – malabsorption of calcium and/or vitamin D. – increased production of specific cytokines and other inflammatory substances due to inflammation in the small intestine. – the autoimmune process that not only damages the intestinal villi but also can directly attack the bones.
	Results in porous, weak and brittle bones that break easily. Common fracture areas are the spine, hips, ribs and wrists.
	Causes bone density readings of 2.5 standard deviations or more below the normal. Is indicated by a bone density reading of 2.5 standard deviations or more below the normal.

Treatment of Bone Disease in Celiac Disease

When celiac disease develops in childhood or adolescence, peak bone mass can be affected, increasing the risk of osteoporosis later in life. However, with early diagnosis and appropriate treatment, decreased bone mass usually can be restored to normal levels, provided the diet contains sufficient nutrients required for bone health. For adults where bone loss resulting in osteopenia or osteoporosis has occurred later in life, correcting the bone abnormalities is more difficult. Nevertheless, it can be managed by diet and nutrient supplementation and, if necessary, by bone-enhancing medications.

The treatment for osteomalacia is supplemental vitamin D, and usually calcium. Bone structure will improve within several weeks, with complete healing by six months. In children, although the skeletal deformities often can be corrected, some may not reach their full growth potential.

Regardless of the type of bone disease affecting those with celiac disease, consuming enough calcium and vitamin D is absolutely essential in addition to following a strict gluten-free diet for life. Here are some further bone health tips:

- Eat a wide of variety of foods to ensure an adequate intake of nutrients that help build and maintain bone density.

- Limit intakes of alcohol and caffeine (e.g., coffee, cola, tea, energy drinks) and do not smoke: all are risk factors for osteoporosis.

- Stay active. Regular weight-bearing activities such as brisk walking, hiking, stair climbing, dancing and tennis, as well as resistance training with weights, can help maintain bone mass. Consult your physician before starting a regular exercise program, especially if osteopenia or osteoporosis is present or if there is a history of fractures.

Iron

This mineral is needed for the production of hemoglobin and myoglobin. Hemoglobin is the component of red blood cells that carries oxygen throughout the body, whereas the myoglobin protein stores oxygen in the muscle cells. Iron also is needed for the formation of certain enzymes and is involved in many other metabolic functions. The majority of iron is found in hemoglobin, myoglobin and enzymes, with the remaining stored in the liver, bone marrow and spleen.

Iron Deficiency or Iron-Deficiency Anemia

Iron deficiency occurs when the normal stores of iron decline gradually over time. Fatigue and irritability are the most common symptoms when iron levels are diminished. If the amount of iron becomes severely depleted, the production of hemoglobin is impaired and the red blood cells deliver less oxygen throughout the entire body. This state is referred to as iron-deficiency anemia (microcytic hypochromic anemia). Symptoms can include extreme fatigue, weakness and irritability, shortness of breath, pale skin, headache, dizziness, brittle nails, sore tongue, decreased appetite and increased susceptibility to infections. It also can cause reduced attention span in children, resulting in negative behavioral and developmental issues.

The main reasons for iron deficiency are an inadequate dietary iron intake, impaired iron absorption and blood loss. Individuals with celiac disease frequently develop iron-deficiency anemia due to the inability of the small intestinal villi to absorb iron in spite of adequate dietary intakes and/or supplementation. Treatment of iron deficiency or iron-deficiency anemia in celiac disease includes (1) following a strict gluten-free diet so the intestinal damage can be repaired, (2) consuming more iron-rich foods, and (3) taking an iron supplement if necessary (first consult a physician or dietitian).

Table 8.9   Dietary Reference Intake for iron

	Age	Iron (mg/day)
Infants	0–6 mo	0.27*
	7–12 mo	11
Children	1–3 y	7
	4–8 y	10
Males	9–13 y	8
	14–18 y	11
	19–50 y	8
	51–70 y	8
	>70 y	8
Females	9–13 y	8
	14–18 y	15
	19–50 y	18
	51–70 y	8
	>70 y	8
Pregnancy	≤18 y	27
	19–30 y	27
	31–50 y	27
Lactation	≤18 y	10
	19–30 y	9
	31–50 y	9

* Adequate Intake (AI)

Food Sources of Iron

Absorption of iron from dietary sources will vary depending on the body's total iron stores (when iron levels are low, absorption increases), the type of iron in the food and other dietary factors. The two types of iron in foods are heme and non-heme:

Heme Iron

- Is more readily absorbed by the body than is non-heme iron
- Absorption is not changed by other foods in the diet
- Is found only in meat, poultry, fish and shellfish

Non-Heme Iron

- Is not absorbed as well as is heme iron
- Absorption can be increased or decreased by other foods in the diet
- Is found in fruits, vegetables, legumes, grains and eggs
- Is also found in meat, poultry, fish and shellfish

Maximizing Iron Absorption

1. Choose foods high in iron (see pp. 81–84).

2. Eat a source of heme iron with non-heme iron at the same meal, for example:

   - Stir-fried beef, chicken, pork, fish or seafood with vegetables (e.g., broccoli) and rice and toasted almonds or sesame seeds
   - Chili made with meat and beans

3. Vitamin C increases absorption of non-heme iron; therefore, combine a vitamin C-rich food (e.g., citrus fruits and juices, kiwi fruit, strawberries, cantaloupe, broccoli, peppers [green, orange, red and yellow], tomatoes, potatoes, cabbage) with non-heme iron foods at the same meal, for example:

   - Poached egg and glass of orange juice
   - Casserole containing rice, beans and canned tomatoes or tomato sauce
   - Spinach salad with strawberries or orange segments

4. Avoid drinking coffee or tea with meals as these beverages contain tannins that interfere with iron absorption.

Iron Supplements

In addition to consuming iron-rich foods, some individuals with newly diagnosed celiac disease may need supplemental iron until the deficiency has been corrected. Be aware that iron supplements may cause nausea, abdominal pain and constipation. If these side effects occur, it may be helpful to (1) start with a lower dose and gradually increase, (2) take iron with a small amount of food and (3) if constipated, increase fiber intake and drink plenty of water.

Table 8.10 Iron content of flours and starches (highest to lowest)

Flours and Starches	1 cup (weight in grams)	Iron (mg)
Rice Bran (crude)	118	21.9
Lentil Flour (whole)	180	17.0
Corn Flour – Yellow (masa, enriched)	114	9.7
Soy Flour (defatted)	105	9.7
Teff Flour	160	9.7
Black Bean Flour (whole)	129	9.0
Navy Bean Flour (whole)	149	8.9
Amaranth Flour	120	8.2
Pea Flour – Yellow (whole)	166	8.0
Garfava™ Flour	157	7.9
Pinto Bean Flour (whole)	130	7.8
Oat Flour	120	7.7
Soy Flour (low-fat)	88	7.2
Cornmeal – Yellow (degermed, enriched)	157	6.9
Flaxseed Meal / Ground Flax	112	6.4
Chickpea / Garbanzo Bean Flour (whole)	111	6.3
Soy Flour (full-fat)	84	5.4
Hazelnut Flour	112	5.3
Mesquite Flour	146	5.1
Oat Bran (raw)	94	5.1
Buckwheat Flour (whole groat)	120	4.9
Millet Flour	119	4.7
Quinoa Flour	112	4.5
Cornmeal – Yellow (whole grain)	122	4.2
Sorghum Flour – White (whole grain)	121	3.8
Almond Flour (blanched)	112	3.7
Almond Meal (natural with skins)	100	3.7
Chestnut Flour	102	3.5
Rice Flour – Brown	158	3.1
Potato Starch	192	2.9
Corn Flour – Yellow (whole grain)	117	2.8
Peanut Flour (low-fat)	60	2.8
Potato Flour	160	2.2
Corn Bran (crude)	76	2.1
Cornmeal – Yellow (degermed, unenriched)	157	1.7
Sorghum Flour – White (refined, unenriched)	161	1.6
Peanut Flour (defatted)	60	1.3
Corn Flour – Yellow (degermed, unenriched)	126	1.2
Cornstarch	128	0.6
Rice Flour – White	158	0.6
Arrowroot Starch/Flour	128	0.4
Rice Flour – Sweet	160	0
Tapioca Starch/Flour	120	0

Table 8.11 Iron content of grains (highest to lowest)

Grains (cooked)	1 cup (weight in grams)	Iron (mg)
Amaranth	246	5.2
Teff	252	5.2
Rice – White (long grain, parboiled, enriched)	158	2.9
Oats – Steel-Cut	245	2.8
Quinoa	185	2.8
Sorghum – White (whole grain)	170	2.2
Oatmeal – Regular, Quick, Rolled Oats	234	2.1
Rice – White (long grain, enriched)	158	1.9
Buckwheat Groats (roasted)	168	1.3
Millet	174	1.1
Rice – Brown (long grain)	202	1.1
Rice – Wild	164	1.0
Sorghum – White (refined/pearled)	187	0.5
Rice – White (long grain, parboiled, unenriched)	158	0.4
Rice – White (long grain, unenriched)	158	0.3

Table 8.12 Iron content of meats and alternatives (highest to lowest)

Meat, Fish and Poultry	Amount	Iron (mg)
Chicken Liver (cooked)	3.5 oz.	11.6
Oysters (canned)	3.5 oz.	6.6
Beef Liver (cooked)	3.5 oz.	6.5
Beef Tenderloin Steak (cooked)	3.5 oz.	3.6
Ground Beef – Extra Lean (cooked)	3.5 oz.	3.2
Sardines (canned in oil)	8 small	2.8
Clams (cooked)	10 small	2.7
Roast Beef (cooked)	3.5 oz.	2.3
Lamb – Loin (cooked)	3.5 oz.	2.2
Shrimp (canned)	3.5 oz.	2.1
Tuna – Light (canned in water, drained)	3.5 oz.	1.6
Turkey – Dark Meat (cooked)	3.5 oz.	1.4
Chicken – Dark Meat (roasted)	3.5 oz.	1.3
Pork Tenderloin (cooked)	3.5 oz.	1.2
Chicken Breast (cooked)	3.5 oz.	1.0
Pork – Loin Roast (cooked)	3.5 oz.	0.9
Egg (whole, cooked)	1 large	0.6
Salmon – Sockeye (cooked)	3.5 oz.	0.5
Shrimp (cooked)	3.5 oz.	0.5

Legumes (cooked)	Amount	Iron (mg)
Soybeans – Mature	1 cup	8.8
Lentils	1 cup	6.6
White Beans	1 cup	6.6
Kidney Beans – Red	1 cup	5.2
Chickpeas / Garbanzo Beans	1 cup	4.7
Navy Beans	1 cup	4.3
Cranberry/Romano Beans	1 cup	3.7
Black Beans	1 cup	3.6
Pinto Beans	1 cup	3.6
Soybeans – Edamame	1 cup	3.5
Fava/Broad Beans	1 cup	2.6
Split Peas	1 cup	2.5

Nuts and Seeds	Amount	Iron (mg)
Chia Seeds	1 cup	17.5
Hemp Seeds (hulled)	1 cup	12.7
Pumpkin Seeds (kernels, dried)	1 cup	11.4
Flaxseeds	1 cup	9.6
Sesame Seeds (kernels, dried, decorticated)	1 cup	9.5
Flaxseed Meal / Ground Flax	1 cup	6.4
Hazelnuts/Filberts	1 cup	6.3
Almonds (whole, natural with skins)	1 cup	5.3
Sunflower Seeds (hulled, kernels, dry-roasted)	1 cup	4.9
Almonds (whole, blanched)	1 cup	4.8
Brazil Nuts (unblanched)	1 cup	3.2
Walnuts – English (shelled, halves)	1 cup	2.9
Pecans (halves)	1 cup	2.5
Peanuts (dry-roasted)	1 cup	2.3

Table 8.13   Iron content of fruits, vegetables and miscellaneous
(highest to lowest)

Fruits	Amount	Iron (mg)
Prune Juice	1 cup	3.0
Raisins (seedless)	½ cup	1.4
Apricots (dried, halves)	6 halves	0.6
Prunes (dried, pitted)	6 prunes	0.5

Vegetables	Amount	Iron (mg)
Spinach (cooked)	1 cup	6.4
Peas – Snow (cooked)	1 cup	3.2
Mushrooms (cooked)	1 cup	2.7
Peas – Green (cooked)	1 cup	2.5
Acorn Squash (cooked)	1 cup	1.9
Brussels Sprouts (cooked)	1 cup	1.9
Collards (frozen, chopped, cooked)	1 cup	1.9
Broccoli (chopped, cooked)	1 cup	1.1
Potato – White (baked with skin)	1 medium	1.1
Spinach (raw)	1 cup	0.8
Asparagus (cooked)	4 spears	0.6

Miscellaneous	Amount	Iron (mg)
Blackstrap Molasses	1 Tbsp.	2.8

Folate

This B vitamin is necessary for the formation of DNA and RNA (the building blocks of all cells) as well as red blood cells. In addition, it is required for protein metabolism and enzyme reactions. Because of its role in the development of new cells, folate is crucial during pregnancy. Women of child-bearing age who may become pregnant need to consume adequate amounts of folate prior to and during the first few months of pregnancy in order to reduce the risk of neural tube defects such as spina bifida and anencephaly in the fetus.

Folate Deficiency and Folate-Deficiency Anemia

A deficiency of folate can lead to macrocytic megaloblastic anemia, which is characterized by a reduced number of red blood cells that also are very large and immature. As a result, the oxygen-carrying capacity of these underdeveloped cells is impaired. Symptoms are similar to those of iron-deficiency anemia but also can include tinnitus (ringing in the ears), cracked lips, trouble concentrating, an irregular heartbeat and chest pain.

The two main reasons for folate deficiency are an inadequate intake and a decreased absorption of folate in the small intestine. Additionally, some medications can deplete folate levels or interfere with its action. Individuals with celiac disease may present with folate deficiency, although folate-deficiency anemia is not as common as iron-deficiency anemia. Treatment of folate deficiency or folate-deficiency anemia in celiac disease includes (1) following a strict gluten-free diet, (2) eating more folate-rich foods and (3) taking a folic acid supplement if necessary (first consult a physician or dietitian).

Table 8.14 Dietary Reference Intake for folate

	Age	Folate (mcg/day)
Infants	0–6 mo	65
	7–12 mo	80
Children	1–3 y	150
	4–8 y	200
Males	9–13 y	300
	14–18 y	400
	19–50 y	400
	51–70 y	400
	>70 y	400
Females	9–13 y	300
	14–18 y	400*
	19–50 y	400*
	51–70 y	400
	>70 y	400
Pregnancy	≤18 y	600**
	19–30 y	600**
	31–50 y	600**
Lactation	≤18 y	500
	19–30 y	500
	31–50 y	500

* In view of evidence linking folate intake with neural tube defects in the fetus, it is recommended that all women capable of becoming pregnant consume 400 micrograms (mcg) from supplements or fortified foods in addition to intake of food folate from a varied diet.

** It is assumed that women will continue consuming 400 micrograms from supplements or fortified food until their pregnancy is confirmed and they enter prenatal care, which ordinarily occurs after the end of the periconceptional period – the critical time for formation of the neural tube in the fetus.

Food Sources of Folate

The terms "folate" and "folic acid" are used interchangeably for this water-soluble B vitamin, even though technically they are not the same. Folates are found naturally in foods such as asparagus, broccoli, beets, orange juice, sunflower seeds and liver, as well as edamame and dried beans, lentils and peas. Folic acid is the synthetic form used in supplements and fortified foods, and is more readily absorbed by the body than are folates. In North America, fortified grains and grain-based products (e.g., breads, cereals, pastas) are the main sources of folic acid; however, gluten-free products typically are not fortified.

Here are some tips for getting enough folate: (1) eat foods rich in folate on a daily basis (see pp. 86–88), (2) choose gluten-free cereals, breads, pasta, baking mixes, cornmeal, corn flour, rice and other foods that are enriched/fortified with folic acid and (3) take a multivitamin and mineral supplement. Most brands contain 400 micrograms; prenatal supplements range between 600–1000 micrograms.

Table 8.15 Folate content of flours and starches (highest to lowest)

Flours and Starches	1 cup (weight in grams)	Folate (mcg)
Cornmeal – Yellow (degermed, enriched)	157	526
Corn Flour – Yellow (masa, enriched)	114	382
Amaranth Flour	120	344
Soy Flour (defatted)	105	320
Chickpea / Garbanzo Bean Flour (whole)	111	309
Quinoa Flour	112	308
Soy Flour (full-fat)	84	290
Soy Flour (low-fat)	88	254
Black Bean Flour (whole)	129	245
Pinto Bean Flour (whole)	130	242
Lentil Flour (whole)	180	215
Navy Bean Flour (whole)	149	161
Peanut Flour (defatted)	60	149
Teff Flour	160	139
Hazelnut Flour	112	127
Chestnut Flour	102	111
Flaxseed Meal / Ground Flax	112	97
Peanut Flour (low-fat)	60	80
Rice Bran (crude)	118	74
Buckwheat Flour (whole groat)	120	65
Oat Flour	120	65
Corn Flour – Yellow (degermed, unenriched)	126	60
Almond Flour (blanched)	112	55
Millet Flour	119	50
Oat Bran (raw)	94	49
Cornmeal – Yellow (degermed, unenriched)	157	47
Almond Meal (natural with skins)	100	44
Potato Flour	160	40
Cornmeal – Yellow (whole grain)	122	30
Sorghum Flour – White (whole grain)	121	30
Corn Flour – Yellow (whole grain)	117	29
Mesquite Flour	146	26
Rice Flour – Brown	158	25
Pea Flour – Yellow (whole)	166	23
Arrowroot Starch/Flour	128	9
Rice Flour – White	158	6
Corn Bran (crude)	76	3
Cornstarch	128	0

Table 8.16 Folate content of grains (highest to lowest)

Grains (cooked)	1 cup (weight in grams)	Folate (mcg)
Rice – White (long grain, parboiled, enriched)	158	215
Rice – White (long grain, enriched)	158	153
Quinoa	185	78
Amaranth	246	54
Teff	252	45
Rice – Wild	164	43
Oats – Steel-Cut	245	34
Millet	184	33
Buckwheat Groats (roasted)	168	24
Rice – Brown (long grain)	202	18
Oatmeal – Regular, Quick, Rolled Oats (unenriched)	234	14
Sorghum – White (whole grain)	170	13
Rice – White (long grain, parboiled, unenriched)	158	5
Rice – White (long grain, unenriched)	158	5

Table 8.17 Folate content of meats and alternatives (highest to lowest)

Meat, Poultry, Fish and Seafood	Amount	Folate (mcg)
Chicken Liver (cooked, simmered)	3.5 oz.	578
Beef Liver (cooked, braised)	3.5 oz.	253
Clams	9 small	25
Egg (whole, raw)	1 large	22

Legumes (cooked)	Amount	Folate (mcg)
Soybeans – Edamame	1 cup	482
Cranberry/Romano Beans	1 cup	366
Lentils	1 cup	358
Pinto Beans	1 cup	294
Chickpeas / Garbanzo Beans	1 cup	282
Black Beans	1 cup	256
Navy Beans	1 cup	255
Kidney Beans – Red	1 cup	230
Fava/Broad Beans	1 cup	177
White Beans	1 cup	145
Split Peas	1 cup	127
Soybeans – Mature	1 cup	93

Nuts and Seeds	Amount	Folate (mcg)
Sunflower Seeds (hulled kernels, dry-roasted)	1 cup	303
Hemp Seeds (hulled)	1 cup	176
Sesame Seeds (kernels, dried, decorticated)	1 cup	172
Hazelnuts/Filberts	1 cup	153
Flaxseeds	1 cup	146
Peanuts (dry-roasted)	1 cup	142
Walnuts – English (shelled, halves)	1 cup	98
Flaxseed Meal / Ground Flax	1 cup	97
Pumpkin Seeds (kernels, dried)	1 cup	75
Almonds (whole, blanched)	1 cup	71
Almonds (whole, natural with skins)	1 cup	63
Brazil Nuts (unblanched)	1 cup	29
Pecans (halves)	1 cup	22

Table 8.18   Folate content of fruits and vegetables (highest to lowest)

Fruits	Amount	Folate (mcg)
Mango	1 cup	71
Orange	1 medium	48
Orange Juice (chilled, from concentrate)	1 cup	47
Strawberries (sliced)	1 cup	40
Melon – Cantaloupe or Honeydew (diced)	1 cup	33
Pineapple (chunks, raw)	1 cup	30
Banana	1 medium	24

Vegetables	Amount	Folate (mcg)
Spinach (cooked)	1 cup	263
Okra (frozen, cooked)	1 cup	184
Broccoli (chopped, cooked)	1 cup	168
Beets (cooked)	1 cup	136
Collards (frozen, chopped, cooked)	1 cup	129
Peas – Green (cooked)	1 cup	101
Brussels Sprouts (cooked)	1 cup	94
Parsnips (cooked)	1 cup	90
Asparagus (cooked)	4 spears	89
Cabbage – Chinese (cooked)	1 cup	70
Peppers – Red (chopped)	1 cup	69
Potato – White (baked with skin)	1 medium	66
Lettuce – Romaine (shredded)	1 cup	64
Spinach (raw)	1 cup	58
Cauliflower (cooked)	1 cup	55
Tomato Juice	1 cup	49
Acorn Squash (cooked)	1 cup	39
Corn – Yellow (cooked)	1 cup	34
Cabbage (cooked)	1 cup	22

Vitamin B$_{12}$

Vitamin B$_{12}$ is essential for the synthesis of red blood cells, DNA and RNA. It also plays a role in the maintenance of the nervous system and is involved in the formation of myelin, a part of the insulating sheath around the nerves.

Vitamin B$_{12}$ Deficiency and Vitamin B$_{12}$ Deficiency Anemia

A deficiency of vitamin B$_{12}$ can lead to macrocytic megaloblastic anemia. This condition develops slowly after the normal stores of vitamin B$_{12}$ in the liver have become depleted (may take up to three years after depletion). Symptoms of vitamin B$_{12}$ deficiency are similar to those of folate deficiency but also can include depression, peripheral neuropathy (numbness and tingling of the hands and feet), muscle weakness, lack of coordination, balance problems and confusion. Prolonged vitamin B$_{12}$ deficiency can cause irreversible nerve damage.

Vitamin B$_{12}$ deficiency usually is due to impaired absorption, not to an inadequate intake. There are several steps involved in the absorption of this vitamin. Beginning in the stomach, naturally occurring acid and enzymes separate vitamin B$_{12}$ from other components in food. Next, vitamin B$_{12}$ is bound to a substance called "intrinsic factor" (located in the lining of the stomach) and is then transported to the lower part of the small intestine (terminal ileum), which is where the majority of vitamin B$_{12}$ is absorbed. Because this area typically is not affected in celiac disease, deficiency is not common. Nevertheless, vitamin B$_{12}$ deficiency still can occur in celiac disease, although the reasons are not clearly understood. Some possible explanations for this deficiency in individuals with celiac disease are:

- Low stomach acid levels caused by long-term use of gastric acid blocking agents for the treatment of reflux or ulcers. Prior to diagnosis, individuals with celiac disease may have taken over-the-counter and/or prescription medications for various gastrointestinal symptoms that can reduce acid levels.

- Pernicious anemia – an autoimmune disease producing antibodies that destroy the cells in the stomach containing the intrinsic factor.

- Small intestinal bacterial overgrowth (often a consequence of small intestinal damage).

Treatment of vitamin B$_{12}$ deficiency or vitamin B$_{12}$-deficiency anemia in celiac disease includes (1) following a strict gluten-free diet, (2) eating foods that are rich in vitamin B$_{12}$ and (3) vitamin B$_{12}$ supplementation (first consult a physician or dietitian).

Table 8.19 Dietary Reference Intake for vitamin B$_{12}$

	Age	Vitamin B$_{12}$ (mcg/day)
Infants	0–6 mo	0.4
	7–12 mo	0.5
Children	1–3 y	0.9
	4–8 y	1.2
Males	9–13 y	1.8
	14–18 y	2.4
	19–50 y	2.4
	51–70 y	2.4*
	>70 y	2.4*
Females	9–13 y	1.8
	14–18 y	2.4
	19–50 y	2.4
	51–70 y	2.4*
	>70 y	2.4*
Pregnancy	≤18 y	2.6
	19–30 y	2.6
	31–50 y	2.6
Lactation	≤18 y	2.8
	19–30 y	2.8
	31–50 y	2.8

* Because 10 to 30 percent of older people may malabsorb food-bound B$_{12}$, it is advisable for those older than 50 years to meet their requirement mainly by consuming foods fortified with B$_{12}$ or a supplement containing B$_{12}$.

Food Sources of Vitamin B$_{12}$

Vitamin B$_{12}$ is naturally found in meat, fish, seafood, poultry, eggs and dairy products. Additionally, some brands of cereals, non-dairy beverages, nutritional yeasts, veggie "meats" and other non-animal-based food products are fortified with B$_{12}$, although not all of these products are gluten free. For vegans and some vegetarians, a vitamin B$_{12}$ supplement and/or fortified foods are needed in order to meet the daily requirements.

Table 8.20 Vitamin B$_{12}$ content of various foods (highest to lowest)

Foods	Amount	Vitamin B$_{12}$ (mcg)
Clams (cooked)	9 small	84.6
Beef Liver (cooked, braised)	3.5 oz.	70.6
Oysters (canned)	3.5 oz.	19.1
Chicken Liver (cooked, simmered)	3.5 oz.	16.9
Sardines (canned in oil)	8 small	8.6
Nutritional Yeast	¼ cup	7.0
Salmon – Sockeye (canned, drained, solids with bones)	3.5 oz.	5.5
Salmon – Pink (canned, drained, solids with bones)	3.5 oz.	5.0
Beef Tenderloin Steak	3.5 oz.	4.6
Salmon – Sockeye (cooked)	3.5 oz.	4.5
Ground Beef – Extra Lean (cooked)	3.5 oz.	2.8

Foods (cont'd)	Amount	Vitamin B$_{12}$ (mcg)
Lamb – Loin (cooked)	3.5 oz.	2.0
Turkey – Dark Meat (cooked)	3.5 oz.	1.7
Roast Beef (cooked)	3.5 oz.	1.5
Soy Beverage – Plain (fortified)	1 cup	1.5
Tuna – Light (canned in water, drained)	3.5 oz.	1.2
Yogurt – Greek, Vanilla (low-fat)	6 oz.	1.1
Milk (low-fat/1%)	1 cup	0.9
Pork – Loin Roast (cooked)	3.5 oz.	0.9
Cottage Cheese (low-fat/1%)	1 cup	0.7
Ham – Extra Lean (roasted)	3.5 oz.	0.7
Shrimp (canned)	3.5 oz.	0.7
Egg (whole, cooked)	1 large	0.6
Mozzarella Cheese (partially skimmed)	2 oz.	0.46
Chicken – Dark Meat (cooked)	3.5 oz.	0.3

Dietary Fiber

Found in plant-based foods, dietary fiber is a type of carbohydrate that cannot be broken down or absorbed by the human digestive tract. It helps to regulate bowel movements, stabilize blood sugar levels and increase satiety and fullness. Research has shown that a high-fiber diet plays a role in the prevention of certain chronic diseases such as coronary artery disease, diabetes, colon cancer and diverticular disease.

There are two forms of fiber – soluble and insoluble. Soluble fiber dissolves in water, turns into a gel and thereby slows down the digestion and absorption of foods. Insoluble fiber attracts water, bulking and softening the stool, and so causes food to pass through the digestive system more easily. All plant foods contain both forms of fiber but in varying amounts.

Fiber and Celiac Disease

At diagnosis, individuals with celiac disease may present with either diarrhea, constipation or alternation between both. While it is known that diarrhea occurs due to inflammation and malabsorption, it is not clearly understood why some experience constipation in spite of having intestinal damage. Diarrhea generally resolves relatively quickly after gluten has been removed from the diet. Unfortunately, constipation may develop or worsen on the gluten-free diet because (1) high-fiber gluten-containing foods such as wheat bran, whole wheat breads and cereals must be avoided and (2) many gluten-free substitutes are low in dietary fiber. Consuming adequate amounts of dietary fiber is important not only for gastrointestinal health but also in disease prevention.

Table 8.21   Dietary Reference Intake for fiber

	Age	Fiber (grams/day)
Infants	0–6 mo	ND*
	7–12 mo	ND*
Children	1–3 y	19
	4–8 y	25
Males	9–13 y	31
	14–18 y	38
	19–30 y	38
	31–50 y	38
	51–70 y	30
	>70 y	30
Females	9–13 y	26
	14–18 y	26
	19–30 y	25
	31–50 y	25
	51–70 y	21
	>70 y	21
Pregnancy	≤18 y	28
	19–30 y	28
	31–50 y	28
Lactation	≤18 y	29
	19–30 y	29
	31–50 y	29

* **ND** – Not determinable due to lack of data of adverse effects in this age group and concern with regard to lack of ability to handle excess amounts. Source of intake should be from food only to prevent high levels of intake.

Sources of Fiber

Whole grains, fruits, vegetables, legumes, nuts and seeds are rich sources of dietary fiber. Commercial fiber supplements also are available such as Citrucel® (powder), Konsyl® (powder and capsules) and Metamucil® (powder and capsules are gluten free, but wafers are not).

Healthy Tips to Increase Fiber Intake

- Increase fiber intake gradually; start with small amounts to prevent possible abdominal pain and gas.
- Increase consumption of fluids, especially water.
- Eat a variety of high-fiber gluten-free foods on a regular basis.
- Start the day with a bowl of hot cereal (e.g., gluten-free oatmeal or steel-cut oats, buckwheat, quinoa).
- Add ground flax or chia seeds to pancake batter, hot cereals, baked products and smoothies.
- Use brown rice, buckwheat, millet, gluten-free oat groats, quinoa, teff and wild rice in salads, soups and pilafs.

- Extend hamburger patties and meat loaf with ground flax, gluten-free rolled oats or cooked brown rice, lentils, quinoa, amaranth or teff.
- Add cooked chickpeas / garbanzo beans, kidney beans or lentils to salads and casseroles.
- Make vegetable soups with lentils or split peas.
- Choose gluten-free flour mixes or recipes that include high-fiber flours (e.g., almond, amaranth, brown rice, buckwheat, hazelnut, pulses [bean, lentil and pea flours], mesquite, millet, gluten-free oats, quinoa, sorghum, teff).
- Eat high-fiber snacks such as dried fruits, nuts, seeds, popcorn, gluten-free snack bars (made with dried fruits, nuts and seeds), raw fruits and vegetables.
- Choose whole grain crackers containing nuts and seeds instead of rice cakes or crackers made with white rice.
- Add dried fruits, nuts and/or seeds to hot cereals; to muffin, cookie and bread recipes; and to salads and stir-fry dishes.
- Eat whole fruits or vegetables rather than drinking juice.
- Choose pastas made with beans, brown rice, lentils, quinoa and/or wild rice.

Table 8.22 Dietary fiber content of flours and starches (highest to lowest)

Flours and Starches	1 cup (weight in grams)	Dietary Fiber (grams)
Corn Bran (crude)	76	60
Mesquite Flour	146	46
Navy Bean Flour (whole)	149	35
Black Bean Flour (whole)	129	34
Flaxseed Meal / Ground Flax	112	31
Lentil Flour (whole)	180	31
Rice Bran	118	25
Pea Flour – Yellow (whole)	166	21
Pinto Bean Flour (whole)	130	21
Chickpea Flour (whole)	111	18
Soy Flour (defatted)	105	18
Chestnut Flour	102	17
Oat Bran (raw)	94	15
Soy Flour (low-fat)	88	14
Almond Meal (natural with skins)	100	13
Buckwheat Flour (whole groat)	120	12
Garfava™ Flour	157	12
Teff Flour	160	12
Almond Flour (blanched)	112	11
Hazelnut Flour	112	11
Oat Flour	120	11
Amaranth Flour	120	10
Peanut Flour (defatted)	60	10
Peanut Flour (low-fat)	60	10
Corn Flour – Yellow (whole grain)	117	9
Cornmeal – Yellow (whole grain)	122	9

Flours and Starches (cont'd)	1 cup (weight in grams)	Dietary Fiber (grams)
Potato Flour	160	9
Quinoa Flour	112	8
Sorghum Flour – White (whole grain)	121	8
Soy Flour (full-fat)	84	8
Corn Flour – Yellow (masa, enriched)	114	7
Rice Flour – Brown	158	7
Cornmeal – Yellow (degermed, enriched or unenriched)	157	6
Arrowroot Starch/Flour	128	4
Millet Flour	119	4
Rice Flour – White	158	4
Sorghum Flour – White (refined, unenriched)	161	3
Corn Flour – Yellow (degermed, unenriched)	126	2
Rice Flour – Sweet	160	2
Cornstarch	128	1
Potato Starch	192	0
Tapioca Starch/Flour	120	0

Table 8.23 Dietary fiber content of grains (highest to lowest)

Grains (cooked)	1 cup (weight in grams)	Dietary Fiber (grams)
Teff	252	7
Oats – Steel-Cut	245	6
Amaranth	246	5
Buckwheat Groats (roasted)	168	5
Quinoa	185	5
Oatmeal – Regular, Quick, Rolled Oats (unenriched)	234	4
Sorghum – White (whole grain)	170	4
Rice – Brown (long grain)	202	3
Rice – Wild	164	3
Millet	174	2
Sorghum – White (refined/pearled)	187	1
Rice – White (long grain, enriched or unenriched)	158	<1
Rice – White (long grain, parboiled, enriched or unenriched)	158	<1

Table 8.24 Dietary fiber content of legumes, nuts and seeds
(highest to lowest)

Legumes (cooked)	1 cup (weight in grams)	Dietary Fiber (grams)
Navy Beans	182	19
Lentils	198	16
Split Peas	196	16
Black Beans	172	15
Cranberry/Romano Beans	177	15
Pinto Beans	171	15
Chickpeas / Garbanzo Beans	164	13
Kidney Beans – Red	177	13

Legumes (cooked) (cont'd)	1 cup (weight in grams)	Dietary Fiber (grams)
White Beans	179	11
Soybeans – Mature	172	10
Fava/Broad Beans	170	9
Soybeans – Edamame	155	8

Nuts and Seeds	1 cup (weight in grams)	Dietary Fiber (grams)
Chia Seeds	227	78
Flaxseeds	168	46
Flaxseed Meal / Ground Flax	112	31
Almonds (whole, natural with skins)	143	18
Sesame Seeds (kernels, dried, decorticated)	150	17
Almonds (whole, blanched)	145	14
Sunflower Seeds (hulled kernels, dry-roasted)	128	14
Hazelnuts/Filberts	135	13
Peanuts (dry-roasted)	146	12
Brazil Nuts (unblanched)	133	10
Pecans (halves)	99	10
Pumpkin Seeds (kernels, dried)	129	8
Walnuts – English (shelled halves)	100	7
Hemp Seeds (hulled)	160	6

Table 8.25 Dietary fiber content of fruits (highest to lowest)

Fruits	Amount	Dietary Fiber (grams)
Raspberries	1 cup	8
Blackberries	1 cup	8
Pear	1 medium	6
Rhubarb (frozen, cooked, with sugar)	1 cup	5
Cranberries – Sweet (dry)	½ cup	4
Apple (raw with skin)	1 medium	4
Blueberries	1 cup	4
Cherries – Sweet (raw)	24	4
Kiwifruit	2 small	4
Prunes (dried, pitted)	6	4
Raisins (seedless)	½ cup	3
Strawberries (sliced)	1 cup	3
Banana	1 medium	3
Orange	1 medium	3
Applesauce (unsweetened)	1 cup	3
Mango	1 cup	3
Figs (dried)	4	3
Apricots (dried, halves)	6 halves	2
Prune Juice	¾ cup	2
Pineapple (chunks, raw)	1 cup	2
Nectarine	1 medium	2
Peach	1 medium	2

Fruits (cont'd)	Amount	Dietary Fiber (grams)
Plums	2 medium	2
Apricots (fresh)	3	2
Melon – Cantaloupe or Honeydew (diced)	1 cup	1
Grapes – Red or Green (seedless)	20	1

Table 8.26 Dietary fiber content of vegetables (highest to lowest)

Vegetables	Amount	Dietary Fiber (grams)
Acorn Squash (cooked)	1 cup	9
Peas – Green (cooked)	1 cup	9
Parsnips (cooked)	1 cup	6
Broccoli (chopped, cooked)	1 cup	5
Collards (frozen, chopped, cooked)	1 cup	5
Carrots (cooked)	1 cup	5
Turnips (cooked, mashed)	1 cup	5
Peas – Snow (cooked)	1 cup	5
Spinach (cooked)	1 cup	4
Brussels Sprouts (cooked)	1 cup	4
Beans – Green (cooked)	1 cup	4
Sweet Potato (baked with skin)	1 medium	4
Corn – Yellow (cooked)	1 cup	4
Potato – White (baked with skin)	1 medium	4
Pumpkin (canned)	½ cup	4
Beets (cooked)	1 cup	3
Mushrooms (cooked)	1 cup	3
Carrots (baby, raw)	10	3
Cauliflower (cooked)	1 cup	3
Cabbage (cooked)	1 cup	3
Eggplant (cooked)	1 cup	3
Peppers – Green or Red (chopped)	1 cup	3
Zucchini (cooked)	1 cup	2
Onions (cooked)	⅓ cup	1
Tomatoes – Cherry	6	1
Asparagus (cooked)	4 spears	1
Celery (raw)	1 stalk	1
Lettuce – Romaine (shredded)	1 cup	1
Tomato Juice	1 cup	1
Spinach (raw)	1 cup	1

Gluten-Free Alternatives
(Grains, Legumes, Seeds and Starches)

9

In many countries around the world, gluten-containing grains, especially wheat, are major staples in the diet. Completely eliminating wheat, barley and rye from the diet is definitely challenging, but the good news is that there are many gluten-free alternatives including grains, legumes, seeds and starches. Many of these are stand-alone foods and also are easily incorporated into other dishes, as well as available in baked goods, cereals, crackers, pasta and other gluten-free specialty products. For information on purchasing these alternatives and how to use them, see the following chapters: Gluten-Free Meal Planning (pp. 115–130), Gluten-Free Shopping (pp. 131–134), Gluten-Free Cooking and Baking (pp. 143–156) and Recipes (pp. 157–204).

Grains

Grains consist of an outer protective layer called the husk (sometimes referred to as the hull) and an inner seed (kernel). During processing, the inedible husk is removed, leaving the edible seed to be used in a variety of ways. Grains can be divided into two categories: whole grains and refined grains.

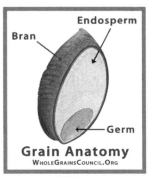

Grain Anatomy
WHOLEGRAINSCOUNCIL.ORG

Courtesy of Oldways and the Whole Grains Council
wholegrainscouncil.org

Whole Grains

A grain kernel is made up of three parts: the outer bran layer, the starchy endosperm and the germ. The term "whole grain" implies that all three edible parts of a kernel have been preserved for its use as a food product.

There are many different types of whole grains (see table 9.1 on p. 98). Most belong to the grass (*Gramineae*) family; however, amaranth, buckwheat and quinoa come from different botanical families and are referred to as "pseudograins." Regardless of their classification, all whole grains are similar in their nutritional profile, preparation and use.

Whole grains provide a wide range of key nutrients such as B vitamins, minerals, protein, fiber, carbohydrates, healthy fats and plant compounds (e.g., antioxidants, phytochemicals). Due to their nutritional composition, regular consumption of whole grains has been linked to many health benefits. Studies have shown these to include reduced risk of heart disease, stroke, type 2 diabetes and certain types of cancers, and as well to play an important positive role in gastrointestinal health and weight management.

Table 9.1 Gluten-free status of whole grains

Gluten-Free	Gluten-Containing †
Amaranth* Buckwheat* Corn Millet Oats** Quinoa* Rice (black, brown, green, purple, red) Sorghum Teff Wild rice	Barley Rye Triticale Wheat (including all types such as durum, einkorn, emmer, farro, kamut and spelt)
* Pseudograins ** Pure, uncontaminated	† For more information on the types and forms of these grains see page 10

Refined Grains

A refined grain has had the nutrient-dense bran and germ removed, leaving only the starchy endosperm. This refining process extends shelf life and results in a finer texture often desired for products such as breads and other baked goods. However, the levels of fiber and other important nutrients are significantly lower compared to those of the whole grain. While some refined grains are subsequently "enriched" with iron and the B vitamins thiamin, riboflavin, niacin and folic acid, they still lack the full range of nutrients found in whole grains.

Gluten-Free Grains

The following section provides a brief descriptive overview of each of the gluten-free grains. See pages 318–320 for the nutrient composition of the various grains. To learn how to cook these grains, see pages 143 and 144. For more information on using gluten-free flours, see pages 147–156. General tips on how to incorporate these gluten-free grains into meals and snacks are on page 112. The recipe section, found on pages 157–204, uses many of these grains and/or their flours. For a list of brands that sell gluten-free grains, see page 243.

Amaranth

Amaranth is a broad-leafed plant that produces florets containing tiny grain-like, tan-colored seeds. This pseudograin has been used as a dietary staple by many ancient civilizations around the world. Globally, areas where amaranth is grown include Mexico, South America, Africa, Asia, Russia and the U.S. Amaranth seeds have a robust, nutty flavor and can be eaten whole, popped (like popcorn), puffed (cereal) or ground and used as flour.

Amaranth seeds are similar in size to poppy seeds.

Amaranth flour is made by finely grinding the whole amaranth seed.

For recipes using amaranth, see pages 158, 174, 176, 180 and 198.

Buckwheat

Buckwheat is thought to have originated in China. The largest producers of buckwheat today are China, Japan, Russia and North America, although it is also grown in Europe, India, Australia and South America. Despite its name, buckwheat is not wheat nor related to wheat. It is botanically classified as a fruit, not a cereal grain, and is closely related to rhubarb. This flowering plant produces triangular-sided seeds covered by a black shell. The outer shell is removed (hulled) and what remains is known as a groat. These groats are available roasted or unroasted.

Unroasted groats range in color from light green to brown, and have a mild taste. They are packaged whole or ground.

Roasted groats, also known as "kasha," are darker in color and have a stronger, distinctive, nutty flavor compared to unroasted groats. Kasha is packaged in four granulations (whole, coarse, medium and fine).

Buckwheat grits are ground unroasted groats and often are labeled as "cream of buckwheat" hot cereal.

Buckwheat flour (light, medium and dark) is made from ground unroasted groats and may be blended with varying levels of finely milled black buckwheat hulls. The medium and dark flours contain higher percentages of the hulls, which give them a more robust flavor. The light flour has a milder, mellow flavor because it usually does not contain added buckwheat hulls. Some brands of what may be labeled buckwheat flour or pancake mix actually are a blend of buckwheat flour and wheat flour, so be sure to check the label for pure buckwheat flour.

Buckwheat pasta can be made from buckwheat flour alone or in combination with other ingredients such as corn, rice, lentils and/or sorghum. Japanese soba noodles are a type of buckwheat pasta made either from 100% buckwheat flour or from a combination of buckwheat and wheat flours.

For recipes using buckwheat, see pages 158, 174, 198 and 199.

Corn

Corn, also known as "maize," is one of the most frequently cultivated grains worldwide, with the U.S. topping the list as the biggest producer and exporter. Other leading producers include China, Brazil, Argentina and the Ukraine. While the majority of corn produced is used for animal feed and industrial purposes (e.g., ethanol fuel), it also is used extensively as a stand-alone food or as an ingredient or component in food and beverages (e.g., starches, sweeteners, oils, alcohol). There are numerous varieties of corn and they come in an array of colors (white, yellow, pink, red, blue, purple and black). Corn kernels are processed into many different forms.

Corn grits are coarsely ground dried corn kernels (whole grain or refined) that when cooked are eaten as a breakfast cereal or side dish. Refined corn grits may be enriched with iron and B vitamins.

Hominy is dried whole corn kernels that have been soaked in an alkaline liquid and then cooked. This process removes the hulls and softens the kernels, making them easier to grind. It also makes some nutrients, especially niacin, more readily available to be absorbed by the digestive system. When limewater is used as the alkaline solution, the calcium content of the hominy is increased. Hominy is available as whole kernels, coarsely ground into hominy grits or finely ground into masa harina.

Masa harina, the flour milled from finely ground hominy, traditionally is used to make corn tortillas.

Cornmeal, made from dried ground corn kernels (yellow, white, red or blue varieties), is available in coarse, medium or fine grind. Most cornmeal is made from refined corn kernels (i.e., the bran and germ have been removed) and if so is often labeled "degerminated." Some brands of refined cornmeal may be enriched with iron and B vitamins to compensate for nutrient loss during processing; however, whole-grain cornmeal is higher in fiber in comparison to refined cornmeal.

Corn flour is more finely ground than cornmeal. It can be milled from either whole-grain or refined corn kernels.

Cornstarch is produced from the starchy endosperm of the corn kernel.

Corn bran, made from the outer layer of whole-grain corn kernels, is extremely high in insoluble fiber.

Corn pasta is made either from corn flour and/or cornmeal alone or in combination with other gluten-free ingredients (e.g., buckwheat, lentil, millet, potato, quinoa, rice). This pasta also may be enriched.

Corn polenta, a traditional Italian dish, is a smooth creamy porridge usually made from boiled cornmeal and often topped with cheese or sauce. Cooked polenta also can be placed in a baking dish to cool then cut into squares that can be pan-fried, grilled or baked. Precooked polenta in plastic tubes can be purchased plain or flavored with other ingredients. Both "made-from-scratch" and purchased precooked polenta can be either 100% cornmeal or in a cornmeal/quinoa or cornmeal/potato blend, and also are sometimes made just from semolina wheat.

Popcorn is a variety of corn with kernels that burst open when heated. It is considered a whole grain.

Corn oil is extracted from the corn germ and can be purchased as 100% corn oil or mixed with other types of vegetable oils.

For recipes using corn (not including cornstarch or cornflakes), see pages 161, 183, 197 and 202.

Millet

The word "millet" refers to various grasses that grow in semi-arid regions of the world. The six species of major importance are proso, finger, foxtail, barnyard, browntop and pearl. Although most millet is cultivated for animal feed or birdseed, the pearl, finger and proso varieties are more commonly used in foods and beverages (e.g., beer).

Closely related to corn, millet seeds are very small and round in shape, and can be yellow, white, grey or red. The major variety found in North America is the light yellow millet which has a slightly corn-like, sweet, nutty flavor. Food-grade millet is hulled and the inner seed is sold whole, puffed, coarsely ground into grits/meal or finely ground into flour.

Millet has the outer inedible husk (hull) removed and the remaining kernel (which contains the bran, germ and endosperm) is packaged either whole or ground into flour.

Millet grits are made from grinding whole-grain millet to a coarse texture, and when cooked is most often eaten as a breakfast cereal or side dish.

Millet flour is finely ground whole-grain millet.

For recipes using millet, see pages 174, 185, 192 and 198.

Oats

Oats have been cultivated for thousands of years and were initially used for medicinal purposes and animal feed prior to becoming a widespread dietary staple. A popular crop in Scotland and Ireland, oats were brought to North America in the early seventeenth century by Scottish settlers. Today, the largest commercial producers of oats are the European Union (mainly Finland and Sweden), Russia, Canada, Australia and the U.S. Oats are a naturally gluten-free grain, rich in fiber, protein and other nutrients.

For a number of reasons, oats frequently are contaminated with gluten-containing grains. Oats often are grown alongside or in rotation with wheat, barley and/or rye; therefore, contamination happens by proximity to or by intermingled volunteer growth of the contaminant grain. In addition, oats can be contaminated due to shared equipment used for planting, harvesting, storage, transportation and milling. Fortunately, there are companies that produce gluten-free oats. More information on the safety of oats for the gluten-free diet can be found on pages 27–30.

For a listing of companies with gluten-free oat products, see appendix A on page 305.

Oats have a sweet, nutty flavor, making them a popular choice for breakfast dishes, baked goods and desserts. Whole-grain oats are available in several different forms.

Oat groats are the oat kernels that remain once the inedible outer hull is removed. They are long and thin with a deep indent running down the centre of the kernel. Compared to other forms of oats, the groats take the longest to cook.

Steel-cut and **stone-ground oats** are whole oat groats that have been cut into smaller pieces, a process that enables a reduced cooking time. The kernels of steel-cut oats, sometimes called "Irish oatmeal," usually are cut into two or three pieces. Stone-ground oats, known as "Scottish oatmeal," comprise smaller, various-sized pieces and produce a smoother, creamier hot cereal.

Rolled oats are oat groats that have been steamed and then rolled to flatten into flakes of various thicknesses. While the nutrient composition remains the same, texture and cooking times vary based on the flake size and thickness. From largest to smallest size and thickness, rolled oats include large flake (also known as old-fashioned), quick-cooking and instant. Some rolled oats are roasted during processing to enhance the flavor. Rolled oats are available either plain or flavored with various ingredients and/or sweeteners.

Oat bran is the outermost layer of the whole oat groat. While all forms of oats contain this nutritious part of the kernel, milling specifically for oat bran separates the fiber-rich layer from the other parts of the kernel. Oat bran is high in the soluble fiber called beta-glucan, which is known to have cholesterol-lowering effects.

Oat flour is made by finely grinding whole-grain oat groats.

Oat beverages are non-dairy alternatives derived from oat-based ingredients (but usually not from gluten-free oats). Some brands also may contain barley. They are available plain or flavored, and often enriched with vitamins and minerals. The various fruit-based drinks containing oats may or may not be gluten-free.

For recipes using oats, see pages 163, 169, 170, 177 and 191.

Quinoa

Quinoa, originating in South America, was a staple of the Incas, who called it "the mother grain." It is not actually a grain but the seed of a broad-leafed plant that is a close relative to spinach. There are hundreds of varieties of quinoa, ranging in color from white to red and purple to black, and some varieties are now grown in North America and Europe. The seed looks like a cross between sesame seed and millet and has a distinct nutty flavor. Quinoa seeds are naturally covered with saponin, an extremely bitter substance that protects them from consumption by birds and insects. For the seed to be edible, the saponin must be removed. While most companies specially process quinoa to remove this bitter coating, rinsing quinoa before cooking will help to remove any remaining saponin residue. Quinoa is sold in several forms including seeds, flakes, puffs and flour.

Kañiwa is a close relative of quinoa and also originated in South America. Its seed is about half the size of those of quinoa and it often is referred to as "baby quinoa." Compared to the mother grain, kañiwa has a milder flavor, is slightly higher in protein and fiber and does not contain the bitter saponin coating. Kañiwa varieties are available in red, grey and beige colors, and sold as whole seeds or ground into flour. Interestingly, kañiwa seeds turn a dark reddish-brown color once cooked.

Quinoa and **kañiwa** are the whole seeds.

Quinoa flakes are made from whole quinoa seeds that have been steamed and then rolled to flatten into flakes. They are consumed as a breakfast cereal similarly to rolled oats.

Quinoa and **kañiwa flours** are produced from finely grinding the seeds.

Quinoa pasta usually is made from a combination of quinoa flour and other ingredients such as amaranth, beans, corn, lentils, potatoes and/or rice.

Quinoa polenta is made from quinoa flour and cornmeal. It also may be seasoned so check for gluten-containing ingredients.

Quinoa beverages are non-dairy alternatives that also may contain other ingredients (e.g., chia) and may be enriched/fortified with vitamins and minerals.

For recipes using quinoa, see pages 158, 160, 163, 170, 172, 174, 185, 187, 198 and 200.

Rice

Rice is considered a major dietary staple worldwide, particularly in Asian, Mediterranean and South American cuisines. Native to Asia and Africa, after years of trade and exportation rice now is grown all over the globe. Several thousand varieties of rice exist and are available in different colors ranging from black, brown, red, purple and green to white.

Rice usually is categorized by grain size (long, medium and short) and texture. Long-grain rice has long slender kernels and becomes light and fluffy once cooked, making it a suitable choice for side dishes and pilafs. The kernels of medium- and short-grain rices are shorter and wider. When cooked, they retain more moisture than do long-grain types and have a greater tendency to stick together, appropriate for dishes such as sushi, risotto and rice pudding.

In addition to the more traditional types of rice found on the market, some unique varieties of specialty rice also are available. Aromatic rices such as basmati, jasmine and texmati have unique flavors and aromas, and usually are long-grained. Arborio, an Italian short-grain rice, commonly is used for recipes that call for a creamy consistency, such as risotto. Glutinous/sweet rice is a sticky type of short-grain rice; however, despite its name, glutinous/sweet rice does not contain gluten.

After rice is harvested, it is dried and cleaned then is processed in a variety of ways. Rice is available in many different forms.

Whole-grain rice (brown, black, green, purple, red) has the outer inedible husk removed and the remaining kernel (which contains the bran, germ and endosperm) then is packaged either whole or ground into flour.

Refined rice (white) is brown rice with the bran and germ removed, leaving only the starchy endosperm. Some brands of white rice may be enriched with iron and B vitamins (thiamin, riboflavin, niacin and folic acid).

Instant dry rice, either **whole-grain or white**, is precooked then dried in order to reduce final cooking time. White rice is available enriched or unenriched.

Ready-to-eat rice, packaged in shelf-stable and frozen formats, is made either from whole-grain or from refined white rice.

Parboiled (converted) white or brown rice are kernels that have been soaked, steamed under pressure then dried while still within the outer inedible husk. This process transfers certain nutrients from the husk and bran into the inner kernel of the rice. The husk then is removed, resulting in parboiled brown rice. Parboiled white rice results from further milling that removes the bran and germ, and is available enriched or unenriched.

Rice flour is milled from either whole-grain or refined rice kernels. Brown rice flour contains the bran, germ and endosperm, and is higher in fiber and other nutrients compared to white and sweet white rice flours (which have the bran and germ removed).

Rice bran is the outer layer of the whole-grain rice kernel, and often is blended with the germ and stabilized using heat, water and pressure to increase the shelf life. It is very high in fiber.

Rice polish consists of a portion of bran and germ from the brown rice kernel. Lighter in color than pure rice bran, it is high in fiber and can be substituted for rice bran in recipes.

Rice bran oil is extracted from the bran and/or germ. In Asian countries, this oil is commonly used for cooking.

Rice vinegar usually is produced from fermented rice; however, it also may comprise other grains (e.g., barley, millet, sorghum, wheat). It may or may not be distilled, and can be purchased either plain or seasoned with a variety of different ingredients. Check the label for gluten-containing ingredients.

Cream of rice cereal, also known as cream of rice farina, is made from coarsely ground whole-grain brown or refined white rice and is gluten free. However, farina made from wheat contains gluten.

Rice pasta is produced either solely from brown and/or white rice or in combination with other gluten-free ingredients (e.g., amaranth, corn, flax, millet, potatoes, quinoa, soy, rice bran, pea protein, vegetable powders, wild rice, eggs). It may be enriched/fortified with vitamins and minerals.

Rice beverages are a non-dairy alternative made from white or brown rice and other ingredients. They are available unsweetened or sweetened, in plain or flavored varieties and in refrigerated or shelf-stable packages, as well as in dry powder form. They may be enriched/fortified with vitamins and minerals.

For recipes using rice, see pages 158, 161, 163, 166, 168, 175, 176, 179, 185, 186, 188, 189, 191, 195, 200 and 203.

Sorghum

Sorghum, also referred to as milo, is a major cereal grain that grows in hot semi-arid tropical and dry temperate areas of the world including the U.S., Mexico, Africa, India and China. Used as a feed for livestock and in ethanol fuel production, it also is gaining in popularity as a dietary food staple. Slightly smaller than peppercorns, sorghum grains are available in an array of colors including white, yellow, red, burgundy and black. Although white sorghum traditionally has been the most common type found in food products, darker varieties (black and burgundy) are now being introduced into the market as they are higher in fiber, phytochemicals (naturally occurring components in plants) and other nutrients.

There are significant differences among the varieties of sorghum, resulting in a wide range of cooking times and water quantity requirements as well as cooked textures (chewy to soft).

Sorghum grain is fairly neutral in flavor, can be flaked, popped, puffed or milled into flour and is used in many foods and beverages. The stalks of certain varieties of sorghum can be squeezed to extract the juice for making a dark syrup.

Whole-grain sorghum has the outer inedible husk removed and the remaining kernel (containing the bran, germ and endosperm) is packaged either whole or ground into flour. It has a slightly nutty flavor and chewy texture.

Pearled (polished) sorghum has some of the outer bran layer removed from the whole-grain sorghum kernel and therefore is lower in fiber.

Sorghum flour is milled from whole-grain or pearled sorghum. The whole-grain flour is available in light tan, black or burgundy colors.

Sorghum bran is the outer layer of the whole sorghum kernel and is an excellent source of fiber.

For recipes using sorghum, see pages 160, 165, 167, 175, 176, 179, 190 and 200.

Teff

A grass native to Ethiopia, today teff also is grown in India, Australia and northwestern U.S. It is the smallest of all grains in the world (about 100–150 teff grains equal the size of 1 wheat kernel). In color, the grains range from milky white to almost black. White, red and brown are the most common types grown in Ethiopia, while the U.S. produces brown and ivory types.

Teff seeds are more nutritious than the major cereal grains, as its small seed size means the germ and bran (the outer portions where nutrients are concentrated) account for a higher proportion of the seed than do those of other grains. It has a unique, nutty, molasses-like flavor, and is sold as both a whole grain and a flour. In Ethiopia, this major cereal crop is ground into flour that is used to make "injera," a sourdough-type moist and chewy flatbread. Authentic injera usually is made from pure teff flour; however, many North American restaurants prepare it using a combination of teff flour with wheat flour or barley flour, so the resulting bread is not gluten-free. Injera traditionally is served with "wot," a spicy sauce or stew made of meat or ground legumes.

Teff is the whole-grain kernel containing the bran, germ and endosperm.

Teff flour is finely ground from whole-grain teff.

For recipes using teff, see pages 158, 162, 164, 173, 174 and 198.

Wild Rice

Despite its name, wild rice is not a member of the rice family but rather the seed of an aquatic grass. Wild rice, native to North America, grows mainly in shallow lakes and streams in northern Saskatchewan and Manitoba (Canada), as well as in many American states, most notably California and Minnesota. Wild rice has a distinct, nut-like, roasted flavor and a chewy texture. It is sold either plain, mixed with other types of rice, as flour or as an ingredient of pasta.

Wild rice is a whole grain with a long, slender, brownish-black kernel.

Quick-cooking wild rice is whole-grain wild rice that has been processed in order to reduce cooking time. Usually the processing involves precooking and drying; however, alternatively, some processors do not precook but instead simply "scratch the surface" of the kernels.

Ready-to-eat wild rice is packaged in shelf-stable or frozen formats.

Wild rice flour is milled from finely ground wild rice.

Wild rice pasta is made from wild rice and brown rice.

For recipes using wild rice, see pages 188, 191 and 195.

Legumes

Legumes are plants that contain seeds within a pod. There is a broad range of leguminous plants that fall into different categories such as vegetables (green peas, green and yellow beans), pulses (dried beans, chickpeas, lentils, peas), soybeans, peanuts and mesquite.

The following section provides a brief descriptive overview of soybeans, pulses and mesquite. See pages 318, 319 and 321 for the nutrient composition of legumes and legume flours. To learn how to cook pulses and soybeans, see pages 145 and 146. General tips to incorporate legumes into meals and snacks are on page 113. For more information on legume flours, see pages 147–151. The recipe section, found on pages 157–204, uses some of these legumes and/or their flours.

Soybeans

Soybeans, also called soya beans, are leguminous plants whose source can be traced to northern China. They now are grown in many countries around the world and are a major crop in the U.S. An excellent source of complete protein (containing all the essential amino acids), soybeans also are rich in dietary fiber, essential fatty acids, phytochemicals, potassium and folate, as well as other vitamins and minerals.

Whole soybeans are available in green, yellow/tan and black varieties. Edamame, the young green variety of soybeans, is harvested as a fresh whole pod containing large green oval seeds. The yellow/tan and black soybean varieties remain in the field until dry then following harvest, the round seeds are shelled from their pods.

Different forms of soybeans are used extensively in foods and beverages, as well as for animal feed and industrial purposes. Listed below are many common soy-based foods and ingredients.

Edamame is the name given to fresh green soybeans. Available as whole pods with the seeds inside or as individual shelled seeds, edamame is sold fresh (seasonally), frozen, freeze-dried and roasted.

Soybeans (yellow/tan and black) can be purchased either dry or canned (precooked). Yellow soybeans have a mild flavor, whereas black soybeans have a more pronounced flavor. Although similar in nutrients, the black soybeans are higher in antioxidants.

Soynuts are produced by soaking soybeans then oil-roasting or dry-roasting them. They are available either plain, salted or in different flavors.

Soynut butter is made from ground roasted soybeans.

Soy grits are coarsely ground toasted soybeans. Often eaten as a breakfast cereal or side dish, cooked soy grits also can be added to soups, casseroles and ground meat dishes as well as baked goods.

Soy flour is milled from dried ground soybeans and available as full-fat (contains all of the fat in the soybeans), low-fat (contains one-third the amount of fat as full-fat) and defatted (most of the fat removed).

Textured soy protein (TSP), also called textured vegetable protein (TVP), is made from defatted soy flour and is used as a meat substitute. Some brands may contain hydrolyzed wheat protein. Dried TSP can be purchased as chunks, crumbles, bits, slices or flakes; plain or flavored. TSP needs to be rehydrated with hot water or broth before using in recipes.

Soy meat alternatives/analogs are produced from TSP, soy protein isolates and/or soy concentrates. These soy-based alternatives are used to make a variety of vegetarian/meat-free products (e.g., burgers, hot dogs, sausage links, steaks). They are sold refrigerated, frozen or in shelf-stable packaging, and require only heating. Many of these meat substitutes also contain added wheat gluten, hydrolyzed wheat protein, barley malt and/or soy sauce containing wheat.

Soy protein isolate is a dry powder used extensively in food products such as snack bars, soymilk and meat alternatives. The majority of the carbohydrate, fat and fiber have been removed, resulting in a high-protein-content ingredient.

Soybean oil, the fat component extracted from soybeans, is used both as cooking oil and as an ingredient in food products.

Soy beverages usually comprise the liquid resulting from ground whole soybeans that have been water-soaked, cooked then filtered. They also can be produced from full-fat soy flour or soy protein solids. Plain or flavored soy beverages are available both sweetened and unsweetened in full-fat, low-fat or fat-free options. These drinks are sold in both refrigerated and shelf-stable packages, as well as in dry powder form, and may be fortified/enriched with vitamins, minerals and other nutrients.

Other non-dairy soy products such as cheese, yogurt, cream cheese, sour cream and frozen desserts are made from various forms of soybeans and other ingredients.

Soy tofu is made from the liquid of ground whole soybeans that has been coagulated (changed to a firm gelled state). Textures of tofu range from soft/silken to extra-firm and can be purchased plain or flavored. Gluten-containing ingredients such as hydrolyzed wheat protein and/or soy sauce made with soy and wheat may be present in flavored tofu.

Soy tempeh, a cake-like meat substitute, is produced from fermented soybeans and/or grains (e.g., rice, millet, wheat, barley), seeds and other legumes. Sold in the refrigerated or frozen-food sections, soy tempeh may be seasoned with gluten-containing ingredients.

Natto is a traditional Japanese dish made from fermented soybeans and has a very strong taste.

Miso is an intensely flavored condiment used in Asian cooking to season a variety of foods, and usually is derived from fermented soybeans and grains including barley, wheat and/or rice.

Soy sauces, including regular, tamari and shoyu, are produced by fermenting soybeans and often wheat; however, there are some gluten-free varieties available made from only soybeans.

Soy pasta is made either solely from soybeans (dried whole or edamame) or in combination with other ingredients that usually are gluten free, such as corn and potato.

For recipes using soy, see pages 180 and 200.

Pulses

Globally, the leading pulse crop producers are Canada and India. This popular category of legumes is consumed by millions of people around the world. Pulses have an outer seed coat called the hull and an inner seed kernel. They come in assorted sizes, shapes and colors, and are available whole, split or ground into flour. In addition, pulses can be separated into protein, fiber and starch fractions. Dehulled whole chickpeas, lentils and peas have either had the outer coating removed or been split (which removes the outer coating). This process reduces cooking time and also makes for easier milling into flour. However, whole pulses (not dehulled or split) also can be milled into flour.

Pulses are used in many different foods including soups, entrées, pasta dishes, casseroles and other savory and sweet baked goods. Cooked chickpeas / garbanzo beans and peas can be roasted with oil and/or salt or other seasonings, and eaten as a snack.

Key nutrients found in pulses include protein, fiber, complex carbohydrates, folate and other B vitamins, minerals (e.g., iron, magnesium, phosphorus, potassium, zinc) and phytochemicals (naturally occurring plant compounds). When pulses have been dehulled, some of the fiber, vitamins, minerals and other important plant components are lost. For this reason, choose whole pulses and whole pulse flours.

Regular consumption of pulses has been linked to a reduced risk of diabetes, heart disease and certain cancers. In addition, research studies have found that pulses can increase satiety (the feeling of fullness) and thereby help with weight control.

Pulses are grouped into four categories: beans, chickpeas, lentils and peas. Some individual pulses within these categories are referred to by other names (see table 9.2).

Table 9.2 Types of pulses

Category of Pulse	Name	Alternate Name
Beans	Adzuki	–
	Baby Lima	–
	Black	Black Turtle, Preto
	Cranberry	Romano, Speckled Sugar, Borlotti
	Great Northern	Large White
	Kidney – Dark Red	–
	Kidney – Light Red	–
	Kidney – White	Cannellini
	Lima – Baby	–
	Lima – Large	–
	Navy	White Pea, Alubia Chica
	Pink	–
	Pinto	–
	Small Red	–
Chickpeas (round)	Garbanzo	Kabuli, Bengal Gram, Kabuli Chana
	Desi	Kala Chana
	Desi – Split	Chana Dal
Lentils (flat, disc-shaped)	Black	Beluga
	French Green	Dark Speckled, Dupuy
	Large Green	Laird, Masoor Large Green
	Large Green – Split	Yellow Split
	Red	Masoor
	Red – Dehulled	Football
	Red – Split	–
Peas (round)	Green	–
	Green – Split	–
	Yellow	–
	Yellow – Split	–

Mesquite

Mesquite is the North American name for a woody leguminous plant yielding wood chips that are dried and used to impart the unique mesquite flavor to grilled foods. There are over 45 species native to North and South America, Africa and southern Asia, ranging from eight-foot shrubs to sixty-foot trees.

These trees produce bean pods that come in different sizes depending on the specific variety of mesquite tree, and are harvested for various purposes. In some countries, the pods are processed into syrup, jelly, tea and/or coffee. The entire pod also can be ground into coarse mealy flour that has a cinnamon-mocha aroma and sweet, chocolate, molasses-like flavor with a hint of caramel. Alternatively, a combination of milling and sieving techniques using only the inside pulp of the bean pod produces a finer flour that has a sweeter and more concentrated aroma and flavor than does the whole bean pod flour. Mesquite flour, which is light tan in color, recently has been introduced to the North American market. It is best combined with other gluten-free flours to make pancakes and baked products such as breads, muffins, brownies, cakes, cookies and pie crusts. Mesquite flour also can be added to hot cereal (e.g., cream of brown or white rice), meat dishes, soups and gravies.

The nutritional composition of mesquite flour varies considerably depending on the variety of mesquite plant, the soil type in which it grows and whether the whole pod or only the pulp of the pod is used. Whole-pod flour is higher in protein and calcium than that made from only the pulp. However, both types of flours are very high in fiber.

Seeds

Chia, flax, hemp, pumpkin, sesame and sunflower seeds are nutritious additions to the gluten-free diet. These seeds are rich in nutrients, especially fiber, protein, healthy fats, minerals and phytochemicals. Different forms of seeds can be incorporated into many food products.

The following section provides a brief overview of some seeds. See pages 318 and 321 for the nutrient composition of seeds. General tips for incorporating seeds into meals and snacks are on page 114. The recipe section, found on pages 157–204, uses some of these seeds as ingredients.

Chia

Chia, a flowering plant belonging to the mint family, played a prominent role in the diet of the ancient Aztec and Mayan civilizations. Grown in Central and South America, the plant produces small seeds ranging in color from white to brown to black. This mildly flavored seed is very high in omega-3 fatty acids, fiber, protein and many other nutrients such as calcium, iron, magnesium and zinc. Chia seeds can be purchased whole or ground, and they also are found in beverages, cereals, puddings, snack bars and other foods.

Whole chia seeds do not need to be ground and can be added directly to foods and beverages.

Ground chia, also known as milled chia, can be purchased in vacuum-sealed packages. Alternatively, whole chia seeds can be ground in a coffee/spice grinder or food processor for use in cooking and baking. Chia should be stored in the refrigerator to retain optimum freshness.

Chia seed oil is found in omega-3 supplements and also is used as a cooking oil.

For a recipe using chia seeds, see page 177.

Flax

Flax is grown across the Canadian prairies and the northern U.S. This glossy flat oval seed, available in brown or yellow colors, is about the size of a sesame seed and has a pointed tip. Various components of lower-grade qualities of flax are processed for industrial purposes (e.g., paint, flooring) and paper products, as well as incorporated into pet foods. Higher-quality food-grade flaxseeds are used for human food consumption.

Regardless of the color of the flaxseed, the nutritional composition is very similar. Flax is rich in alpha-linolenic acid (an essential omega-3 fatty acid), fiber (soluble and insoluble) and plant lignans (a type of phytochemical). The seed also contains protein and many vitamins and minerals. Due to its very high fiber content, flax helps promote bowel regularity. Researchers have found it may help protect against coronary heart disease, as well as breast and colon cancers. Flax also is being studied for its positive nutritional effects in many autoimmune and chronic diseases.

Flax can be purchased either in seed form (whole seeds or ground) or as an oil.

Whole flaxseed is an excellent source of fiber and other nutrients. In order to gain all the nutritional benefits, especially the omega-3 fatty acids, protein, vitamins and minerals, it is important to grind whole flaxseeds before consuming. Grinding breaks the flax kernels' outer protective coating so that the nutrients are more easily accessible for absorption by the body. Whole flaxseeds can be ground in a coffee/spice grinder or food processor to the consistency of finely ground coffee.

Ground flaxseed, also known as flaxseed meal or milled flaxseed, can be purchased in vacuum-sealed packages on store shelves. For optimum freshness, refrigerate ground flax.

Flax hull lignans, contained in the outer coating of the seed, are ground and sold in capsule or in bulk powder form. These plant-derived compounds are a source of fiber but do not contain the fat component found in whole flax.

Flax oil is cold-pressed from the whole flaxseed. It is high in omega-3 fatty acids and contains no fiber and usually no lignans. Some flax oil manufacturers will add back the lignans after the oil is extracted from the seed. Flax oil should be refrigerated once opened. The oil can be used for salad dressings and dips; however, it is not recommended for baking or frying as it breaks down and easily burns when heated.

Flax beverages are a non-dairy alternative made from flax oil, water and other ingredients. They are available unsweetened and sweetened, and may be enriched/fortified with calcium and vitamins.

For recipes using flaxseeds, see pages 158, 160, 165, 169, 173, 176, 177 and 201.

Hemp

Hemp is a variety of the *Cannabis* plant family grown in many countries around the world. Although hemp and marijuana belong to the same botanical family, they differ in their levels of THC (tetrahydrocannabinol), a psychoactive compound. Unlike marijuana, the hemp plant contains no or very low levels of THC. This tall, leafy plant produces edible seeds that are processed in a variety of ways and the fibrous stalks are used for making clothing, bedding, paper and other products.

A hemp seed contains all the essential amino acids, as well as B vitamins, iron, magnesium, potassium, phosphorus, zinc and other nutrients. Hemp seeds also are rich in essential fatty acids and dietary fiber. Both the whole and hulled hemp seeds contain fiber, mainly the insoluble form; however, the hulls are where most of the fiber is located.

Whole hemp seeds have a crunchy outer shell (hull) and are available only dry-roasted.

Hulled hemp seeds, also called "hemp hearts" or "shelled hemp seeds," have the outer hull removed. These soft edible raw seeds are beige in color with a green tinge and have a slightly nutty, earthy flavor.

Hemp powder is made from whole hemp seeds that have had a significant portion of the fat (oil) removed. What remains is milled to create a very fine powder. The fiber and protein contents will vary depending on the ratio of hemp protein to fibrous hulls in the final product.

Hemp oil is cold-pressed from hemp seeds and should be refrigerated once opened. The oil can be used for salad dressings and dips. It is not recommended for baking or frying as it breaks down and easily burns when heated.

Hemp butter is a spread made from processing whole or hulled hemp seeds either with or without hemp oil.

Hemp beverages are non-dairy alternatives made from hulled hemp seeds, water and other ingredients. Plain and flavored hemp beverages are available, both sweetened and unsweetened.

For a recipe using hemp seeds, see page 177.

Pumpkin

Pumpkin is a type of squash with edible flesh (commonly used in cooking and baking) and seeds. The seed comprises a large, semi-soft white edible hull encasing a small green inner kernel known as a pepita. Either the pepita alone or the entire pumpkin seed can be eaten as a snack. Pumpkin seeds are high in zinc, phosphorus, magnesium, copper, iron and protein, as well as a source of fiber.

Whole dry pumpkin seeds are available raw or roasted, and also may be salted or seasoned.

Pepitas, the flat, oval-shaped green inner kernels, are sold either raw or roasted, with or without salt and other seasonings.

Pumpkin seed butter is made from finely ground pepitas and also may be combined with other ingredients such as oil, salt, sugar and/or spices.

Pumpkin seed oil, extracted from the pepita kernel, is used in some salad dressings.

For recipes using pumpkin seeds, see pages 163, 167, 182, 192 and 200.

Sesame

The sesame plant is a tall herb grown predominantly in Asia and Africa. When dried, the pods of the plant pop open to reveal tiny seeds. These whole sesame seeds come in a variety of colors (black, brown, white, yellow). Each whole seed consists of an outer coating (hull) surrounding a soft white kernel. Sesame seeds usually are dehulled (decorticated); however, whole sesame seeds also can be found in the marketplace. When toasted, sesame seeds have a more distinct nutty flavor than those in raw form.

Sesame seeds are a good source of minerals (e.g., copper, iron, magnesium, zinc), protein, fiber and other nutrients. Although whole sesame seeds are very high in calcium compared to the dehulled seed, the calcium is absorbed less efficiently by the body than it is from most other calcium sources.

Whole sesame seeds have the outer hull intact.

Dehulled/decorticated sesame seeds are the most common form available.

Sesame seed butter/paste, also known as "tahini," is made from finely ground raw or roasted sesame seeds (either whole or dehulled). Salt and/or sugar may be added.

Sesame oil is extracted from sesame seeds. There are two types of oil: the light oil is extracted from raw sesame seeds and is used for frying, while the dark oil is produced from toasted sesame seeds, has a stronger flavor and burns easily, so is used primarily as an ingredient in sauces and dressings.

For recipes using sesame seeds, see pages 186 and 187.

Sunflower

Sunflowers are grown across North America and in parts of Europe. The seeds of these tall plants are embedded in a broad flat face surrounded by bright yellow petals. There are two main varieties of sunflowers, each grown for different purposes. The small black seeds of the oilseed variety are used to make sunflower oil and bird feed. The "confectionary" or non-oil variety produces larger black-and-white-striped seeds that are used both as a popular snack and in other food products. This latter variety of sunflower seed is available with the inedible outer hull either intact or removed.

Sunflower seeds are one of the highest sources of vitamin E (an antioxidant). They also are rich in folate, magnesium, phosphorus and thiamin.

Whole sunflower seeds have an inedible rigid outer hull (shell). In order to access the soft inner kernel, the outer shell must first be cracked open. Whole seeds are available both raw and roasted and may be seasoned. The seasoning blends may contain hydrolyzed wheat protein, wheat flour or wheat starch.

Shelled sunflower seeds, also called sunflower kernels, are available raw or roasted and also may be seasoned. Some seasoning blends may have gluten-containing ingredients.

Sunflower oil is extracted from the oilseed variety of the sunflower. This mildly flavored oil is suitable for frying or as an ingredient in salad dressings and sauces.

Sunflower seed butter, made from ground shelled sunflower seeds, is available in both smooth and crunchy styles, and also may contain sugar, salt and/or other ingredients.

For recipes using sunflower seeds, see pages 163, 167, 178, 182, 185, 187 and 192.

Starches

Starches are derived from the roots of plants (arrowroot, tapioca), from grains (amaranth, corn) and from vegetables (potato), which are dried then ground into fine powders. These versatile ingredients are used extensively in food products as well as in cosmetics, medications and other items. Unlike whole grains, legumes and seeds, starches contain minimal amounts of nutrients. Nevertheless, starches are excellent thickeners and can be used for coating and breading meats, poultry and fish. Also, they are combined with other gluten-free flours to improve the texture of baked goods by lightening and adding a more chewy and elastic consistency to the finished product.

Types of Starches

The most common starches are listed below. See pages 318 and 319 for the nutrient composition of starches, and to learn about how to use these starches in cooking and baking, see pages 147–156.

Arrowroot starch, also known as "arrowroot flour" or "arrowroot starch flour," is ground from the root of a tropical plant.

Cornstarch is made from the starchy endosperm of the corn kernel.

Potato starch is produced from only the starch portion of the potato, whereas potato flour is made from the whole potato. Potato starch and potato flour cannot be substituted for one another in recipes.

Tapioca starch, also called "tapioca flour" or "tapioca starch flour," is derived from the tuberous roots of the tropical cassava (manioc) shrub.

Using Gluten-Free Alternatives

Whole grains, legumes and seeds add variety to the diet while improving the nutritional profile. Because many of these alternatives are high in fiber, it is important to increase intake gradually and to drink more fluids than usual to minimize potential digestive symptoms. When trying a new whole grain for the first time, some people may prefer a half-and-half combination of the grain with white rice as they adjust to the different taste and texture.

Ideas for incorporating these gluten-free alternatives are featured on the following pages. To learn more about how to cook and bake with these nutritious alternatives, see chapter 13 on pages 143–156 as well as recipes on pages 157–204.

Table 9.3   Ideas for incorporating whole grains into the gluten-free diet

Breakfast	For a hot porridge, cook gluten-free whole grains in water or milk of choice and top with fresh or dried fruit, nuts and/or seeds. Examples include: • Whole grains: amaranth, brown rice, millet, quinoa, teff, gluten-free oat groats (steel-cut, stone-ground) • Cream of brown rice or buckwheat cereal • Grits: buckwheat, corn, millet • Rolled or flaked cereal: gluten-free oatmeal, quinoa
	Choose gluten-free whole-grain cereals (flaked or puffed) or granola and serve with milk or yogurt and fresh fruit.
	Heat whole-grain tortillas/wraps (corn or teff) and top with scrambled eggs, low-fat cheese, black beans, salsa and chopped avocado.
	Spread a nut or seed butter on whole-grain toast.
	Make pancakes using pure buckwheat, oat or teff flour.
	Bake muffins using a combination of flours, e.g., whole-grain corn, brown rice, gluten-free oat, quinoa, sorghum or teff.
Lunch/Dinner	Sprinkle cooked whole grains over mixed green salads.
	Dress cold cooked whole grains with pesto or a zesty salad dressing to make tabbouleh.
	Add cooked brown rice, buckwheat, gluten-free oat groats, quinoa, sorghum or wild rice to homemade or purchased soups.
	Serve whole grains as a side dish to replace potatoes, pasta or white rice. Combine with herbs and/or spices.
	Toss cooked whole grains with gluten-free pasta.
	Blend cooked brown rice or gluten-free oat groats with black beans or pinto beans in Southwestern dishes.
	Stuff peppers with cooked amaranth, brown rice, millet, quinoa or teff, and steam or bake.
	Add cooked buckwheat, gluten-free oat groats, quinoa, sorghum or wild rice to rice pilaf.
	Extend hamburger patties or meat loaf with raw gluten-free rolled oats or cooked brown rice, quinoa, amaranth or teff.
	Serve chili over a bed of cooked amaranth, brown rice, millet or quinoa.
	Replace one-quarter of the cornmeal with teff grains for a cornmeal-teff polenta.
	Thicken soups and stews with uncooked amaranth, buckwheat, quinoa, sorghum or teff.
	Use brown rice, buckwheat groats, millet, quinoa, sorghum or wild rice alone or in combination to make a gluten-free stuffing. Add herbs, spices, onions, celery and/or dried fruit.
	Make your own vegetarian burger using cooked amaranth, buckwheat, millet, quinoa or teff with beans, seeds and/or tofu. Add garlic, herbs, spices and onions. Bind with an egg or egg substitute.
	Choose pasta that is made from amaranth, brown rice and/or quinoa and top with cooked vegetables and/or gluten-free sauce.
Snacks	Serve whole-grain crackers with nut or seed butters (almond, sesame, peanut, sunflower, pumpkin).
	Pop amaranth, sorghum or corn. Amaranth and sorghum are best done in a frying pan or stovetop popper (not a hot-air popper) and in small batches.
Baking and Desserts	Use whole-grain rice (black or brown), buckwheat groats, quinoa or wild rice to make a sweet rice-type pudding.
	Use quinoa flakes, gluten-free rolled oats or gluten-free cold cereals and granolas to top baked fruit crisps and cobblers.
	Choose baking mixes or recipes using whole-grain flours (e.g., amaranth, brown rice, buckwheat, millet, gluten-free oats, quinoa, sorghum, teff or wild rice).

Some of the information above is adapted from *Whole Grains and the Gluten-Free Diet* by Carol Fenster, PhD and Shelley Case, RD.

Table 9.4   Ideas for incorporating legumes into the gluten-free diet

Baked Goods	Add puréed cooked lentils and black or white beans to baked goods such as squares, cakes, cookies, granola bars and muffins.
	Legume flours can be used in a variety of baked goods such as biscuits, breads, cakes, cookies, cupcakes, loaves, muffins, squares and pie and pizza crusts, as well as crêpes, pancakes and waffles.
Entrées and Side Dishes	Add canned beans, chickpeas, lentils or soybeans to chili, lasagna, taco meat or spaghetti sauce and reduce the amount of ground beef used in the recipe.
	Top gluten-free pizza with cooked black beans or lentils.
	Cook legume-based pasta instead of white rice pasta.
	Serve cooked black beans and salsa with an omelet or fried eggs.
	Mix mashed cooked white beans into chicken, egg or tuna salad for sandwiches.
	Sprinkle roasted cooked chickpeas, peas or soybeans (soynuts) into stir-fries.
	Make a vegetarian curry using chickpeas and/or lentils.
	Add cooked beans, chickpeas, lentils and/or shelled edamame to cooked grains.
Salads and Soups	Rinse and drain canned black beans or chickpeas and toss with any salad.
	Add cooked beans, chickpeas, lentils or edamame to broth-style soups.
	Make soup using split green or yellow peas.
	Add cooked lentils or chickpeas to cooked chilled grains (e.g., quinoa, sorghum, millet, rice) or to a green or pasta salad and toss with a gluten-free salad dressing.
	Combine cooked red kidney beans, chickpeas, cannellini beans and/or shelled edamame with chopped onion and bell peppers plus seasonings; mix with vinaigrette and let marinate for several hours.
	Mix cooked navy beans with chopped green pepper, canned mandarin orange slices and chopped green onion. Dress with juice from mandarin oranges, white wine vinegar, oil and black pepper. Marinate for two hours.
Snacks, Spreads and Dips	Serve hummus with raw vegetables or spread on gluten-free crackers.
	Steam or microwave edamame; serve warm or cold in pods as a snack or appetizer.
	Mix cooked black beans into gluten-free salsa, and add chopped cilantro and lime juice for an easy dip. Serve with raw vegetables or gluten-free crackers.
	For a variation on guacamole, mash cooked cannellini or white beans with avocado, garlic, cilantro and chopped red onion.
	Drain and purée canned black beans or lentils with herbs and spices and spread on toasted gluten-free bread, bagels or gluten-free English muffins.
	Cooked chickpeas, peas or soybeans can be tossed with oil and/or salt and other seasonings, roasted, then eaten as a snack or sprinkled on top of salads.

Some of the information above was adapted from *Pulses and the Gluten-Free Diet: Cooking with Beans, Peas, Lentils and Chickpeas* by Pulse Canada. www.pulsecanada.com

Table 9.5   Ideas for incorporating nuts and seeds into the gluten-free diet

Baked Goods	Add seeds (e.g., sesame, sunflower kernels, whole or ground flax or chia seeds) to breads, cookies and muffins.
	Pepitas or sunflower kernels (unsalted), sesame seeds and/or flaxseeds can be sprinkled on bread dough or muffin batter before baking.
	Use almond flour or meal to make a dessert crust (e.g., cheesecake, pie) or in cake, cookie or muffin recipes.
Entrées and Side Dishes	Sprinkle toasted sesame seeds, cashews and/or slivered almonds onto stir-fries.
	Top salads with pepitas, shelled sunflower seeds, sesame seeds, slivered almonds or walnuts.
	Mix ¼ cup chia with 1 cup water or milk and ½ tablespoon honey, let sit for at least 30 minutes and top with berries and pepitas for breakfast or a snack.
	Add hemp hearts, chia seeds, ground flax and/or chopped nuts to cold or hot cereal, yogurt and smoothies.
	Add chia seeds or ground flax to homemade burgers to help bind the other ingredients.
	Coat chicken or fish with sesame seeds before baking/frying/grilling.
Snacks, Spreads and Dips	Mix sunflower, sesame or flax oil with balsamic or red wine vinegar for a quick salad dressing.
	Make a pesto by blending olive oil, pine nuts, basil, lemon juice, garlic and Parmesan cheese. Use as a spread or on pasta.
	Spread nut or seed butters (e.g., almond, cashew, peanut, sesame, sunflower) on gluten-free toast, English muffin or bagel. Top with sliced bananas or fruit purée.
	Add pepitas, sunflower kernels and/or nuts to homemade trail mix.
	Combine tahini, lemon juice, garlic, onion powder and water to make a dip. Serve with raw vegetables or crackers.
	Eat a handful of whole hemp seeds, sunflower seeds, pepitas, almonds, pistachios or walnuts for a snack.
	Combine seeds, nuts and dried fruits for a trail mix.
	Roast whole pumpkin seeds and season with salt or other gluten-free seasonings.
	Spread tahini instead of mayonnaise on wraps and sandwiches.
Miscellaneous	Add nut butter to smoothies.

Gluten-Free Meal Planning

10

Getting Started

Successful gluten-free meal planning requires a positive attitude, a little creativity and learning how to make substitutions in "old familiar" favorite recipes and meals. But this is not as difficult as one might think! First of all, many foods are naturally gluten free, including plain meats, fish, seafood, poultry, eggs, milk, cheese, yogurt, legumes, nuts, seeds, fruits, vegetables and grain alternatives such as amaranth, buckwheat, corn, millet, quinoa, rice, sorghum and teff. Also, there is a wide selection of gluten-free specialty products available (e.g., baked goods, cereals, crackers, pastas, sauces, soups) that can replace traditional gluten-containing similar items (see chapter 15 on pp. 205–262).

In the beginning, plan simple meals and snacks with plain foods so you don't become overwhelmed with the new gluten-free lifestyle. Once the basics are mastered, gradually incorporate new items and try more complex dishes with multiple ingredients. If cooking for a family, save time and energy by preparing gluten-free recipes and menu items that everyone can eat, rather than "cooking twice." Other family members can supplement their meals with gluten-containing bread or dessert items if desired.

This chapter includes guidelines for healthy eating, additions and substitutions for the gluten-free diet, meal planning ideas and a sample seven-day gluten-free menu. In addition to this book, gluten-free cookbooks and other resources (see pp. 294–300) offer an abundance of tips for menu planning and recipes.

A Healthy Gluten-Free Diet

When planning meals and snacks, it is important to focus on nutrition. The foundation of the diet should be a wide selection of naturally gluten-free foods that contain an extensive range of nutrients essential for good health. Although not necessary, gluten-free specialty products can be included in the diet to provide greater variety. However, choose these items less often and in smaller portions because many of them are relatively high in simple carbohydrates and fats, and low in fiber, vitamins and minerals. Plus, they usually are more expensive than their gluten-containing counterparts. The tables on the following pages provide some guidelines and tips to help you make healthy food choices.

Table 10.1 General guidelines for healthy gluten-free eating

Food Group	Examples	Healthy Tips and Nutrition Facts
Grains and Grain-Based Foods	GF grain alternatives (e.g., amaranth, buckwheat, cornmeal, millet, oats*, quinoa, rice [black, brown, green, purple, red, white], sorghum, teff, wild rice)	1. Choose GF whole grains more often (e.g., amaranth, buckwheat, cornmeal [whole grain – not degermed], millet, oats*, quinoa, rice [black, brown, green, purple, red], sorghum, teff, wild rice).
	GF bagels, breads, rolls, muffins	2. Choose enriched GF products more often. Not all GF baked products, cereals, pastas and flours are enriched with iron and B vitamins, and many of these are relatively low in fiber because they are made with refined flours and starches.
	GF ready-to-eat cold cereals	
	GF hot cereals (e.g., amaranth, buckwheat grits [cream of buckwheat], corn grits, cornmeal, cream rice [brown, white], hominy grits, millet grits, oats [rolled/oatmeal, steel-cut]*, quinoa, quinoa flakes, rice flakes, soy flakes, soy grits)	3. Choose GF bagels, breads, rolls, muffins, cereals, pastas, tortillas/wraps, pancakes and waffles made with flours and ingredients that are high in fiber, protein, vitamins and minerals (e.g., amaranth, brown rice, buckwheat, flaxseed, legumes, mesquite, millet, oats*, quinoa, sorghum, teff and wild rice).
	GF pasta (e.g., bean, 100% pure buckwheat, corn, pea, potato; quinoa and corn; quinoa and rice; rice [brown, white, wild], soy)	**Note:** Whole grains contain the entire grain seed (usually called the kernel) and consist of three parts – the bran, germ and endosperm.
	GF tortillas and wraps	
	GF pancakes and waffles	
	Popcorn	
Meats and Alternatives	Meats, poultry, fish, seafood, eggs	1. Poultry without the skin and lean meats are lower in fat.
	Legumes (dried beans, lentils, peas, soybeans)	2. Choose eggs, fish, seafood and legumes. 3. Flaxseeds and walnuts, along with some fish (e.g., herring, salmon, trout), are high in omega-3 fatty acids, which play a positive role in heart health.
	Nuts and seeds	
	GF tofu, GF tempeh, GF texturized vegetable protein, GF veggie burgers	4. Some seeds and nuts (almonds, hazelnuts, sunflower) are good sources of vitamin E.

"GF" = Gluten Free

* = Gluten-free oats

Food Group	Examples	Healthy Tips and Nutrition Facts
Fruits	Fresh, frozen and canned fruits and fruit juices Dried fruits	1. To get more fiber, choose whole fruit instead of juice. 2. Choose unsweetened frozen fruit or fruit canned in 100% fruit juice or water. 3. Select orange-colored fruits (e.g., apricot, cantaloupe, orange, mango, nectarine, peach, red or pink grapefruit) more often as they are high in vitamins, minerals and phytochemicals (naturally occurring healthy plant compounds). 4. Choose 100% fruit juice rather than fruit drinks, which contain less juice and more added sugar. 5. If possible choose juices (e.g., orange) enriched with calcium and/or vitamin D.
Vegetables	Fresh, frozen and canned vegetables and vegetable juices	1. Choose dark green and yellow or orange vegetables (e.g., broccoli, carrot, pumpkin, squash, sweet potato) more often as they are high in vitamins, minerals and phytochemicals. 2. For salads, choose romaine lettuce, spinach and kale instead of iceberg lettuce as they are higher in nutrients.
Dairy Products	Milk (fluid and dried powdered) Milk (lactose-free, lactose-reduced) Cheese Yogurt and yogurt-based beverages Milk-based desserts (e.g., puddings made with milk, ice cream, ice milk, frozen yogurt)	1. Choose low-fat milk and milk products. 2. Milk and some yogurt products are enriched with vitamin D, which is a key nutrient that aids in the absorption of calcium. Cheese, ice cream, commercial pudding cups and some yogurts usually are not enriched with vitamin D. 3. Many brands of non-dairy beverages (e.g., flax, hemp, nut, potato, quinoa, rice, soy) and some orange/other fruit juices may be enriched with calcium and/or vitamin D but often do not provide the other nutrients found in milk products. 4. For individuals with lactose intolerance, see pages 68–70.
Fats and Oils	Oils (e.g., canola, coconut, corn, cottonseed, olive, palm kernel, peanut, safflower, sesame seed, walnut) Solid fats such as butter, beef fat (tallow, suet), chicken fat, pork fat (lard), stick margarine, shortening	1. Choose fats and oils that are high in monounsaturated fatty acids (e.g., canola, olive). 2. Limit solid fats and coconut and palm kernel oils. These are high in saturated fats and trans fats that raise LDL ("bad") cholesterol levels in the blood (a contributing factor in coronary heart disease).

Table 10.2 Healthy additions and substitutions for the gluten-free diet

Breakfast Boosters		
If you eat this	**Add this**	**Or try this instead**
Cream of white rice cereal	Nuts, seeds, ground flax, dried fruits, fresh fruit	Cream of brown rice, cream of buckwheat; amaranth, rolled oats*, quinoa flakes, teff
Puffed rice or corn cereal	Fresh fruit	GF granola with nuts, seeds, ground flax, dried fruits
GF white rice bread or bagel	Nut butter, cheese, poached egg, omelet with chopped vegetables	GF enriched bread or bagel; homemade GF bread with brown rice, ground flax or bean flours substituted for some of the white rice, cornstarch, tapioca starch or potato starch
Fruit beverage or fruit drink	Fresh or frozen fruit or fruit juice plus yogurt or low-fat milk and ground flax to make a fruit smoothie (see p. 128)	Calcium-fortified juice, 100% fruit juice
GF waffles or pancakes with syrup	Cottage cheese, yogurt and fruit	Substitute brown rice, buckwheat, bean, mesquite, oat*, quinoa or teff flour or ground flax for some of the white rice flour, or try GF fiber-rich frozen waffles
Crêpes made with white rice flour and topped with syrup	A filling made of blended ricotta cheese, lemon or orange zest and small amount of sugar or sweetener; a topping of berries, peaches or other fruit and maple syrup	Substitute finely ground almond or oat* flour for some of the white rice flour
Fried egg and bacon	Low-fat mozzarella or feta cheese, vegetables and GF ham, smoked salmon or turkey to make an omelet	Use a non-stick pan; try Canadian bacon or low-fat GF turkey or chicken sausage

"GF" = Gluten Free

* = Gluten-free oats

Power Lunches and Dinners

If you eat this	Add this	Or try this instead
Chicken rice soup	Fresh or frozen vegetables	Soup made with dried beans, lentils or peas and vegetables; substitute brown rice or quinoa for white rice
White rice (homemade) pizza crust topped with salami and cheese	Vegetables (e.g., mushrooms, onions, peppers, zucchini)	Add brown rice flour or whole-grain sorghum flour to dough; use low-fat cheese
White rice pasta with butter or margarine	Low-fat cheese and vegetables	Enriched GF pasta; other GF pasta (e.g., bean, brown rice, lentil, quinoa); use less butter or margarine
Sandwich made of GF white rice bread, butter or margarine, mayonnaise and deli meat	Avocado, shredded carrots, sliced cucumbers, lettuce, sprouts, tomatoes	GF enriched bread or bagel; low-fat mayonnaise, salsa or mustard; salmon, tuna, low-fat GF deli meats such as chicken, ham or turkey
White rice and chicken, fish or meat	Fresh or frozen vegetables	Brown rice or a combination of brown, white, and wild rice; buckwheat, millet, quinoa, sorghum, teff
Baked or mashed potato with butter or margarine	Cheese and chopped veggies such as broccoli (on the baked potato); milk and grated low-fat cheese (in the mashed potato)	Yogurt or low-fat sour cream instead of butter or margarine; a sweet potato (for more vitamin A)
Iceberg lettuce salad, GF croûtons, cucumbers and celery with salad dressing	Tomatoes, peppers, cauliflower, broccoli, mushrooms, shredded carrots, black beans, chickpeas, sunflower seeds	Romaine lettuce or spinach with strawberries or mandarin oranges, toasted slivered almonds and/or sesame seeds with low-fat salad dressing

"GF" = Gluten Free

* = Gluten-free oats

Smart Snacks

If you eat this	Add this	Or try this instead
GF pretzels	Unsalted nuts	Trail mix comprising GF granola, dried fruits, nuts and seeds
Rice cakes or rice crackers	Cheese (cubes or string), hummus, nut or seed butter with apple, banana or pear slices	GF snack bar made with seeds, dried fruits and healthy GF grains such as brown rice, oats*, quinoa; GF high-fiber snack crackers made with nuts and/or seeds
Fried corn chips	Salsa and shredded cheese	Baked corn chips with low-fat cheese and salsa; popcorn
Celery sticks	Peanut butter, cheese spread, low-fat cream cheese with raisins	Raw carrots, green snap peas, cucumbers, peppers, cherry tomatoes, broccoli, cauliflower
GF cookie	Fresh fruit and a glass of low-fat milk or enriched GF non-dairy beverage	Homemade cookie made with almond or oat* flour and chopped nuts
GF brownie	Mug of warm steamed low-fat milk or enriched GF non-dairy beverage	Homemade brownie recipe with puréed black beans, chickpeas or lentils
GF muffin made with white rice flour	Add to batter chopped nuts, mashed banana, dried fruits (raisins, cranberries, apricots, dates), ground flax	Pumpkin, pineapple, carrot or banana muffin made with almond, bean, oat* and/or sorghum flour and ground flax
Fruit-flavored yogurt	Fresh fruit and nuts	Plain low-fat yogurt with chopped fruits, nuts and/or seeds

"GF" = Gluten Free

* = Gluten-free oats

Reprinted and adapted with permission from *Rate Your Plate, Living Without* magazine, Fall 2003, pg. 26.
Article by Julie Rothschild Levi; table prepared by Shelley Case, RD.

Gluten-Free Meal-Planning Ideas

The following ideas for specific breakfast, lunch and dinner foods, coupled with the recipes and gluten-free specialty products listed in this book, can be used as a starting point to create your own customized meal plans and delicious meals.

"GF" = Gluten Free   * = Gluten-free oats

Breakfast

Cereals
- GF cold cereal or granola (pp. 208–211), berries and milk or yogurt

- GF hot cereal (e.g., brown rice, buckwheat, oats*, quinoa) with chopped apricots, dates or raisins; cinnamon; brown sugar or maple syrup; and milk or non-dairy beverage

- Spiced Apple Cranberry Buckwheat Cereal (recipe p. 174) with chopped almonds

- Mix rolled oats* with milk or non-dairy beverage, cinnamon and pumpkin seeds. Let sit in the fridge for at least two hours or overnight, top with chopped apples and raisins

Bagels, Breads, English Muffins and Muffins
- GF toast and yogurt with fruit, chopped nuts and/or ground flax

- GF toasted Oatmeal Bread (recipe p. 163), bagel or English muffin; nut or seed butter and sliced bananas

- GF muffin (see pp. 215 and 216; recipes pp. 169–171), cheese and fruit

Eggs
- Scrambled eggs, green onion, ham and cheese on a GF English muffin

- Poached egg on GF toast and sliced oranges

- GF wrap filled with scrambled eggs, black beans, avocado and salsa

- Omelet (with chopped green or red peppers, onions, shredded cheese) and fried leftover potatoes

Crêpes, Pancakes and Waffles
- GF French toast (a great way to use bread that is not fresh or soft), fruit and syrup

- GF waffles (homemade or store-bought), fruit salad and maple syrup

- GF pancakes or crêpes using a GF mix (see pp. 231–237) or make your own (recipes pp. 172, 173) and top with berries and syrup OR nut butter and sliced bananas

Miscellaneous
- High-protein snack bar and an apple

- Fruit smoothie (see p. 128)

Lunch

Soups

- Homemade soup (recipes pp. 183, 184) and melted cheese on GF roll
- GF heat-and-serve soup (see pp. 257–260), GF whole-grain crackers and raw vegetables
- GF cheese bread or GF grilled cheese sandwich with GF tomato soup (canned or homemade)

Salads

- Dark green leafy salad with vegetables plus chopped chicken, canned shrimp, tuna or salmon with GF whole-grain roll
- GF pasta salad with black beans, chopped vegetables, cheddar cheese plus cubed chicken or GF ham and fresh fruit
- Spinach salad with sunflower seeds, chickpeas, feta cheese and strawberries with GF whole-grain crackers
- Quinoa Salad (recipe p. 187) and yogurt with fresh fruit
- Wild Rice Salad (recipe p. 188) with grilled chicken
- Moroccan Salad (recipe p. 185) on a bed of fresh spinach
- Brown Rice Chickpea Kale Salad (recipe p. 186) and yogurt
- Tabbouleh with Shrimp on Mixed Greens (recipe p. 200)

Pizzas and Pastas

- GF pasta and cheese dinner (see pp. 253–255) and raw vegetables
- GF pasta with GF tomato-based or cheese sauce (homemade or store-bought) and salad
- Homemade mini pizzas (GF English muffin with tomato sauce, shredded cheese, chopped ham and drained pineapple chunks)
- Pepperoni Pizza (recipe p. 203) and tossed green salad
- GF pre-baked frozen crust (see p. 221) with GF pizza sauce, grated cheese and favorite toppings (e.g., peppers, onions, mushrooms)

Legumes

- Canned GF baked beans, coleslaw and GF Cornbread (recipe p. 161)

- Black Bean Chili (recipe p. 197) served over a baked potato or toasted GF bun; top with grated cheese

- Hoisin Lentil Lettuce Wraps (recipe p. 194)

- Lentil vegetable curry (lentils, spinach, cauliflower, onions, sweet potato, curry spice powder and light coconut milk)

Miscellaneous

- Baked stuffed potato topped with cheese and broccoli OR cheese and GF ham (make ahead, freeze and heat in microwave) and fresh fruit

- Wild Rice, Chicken & Vegetable Casserole (recipe p. 195)

- Fresh Rolls with Peanut Dipping Sauce (recipe p. 189)

- GF hot dog or sausage on a GF bun, raw vegetables and yogurt-based dip or GF salad dressing

- GF crackers, cheese cubes, GF deli meat or pepperoni sticks; raw vegetables (cucumbers, red pepper and carrots)

- Leftovers (e.g., casseroles, chili, stew, meat and potatoes, chicken and rice)

- GF tortilla chips topped with black beans, tomatoes, peppers, black olives and light cheddar cheese (warm in the oven until cheese is melted)

- GF pancakes, waffles or French toast (see breakfast ideas) and GF sausages

- GF toast and omelet with chopped onions, mushrooms, peppers and shredded cheese

- Soft GF soft corn tortillas stuffed with:

    - cooked mung bean noodles or rice noodles plus meat or shrimp with vegetables (e.g., sprouts, tomatoes, cucumber, green pepper) and sauce (GF soy sauce, honey, ginger and garlic powder)

    - cooked kernel corn plus brown rice and ground beef with pesto sauce and shredded mozzarella cheese

    - grilled fish (e.g., tuna) plus shredded cabbage or lettuce and carrots, topped with guacamole

Sandwiches, Rolls and Wraps

- GF sandwich, roll or wrap with fruit and/or yogurt
- Some suggested fillings:

    - Chicken, egg, salmon or tuna salad with chopped celery, onion and/or herbs

    - Turkey, lettuce, tomato, sprouts and avocado

    - Hummus, spinach, cucumbers, tomato, red onion, peppers and shredded carrots

    - Roast beef, lettuce and cheese

    - Nut butter (e.g., almond, cashew, peanut butter) and jam or jelly

    - Mashed avocado, tomato and red onion

    - GF ham and Swiss cheese

    - Pure crab meat with melted mozzarella cheese

    - Chicken, lettuce and GF Caesar dressing

Sandwich and Wrap Tips

Gluten-free breads and wraps can become dry and/or crumbly relatively quickly so here are a few tips:

- Toasting bread improves flavor and helps keep it from crumbling. Make a sandwich on lightly toasted bread.

- Place GF wrap or tortilla in moist paper towel or a damp clean cloth; heat in the microwave until slightly warm (approximately 15–20 seconds).

- Lightly spread a small amount of salad dressing, mayonnaise or mustard on a wrap to make it moist.

- Consider buying a bread machine, as homemade gluten-free breads are much fresher and more economical than ready-made GF breads.

- Try open-face sandwiches grilled under a broiler. (e.g., tuna or pure crab meat with shredded cheese). Top with sliced tomatoes.

Dinner

Pasta meals served with a tossed green salad

- GF pasta (see pp. 250–253) with GF meat or tomato sauce (homemade or store-bought) sprinkled with Parmesan cheese

- Fettuccini Alfredo (toss together cooked GF pasta, olive oil, fresh garlic or garlic powder, Parmesan cheese, milk)

- Vegetable & Beef Lasagna (recipe p. 196)

Meat, poultry and fish meals

- Barbecued chicken (GF barbecue sauce), grilled vegetables and rice pilaf (brown or wild) OR Multi-Grain Pilaf (recipe p. 191)

- Meat loaf (ground meat plus GF rolled oats OR GF bread crumbs, egg, ketchup or tomato sauce, herbs and/or spices), spaghetti squash and steamed broccoli

- Grilled pork chops with oven-roasted vegetables (butternut squash, carrots, parsnips, onions)

- Baked salmon, wild rice and green beans with slivered almonds

- Roast chicken or turkey with dressing made with GF bread crumbs or Wondergrain Sorghum Stuffing (recipe p. 190), mashed potatoes, gravy (thickened with GF starch) and glazed carrots

- Chicken, pork or lamb kabobs served over pilaf (millet, quinoa or buckwheat with nuts and dried fruits) and GF Greek salad

- Turkey Meatballs with Lemon Sauce (recipe p. 199), brown rice or kasha and green peas

- Steak, baked potato and Greek salad

- Crunchy baked chicken or fish, oven-baked potato fries (homemade) and coleslaw
    - Crunchy coating: crushed GF cereal, GF bread crumbs, ground nuts or cornmeal

- Roast pork, applesauce, baked sweet potato and steamed green snap peas

- Shrimp skewers with grilled mushrooms, peppers and onions over brown rice

- Sweet and sour meatballs served over rice; stir-fried vegetables

- Oven-Fried Chicken (recipe p. 201), mashed potatoes and asparagus

- GF burger (beef, chicken, turkey, salmon, veggie), corn on the cob and watermelon wedges
    - Spicy Sweet Potato Bean Burgers (recipe p. 193)

- GF chicken curry served over rice and topped with Greek yogurt

- Pan-seared halibut, sautéed spinach and roasted beets

Casseroles, stews and miscellaneous

- Sahara Stew over Superblend Grains (recipe p. 198)

- GF corn tacos or tortillas (stuffed with ground beef and flavored with GF taco seasoning, grated cheese and chopped lettuce, tomatoes and avocado; served with salsa and sour cream)

- Chili con carne, GF Cornbread (recipe p. 161) and raw vegetables

- Stir-fry beef, pork, chicken or seafood and vegetables (mix GF soy sauce, arrowroot or tapioca starch, garlic and ginger with water to make a stir-fry sauce OR GF teriyaki sauce) served over rice and sprinkled with toasted almonds and/or sesame seeds

- Bell peppers stuffed with ground turkey, lentils and brown rice or quinoa

- Homemade beef stew (thickened with a GF starch) and Teff Polenta (recipe p. 162)

- Burrito using GF wrap stuffed with mashed black beans, shredded cheese, corn and chopped lettuce, tomatoes, avocado and green peppers

- Moroccan Millet (recipe p. 192) and salad

- Lentil Pizza Squares (recipe p. 202) and tossed salad

- Creamed salmon or tuna (thickened with a GF starch) with green peas served on GF toast
- Lentil Vegetable Soup (recipe p. 183) and GF roll

Snacks

Fruit and Vegetables
- Fresh fruit (e.g., pear, peach, banana, orange, apple, kiwi, melon)
- Dried fruit (e.g., raisins, apricots, cranberries, blueberries, mangoes)
- Canned fruit in water or fruit juice (e.g., pears, peaches, fruit cocktail)
- Applesauce (unsweetened) and string cheese
- Low-fat cottage cheese topped with pineapple or berries
- Sliced apples and nut butter
- Greek yogurt with fruit (berries; apple or pears and cinnamon)
- Small fruit smoothie (see p. 128)
- Baby carrots with hummus
- Celery with peanut butter and raisins
- Raw vegetables (green snap peas, sliced peppers, broccoli, cauliflower) and dip (made with yogurt and herbs or GF salad dressing)

Nuts and Seeds
- Pumpkin or sunflower seeds (plain or GF flavored)
- Plain unsalted nuts (e.g., almonds, walnuts, peanuts, pistachios)
- Soynuts (plain or GF flavored)
- Dried fruit-and-nut mixtures
- Cajun Lentil Trail Mix with Dark Chocolate (recipe p. 182)

Muffins and Quick Breads
- GF bagel (half) with nut or seed butter topped with sliced bananas or apples
- Banana Seed Bread (recipe p. 167)
- Apple Date Bread (recipe p. 166)
- Pumpkin Bread (recipe p. 168)
- GF muffins from a mix (see pp. 231–237) or homemade (recipes pp. 169–171) and cheese
- Sweet Sorghum Banana Date Breakfast Cookies (recipe p. 175)

Snack Bars and Crackers

- GF snack bar or granola bar (see pp. 227–231)
- Carrot Apple Energy Bars (recipe p. 176)
- Fruit n' Nut Bars (recipe p. 177)
- String cheese or cheese cubes with GF whole-grain or lentil crackers
- GF-flavored mini or large rice cakes (see pp. 223, 224) with nut butter
- GF whole-grain or lentil crackers (see pp. 222, 223) with hummus

Miscellaneous

- Popcorn
- GF roasted chickpeas (pp. 224–226)
- Hard-boiled egg and GF whole-grain crackers
- GF beef or turkey jerky (low sodium)
- Coconut & Banana Lentil Bites (recipe p. 178)
- Puddings (homemade or GF prepared)
- GF pretzels (see pp. 224–226)
- Plain bean or corn chips with salsa
- GF granola (see pp. 208–211) and yogurt
- GF cereal and milk

Table 10.3   How to build a smoothie

Step	Amount	Ingredients	
1. Choose a liquid	**1 cup**	• Milk • Lactose-reduced milk • Juice	• Non-dairy beverage (almond, cashew, coconut, rice, soy) • Water
2. Add some fruit	**½ cup each** of one or two choices	• Avocado • Apple • Banana • Blackberries • Blueberries • Cherries • Dates • Mango	• Orange • Peach • Pear • Pineapple • Strawberries • Raspberries • Watermelon
3. Add some vegetables	**1 cup**	• Cucumber • Carrots	• Kale • Spinach
4. Thicken it up	**Varies**	• Chia Seeds (1 Tbsp.) • Flaxseeds (1 Tbsp.) • Hemp seeds (1 Tbsp.) • Ice cubes (3–6)	• Nut butter (1 Tbsp.) • Yogurt (¼ cup) • Dry low-fat milk powder (2 Tbsp.)
5. Add some flavor or sweetness	**Varies**	• Cocoa nibs (1 Tbsp.) • Cocoa (1 Tbsp.) • Coconut (1 Tbsp.) • Cinnamon (¼ tsp.) • Ginger (¼ tsp.)	• Honey or maple syrup (½–1 Tbsp.) • Lemon or lime juice (a squeeze) • Sugar (½–1 Tbsp.) • Fresh mint (1 tsp.) • Vanilla (½–1 tsp.)

Smoothie Pairings

- Milk, blueberries, avocado, spinach, ground flax
- Orange juice, strawberries, yogurt
- Coconut beverage, pineapple, ice, chia seeds
- Milk, banana, orange, yogurt, vanilla
- Water, apple, almond butter, cinnamon, ground flaxseeds
- Water, orange, pineapple, carrots, kale, ground flax
- Water, peaches, spinach, hemp seeds, cinnamon
- Almond beverage, banana, peanut butter, cocoa powder
- Water, kiwi, pear, spinach, lime juice
- Coconut beverage, mango, kale, ground flax
- Watermelon, cucumber, yogurt, mint, lemon juice

Tips

- Experiment with different ingredients to find a favorite combination.
- Depending on the ingredients and individual taste, extra sweetness from honey, syrup or sugar may or may not be needed.
- Thicken smoothies with avocado, nut butters, seeds, frozen fruit and/or ice cubes.
- Add more liquid if smoothie is too thick.
- If the smoothie does not contain milk, milk powder, yogurt or nut butter, add a high-quality protein powder to make it more filling and boost the nutrition.

Sample Seven-Day Gluten-Free Menu

Here is a sample one-week menu to inspire you to eat safely, healthfully and deliciously. Of course, different people have different tastes and nutritional needs, so adapt accordingly. Many of these meals and snacks work well when you're "on the go." For those with lactose intolerance, see pages 69–70 for alternative options.

Monday

Breakfast	Smoothie with fruit, yogurt and ground flax or flaxseeds; GF snack bar
Lunch	Spinach salad with sunflower seeds, chickpeas, feta cheese, strawberries; GF whole-grain crackers **Hint:** Make a homemade salad dressing to keep in the fridge at home and at work.
Snack	Fresh pear and raw almonds
Dinner	GF pasta with seafood or meat sauce and/or grated cheese; grilled vegetables
Treat	Pudding and GF cookie

Tuesday

Breakfast	GF bagel with nut or seed butter; sliced bananas and yogurt
Lunch	Baked white or sweet potato stuffed with broccoli and cheese; fresh fruit **Hint:** Potato can be prepared the night before and reheated prior to eating; bake extra plain potatoes for other dishes throughout the week.
Snack	GF granola with milk
Dinner	Turkey chili; GF cornbread or corn chips; raw vegetables
Treat	Berries (optional: top with yogurt or real whipped cream)

Wednesday

Breakfast	Omelet with vegetables and cheese; leftover fried potatoes; ½ grapefruit
Lunch	Tuna on mixed greens with seasonal fruit; GF puréed vegetable soup (e.g., carrot, squash, potato) topped with grated Parmesan cheese **Hint:** Make soup monthly and freeze in small containers for quick and healthy lunches.
Snack	GF snack bar and yogurt
Dinner	Beef or chicken kabobs; millet or buckwheat pilaf with nuts and dried fruit; steamed asparagus
Treat	Piece of a GF dark chocolate bar

Thursday

Breakfast	GF waffle with pure maple syrup, cottage cheese and peaches
Lunch	GF pasta salad with vegetables and leftover chicken or beef; fresh fruit
Snack	Trail mix of GF cereal, nuts and dried fruit; hot chocolate or decaf latte
Dinner	Poached salmon; brown and/or wild rice; garlic green beans
Treat	Ice cream or sorbet with fresh fruit

"GF" = Gluten Free

Friday

Breakfast	Plain yogurt with fruit and unsweetened coconut; GF toast with nut or seed butter; calcium-fortified orange juice
Lunch	GF bagel with turkey, lettuce, tomato (option: avocado, sprouts); baby carrots; fresh fruit
Snack	String cheese and GF whole-grain crackers
Dinner	Lentil casserole; mixed greens salad
Treat	Baked apple

Saturday

Breakfast	GF cereal with nuts and/or seeds and milk; fresh fruit or leftover baked apple Hint: For a hot and healthy start, try cooked amaranth or quinoa, cream of buckwheat or cream of brown rice.
Lunch	GF grilled cheese sandwich; GF soup; raw vegetables Hint: Use homemade stock or use GF bouillon cubes or broth for a safe and tasty soup base.
Snack	GF whole-grain crackers with hummus
Dinner	Hamburger patty or grilled chicken breast; corn on the cob; coleslaw; watermelon wedges
Treat	Vanilla ice cream with warmed GF brownie or cookie

Sunday

Breakfast	GF blueberry pancakes; GF breakfast sausage; glass of milk or calcium-fortified juice
Lunch	Stir-fry with meat, poultry, seafood or tofu and vegetables; brown rice or quinoa topped with sesame seeds Hint: If eating out, bring your own GF soy sauce and (1) ask the chef to use it in the preparation of your food or (2) when the meal arrives at the table, add it to your food.
Snack	Celery with nut butter and raisins
Dinner	GF pizza; vegetables and dip Hint: Leftover pizza makes a great grab-and-go snack, even when cold.
Treat	Popcorn

Some Ethnic Alternatives:

- Fish or vegetable sushi with GF soy sauce
- Meat or vegetable fajitas (made with GF corn tortillas)
- Seafood paella
- Wild mushroom risotto or polenta
- Veggie, fish, or meat curry over basmati rice
- Pad Thai and Asian fresh rolls made with rice paper

"GF" = Gluten Free

Sample Seven-Day Gluten-Free Menu adapted and reprinted with permission from *Gluten-Free Guidance* by Shelley Case, RD, and Cindy Kaplan. *Today's Dietitian*, March 2003, p. 49. Great Valley Publishing, Inc. **www.todaysdietitian.com**

Gluten-Free Shopping

11

A wide variety of naturally gluten-free foods should form the cornerstone of the gluten-free diet. Fruits, vegetables, nuts, seeds, legumes, milk, yogurt, cheese, meat, poultry, fish, seafood, eggs and gluten-free grains provide an array of nutrients for good health.

Gluten-free products including breads, cereals and many other items are available to replace wheat-based staples in the diet. These products can be purchased in regular supermarkets; in health food, large retail and convenience stores; in gluten-free specialty stores (see pp. 287, 288); and in warehouse clubs and pharmacies, as well as from online retailers and direct from manufacturers. Although the availability of gluten-free products may vary, the number of shelf-stable, refrigerated and frozen items in categories such as baked products, cereals, pastas, baking mixes, snack bars, entrées and soups continues to grow rapidly. For a detailed listing of gluten-free products, see pages 205–262.

Specialty products may be located in designated gluten-free or natural food sections, integrated throughout the store or both. Signs and shelf tags may further identify gluten-free products; however, beware of pitfalls when relying exclusively on signs and tags for determining if a product is gluten-free. For example, gluten-containing items inadvertently may be stocked in a section that corresponds to a gluten-free shelf tag. Therefore, always check the label on the individual product package.

Shopping Tips

At first, learning to read labels and finding safe gluten-free options can be challenging but with time, shopping will get easier and less stressful. Here are some helpful gluten-free shopping tips.

- Create a shopping list before going to the store and/or ordering online. This will ensure that all ingredients for meals and snacks are on hand. Plus, by following a list, one is less likely to make impulse purchases. See the sample shopping list on page 134. In addition to the items on the list, pages 205–262 include more examples of gluten-free products available in the marketplace. After several shopping trips, create a personalized list that will evolve based on individual preferences and what is available in local stores.

- Avoid shopping when hungry. This can lead to impulse purchases and choosing more high-calorie items. Also, shopping on an empty stomach can result in rushing through the grocery store and not taking the time required to adequately read labels.

- Because food companies can and do change the formulations of their products at any time, reading the package label at every time of purchase is essential in order to ensure there are no gluten-containing ingredients. If in doubt about a product, contact the manufacturer (a toll-free number often is on the package) to clarify its manufacturing process and gluten-free status. If possible, call while in the store, as the company service representative usually requires specific information printed on the package in order to answer questions. Also, checking the manufacturer's website on the spot using a cell phone may be helpful.

- The Canadian Celiac Association's *Acceptability of Foods and Food Ingredients for the Gluten-Free Diet* pocket dictionary is an excellent resource covering hundreds of ingredients and food additives. This pocket-sized booklet provides a brief description of each food / food ingredient along with an assessment of its acceptability for the gluten-free diet. See page 295 for how to purchase.

- On product packaging, look for "gluten-free" certification logos from national celiac associations (see pp. 50, 292).

- Some companies have their own gluten-free symbol indicating they have taken precautions to ensure the product is gluten free (e.g., they test ingredients and finished products; have a dedicated gluten-free facility or production line).

- Many products may be gluten free or may make that claim but do not indicate this by a logo or symbol on the package. In such cases, it is especially important to double-check the list of ingredients and, if in doubt, contact the manufacturer.

- Some products may be labeled "wheat free." This is not the same as "gluten free" because wheat-free products may contain barley and rye. Again, be sure to check the label for gluten-containing ingredients.

- For information on gluten-free labeling regulations, precautionary statements and certification programs, see pages 49–64.

- If possible, purchase naturally gluten-free grains, flours and starches that also carry a "gluten-free" claim because inadvertent cross-contamination with gluten-containing grains (e.g., wheat, rye, barley) may occur at any point during planting, growing, harvesting, transportation, processing and packaging.

- Avoid buying gluten-free products from bulk bins, because they easily can become contaminated by

    - scoops that previously have been used with gluten-containing products,

    - being placed in a bin that previously held gluten-containing items and was not thoroughly cleaned, and/or

    - air-borne particles from gluten-containing flours contaminating the general bin area.

- Some in-store and stand-alone bakeries sell gluten-free baked products. However, if the bakery is not a dedicated gluten-free facility, there is a huge risk of cross-contamination due to air-borne wheat flour and the use of shared equipment.

- In smaller centers, availability and selection of gluten-free products may be limited. In that situation, ordering non-perishable items from online retailers is an option. Depending on quantities purchased, free shipping may be offered.

- Take the opportunity to try gluten-free product samples at gluten-free trade shows and celiac association meetings. Retail outlets also have sampling programs; however, ask what precautions have been taken to prevent cross-contamination of the offered product.

- Money-saving coupons for gluten-free products appear both in flyers and in-store, as well as online from manufacturers, celiac associations and other websites (e.g., befreeforme.com and glutenfreecoupons.ca).

- Grocery stores often include a gluten-free section in their flyers (print and online). Compare prices between different stores to find the best deals.

- Pulses (dried beans, lentils and peas) share many texture and taste qualities with meat, yet are healthier and much less expensive. In dishes such as chili, lasagna and spaghetti sauce, replace half or all of the meat with cooked pulses.

- A loaf of purchased gluten-free bread is more expensive and generally smaller in size than its gluten-containing counterpart. Baking gluten-free bread at home usually is more cost-effective and tastes better than store-bought.

- Most gluten-free baked products (e.g., bagels, breads, muffins, rolls) tend to stale quickly; therefore, purchase in smaller quantities and/or freeze immediately.

- If the taste or texture of a purchased or homemade gluten-free product is less than desirable, throwing it out is not the only option. Breads can be combined with spices and herbs to make croûtons, stuffings or bread crumbs. Crush cookies to use in a pie crust recipe.

- Some supermarkets offer shopping tours with a registered dietitian (RD). S/he will provide labeling and nutrition information, budgeting tips and product recommendations. Another option is to contact a private practice dietitian for a personalized shopping tour.

Gluten-Free Shopping List

Bread Products
___ GF bagels, breads, buns, pizza crusts, wraps
___ GF frozen waffles
___ GF muffins

Cereals
___ GF cornflakes, GF crisp rice
___ GF granola (with or without oats*)
___ GF oatmeal / rolled oats*
___ Cream of buckwheat or brown rice, cornmeal

GF Pasta

GF Crackers / Rice Cakes

GF Flours and Starches
___ Almond flour
___ Arrowroot starch
___ Pulse flours (bean, lentil, pea)
___ Cornmeal
___ Cornstarch
___ Oat* flour
___ Potato starch
___ Quinoa flour
___ Rice flour (brown, white)
___ Sorghum flour
___ Tapioca starch

GF Baking Ingredients and Mixes
___ GF bread mix
___ GF muffin mix
___ GF pancake and waffle mix
___ GF baking powder
___ Baking soda
___ Xanthan gum or guar gum

Grains
___ Buckwheat groats
___ Millet
___ Oats*
___ Quinoa
___ Rice (brown, white, wild)
___ Sorghum (whole grain, pearled)

Pulses (Dry or Ready-to-Eat)
___ Beans (e.g., garbanzo [chickpeas], kidney, white)
___ GF canned baked beans
___ Lentils, peas (whole or split)

Nuts and Seeds
___ Almonds, cashews, peanuts, pecans, pistachios, walnuts
___ Chia, flax, hemp, pumpkin, sesame, sunflower seeds
___ Nut and seed butters (almond, cashew, peanut, sesame, sunflower)

Meat, Poultry, Fish and Seafood
___ Fresh or frozen (plain) meat, poultry, fish and seafood
___ GF deli meats

Dairy
___ Milk (non-fat/skim, low-fat/1%, reduced-fat/2%)
___ Yogurt (plain or fruit-based)
___ Cheese
___ Eggs

Produce (Fruits and Vegetables)
___ GF dried fruits
___ Fresh, frozen or canned fruit (plain)
___ Fresh, frozen or canned vegetables (plain)
___ Tomato paste
___ Tomatoes (canned)

GF Bouillons, Broths, Soups and Stocks

Condiments and Sauces
___ Ketchup, plain mustard, relish, mayonnaise
___ GF barbecue sauce
___ GF pizza and pasta sauces
___ GF salsa
___ GF soy sauce

Fats and Oils
___ Butter or margarine
___ Vegetable oil (e.g., canola, olive)
___ GF salad dressings

Miscellaneous
___ Honey, molasses, sugar (brown, white)
___ Jam, jelly, marmalade
___ Vanilla
___ Vinegars (except malt vinegar)

Spices
___ Black pepper
___ Garlic powder, fresh garlic
___ GF seasoning blend
___ Onion powder

* Oats often are cross-contaminated with barley, wheat and/or rye. Purchase only gluten-free oats and oat products. For more information about oats, see pages 27–30.

Cross-Contamination: Home and Away from Home

12

Cross-contamination can occur if gluten-free foods or ingredients come into contact with gluten-containing items. This can happen during production, at the retail store, in the home or restaurant kitchen or in any other locations where food is prepared. As discussed in chapter 6 (pp. 43–48), even small amounts of gluten can be harmful if consumed by those with celiac disease; therefore, it is essential to take precautions to prevent cross-contamination and to avoid purchasing contaminated gluten-free foods and beverages. Prevention know-how is especially important if the person with celiac disease shares the kitchen with others who eat gluten-containing foods, and should be of concern to everyone in the household. This chapter includes tips for setting up a gluten-free kitchen and for eating safely when away from home. For information on cross-contamination of in-store gluten-free products, see page 132.

Preventing Cross-Contamination in the Kitchen

• Store all gluten-free products in labeled containers. Buy brightly colored stickers and place them on everything that is and must remain gluten free, or use a permanent marker and in bold print "GLUTEN FREE" either directly on the storage containers or on labels affixed to them.

• Keep all gluten-free foods together in their own area in the cupboard or pantry. Store them on the shelves *above* gluten-containing items to prevent flour, dust or crumbs (from gluten-containing breads, cookies, crackers, etc.) from falling onto gluten-free items. In the refrigerator, keep gluten-free foods on the top shelves.

• Always make sure that the counter space used for preparing gluten-free foods is freshly washed and thoroughly cleaned to ensure it is free from gluten-containing crumbs or flour dust.

• Pots, pans, bowls and utensils that have been used for preparing gluten-containing foods should be well scrubbed and free of any residues before using for preparation of gluten-free foods. Because removing gluten-containing particles from items made of porous materials or having small crevices and hard-to-clean surfaces is difficult, it is best to have a separate and designated set of those types of items for gluten-free food preparation (e.g., cutting boards, sifter, mixer, food processor, wooden spoons, waffle iron, muffin tins, cookie sheets, cake pans and bread machine).

• Use a separate and dedicated colander to drain gluten-free pasta, as removing all traces of wheat-based pastas from a colander is difficult.

- Have a dedicated gluten-free toaster. If not, use a toaster oven where the rack can be removed and washed if others have used it. Another option is to buy special "toaster bags" that hold slices of gluten-free bread and allow safe toasting in a regular toaster. These reusable bags can be purchased online from Amazon, from some gluten-free specialty companies and at some health food stores.

- Ensure the microwave is cleaned before heating gluten-free foods. Another option is to cover the gluten-free food cooking container with a paper towel or clean microwave-safe lid.

- Clean the barbecue grill thoroughly to remove all residues of previously cooked foods before grilling gluten-free foods. If this is not possible, cook gluten-free foods on aluminum foil laid on top of the grill bars.

- Buy or prepare duplicate containers of "scoopable" items such as peanut butter, jam, butter and margarine and label one "GLUTEN FREE" to prevent its contents from becoming cross-contaminated by others preparing gluten-containing products (e.g., using a same single knife for putting spread on toast, sandwich bread or buns).

- Immediately after preparation or purchase of items such as vegetable dips, hummus, guacamole and salsa, transfer a portion into a separate labeled container for the person(s) eating gluten-free. This will prevent cross-contamination by "dipping" of gluten-containing foods (e.g., chips, crackers, breads).

- Have a separate cutting board that is used for gluten-free foods only.

- Buy condiments such as ketchup, mustard, relish and mayonnaise in squeeze containers, and do not allow nozzles to come into contact with gluten-containing foods.

- In a buffet setting, place the labeled gluten-free items at the beginning of the serving line. All dishes, both gluten free and gluten containing, should have their own separate serving utensils. Let those who need to eat gluten free go through the line first to reduce the possibility of cross-contamination that may occur if others use the serving utensils from gluten-containing dishes for the gluten-free items.

- Bake gluten-free and gluten-containing items on separate days. If done on the same day, do the gluten-free baking first. Be sure to cool and store gluten-free baked goods in bags or containers before starting to bake the gluten-containing items. This ensures that wheat flour particles in the air do not contaminate gluten-free baked goods before or after they have been made.

Eating Away from Home

Once the basics of the gluten-free diet have been mastered, eating "safely" away from home certainly is possible. A positive attitude and a "game plan" are essential for a safe and successful experience. Some resources on the subject of gluten-free eating out and traveling, including guidebooks, dining cards in English and other languages, travel clubs and websites are found on pages 300–303. Following are some helpful tips for dining in restaurants, at social events and when traveling.

Restaurants

Selecting a Place to Eat

- Check the Internet to see if a restaurant's website has a gluten-free menu or offers gluten-free options. If there is no such information available, call the restaurant and ask whether it can accommodate your dietary needs. Telephone the day before or early the same day of the planned occasion, avoiding the peak busy hours, and ask to speak to the chef. Most chefs have at least a general awareness of the gluten-free diet and often can advise which items are safe, suggest ingredient substitutions and/or create an alternative dish.

- Be careful in restaurants where language differences may make communication difficult or unclear. Food service and wait staff may not easily understand questions regarding gluten-free restrictions. International language restaurant cards listing "Allowed" and "Not Allowed" ingredients and foods can be helpful (see p. 301).

- Due to a variety of factors, fast-food and quick-service restaurants may not have ready answers to questions about ingredients and food preparation methods. Fortunately, some restaurants have an ingredients listing for their menu items and/or indicate which ones may be gluten free. This can be helpful when making food selections; however, enquiring whether precautions have been taken to prevent cross-contamination is still essential. Because front-line staff may or may not be properly educated on how to safely prepare and/or handle gluten-free foods, speak to a manager to ensure the order is handled properly.

- Fine dining restaurants usually offer a less hurried atmosphere and will allow more time for accommodating special needs. Remember that it is the right of the paying customer to ask appropriate questions and advocate for a safe meal.

Timing of Meals

- Avoid peak meal times. Dining either "early" or "late" usually will mean a more leisurely meal with easier access to less-harried staff for asking questions and requesting special needs.

- Allow extra time for eating out (e.g., before a concert, etc.) in case it's needed for accommodating a gluten-free meal.

Explain Dietary Restrictions Briefly

- Many in the food industry are now aware of the gluten-free diet. However, restaurant managers, chefs and servers may not fully understand that while for some people a gluten-free diet is a personal choice or preference, for others it is a required necessity for medical reasons. The customer with celiac disease needs to feel confident that the staff realizes that deviation from gluten free can result in serious health consequences, and so will not merely "pay lip service" to enquiries and requests. Therefore, it is critical to clearly explain the importance of ensuring that the foods and beverages are made with safe ingredients and that steps are taken to avoid cross-contamination. Although celiac disease is not a "food allergy," because most servers are more aware of "allergies" as a health concern, it may be helpful to describe the situation as a severe food allergy that will result in extreme sickness if the order is not handled correctly.

- Remember to be pleasant and to smile when making requests. Ask the server and/or chef if s/he could help with selection of safe menu items.

Ask Detailed Questions

- Some servers have limited knowledge of where food comes from, of food storage and preparation methods, and of cooking in general; therefore, any very specific questions should be directed to the manager or, better still, the chef. The only person who really knows what goes into a dish is the person who makes it.

- Ask detailed questions about the ingredients used in the menu items and about preparation and cooking methods.

- Inquire about how the kitchen staff is alerted to a gluten-free order, and whether a manager or one key staff member follows the order from the table to the chef and back to the customer.

- If a restaurant that advertises gluten-free items also bakes with wheat flour, inquire as to what measures are taken to minimize or prevent gluten-free ingredients and meals from becoming cross-contaminated with gluten.

Menu Item Considerations

- **Salads and Salad Dressings**
  - Contamination can occur if the surfaces used to cut, chop and assemble salad ingredients have not first been thoroughly cleaned.

  - Salads may contain croûtons and other wheat-based ingredients (e.g., Asian noodles, won tons, pasta, taco chips and shells). If a salad arrives at the table with any of these prohibited ingredients, send it back. Explain that due to the cross-contamination, merely removing the unsafe ingredient(s) doesn't solve the problem and a fresh salad must be made.

  - Salad dressings may contain unsafe ingredients (e.g., wheat flour, wheat starch, hydrolyzed wheat protein, soy sauce made from wheat). If there are no specifically designated gluten-free dressings, ask for a lemon wedge and oil, or balsamic or wine vinegar and oil, or bring a small container of dressing from home.

- **Marinades**
  - Teriyaki or soy sauce (most often are made with wheat) or beer (barley or wheat-based) may have been used to marinate meat, poultry, fish or seafood.

- **Soups and Sauces**
  - Soups and sauces often are made with commercial soup bases or "flavor" cubes containing wheat flour, wheat starch or hydrolyzed wheat protein.

  - Roux (pronounced "roo") is a combination of butter and flour that commonly is used to thicken sauces. Many restaurants also use commercial canned, frozen or dry sauce mixes that contain gluten-unsafe ingredients. Ask if the chef can use cornstarch to thicken a "from-scratch" sauce; otherwise, it is safest to avoid sauces.

- **Meat, Poultry, Fish and Seafood**
  - These menu choices typically may be dusted, dredged or breaded with flour or bread crumbs before being grilled or fried.

  - Some burgers (meat, poultry, fish or vegetarian) may contain wheat flour, wheat starch, wheat gluten or bread crumbs.

  - Seasonings containing wheat flour or wheat starch may be used in the preparation of meat, poultry, fish or seafood.

  - Prime rib may be cooked or served with an *au jus* (pan juices or some equivalent) that contains unsafe ingredients.

- Steaks, ribs, chicken, and other foods may be cooked on the same flat or charcoal grills where gluten-containing breads and rolls have been toasted.

- Despite your instructions, steak may arrive at your table topped with fried battered or floured onion rings or a burger may come served on a wheat-based bun. If this occurs, ask for a new steak or burger. Remember to cut into the meat before sending it back so it is evident that the return item is "new."

- Imitation crab and other seafood ("surimi") may contain wheat starch.

- Imitation bacon bits may contain hydrolyzed wheat protein.

- Cooked bacon sometimes is placed on top of bread that will soak up the excess fat. This is common at buffet breakfasts.

• Eggs
- Eggs often are cooked on a grill where French toast and pancakes have been or are being prepared. Ask for your eggs to be cooked in a separate clean pan.

- Pancake batter may be added to an omelet to make it fluffier.

• Fried Foods
- Some brands of French fries contain wheat flour or wheat starch used as a coating or in the seasoning blend.

- The menu may indicate an item is gluten free; however, it may be cooked in the same fryer as are gluten-containing foods. For example, the oil used to deep-fry foods may be used for both breaded (e.g., chicken fingers, onion rings, fish) and non-breaded (French fries, corn tortillas, tortilla and taco chips) items, in which case these latter foods should be avoided. In some large restaurants and fast-food establishments, French fries and other gluten-free items may be cooked in separate fryers, reducing the risk of cross-contamination.

• Rice, Hash Browns and Fried Potatoes
- "Rice" pilafs actually may comprise a combination of rice and other grains (e.g., barley, wheat) and/or have added seasonings containing hydrolyzed wheat protein, wheat flour or wheat starch. Also, many restaurants use commercially packaged rice with gluten-containing seasonings. It is best to choose plain steamed rice cooked in water.

- Some frozen hash brown or fried potatoes may contain wheat starch, wheat flour or hydrolyzed wheat protein. Even if these potato dishes do not contain any prohibited ingredients, they frequently are cooked on grills or in fryers where gluten-containing items have been prepared.

• Pasta
- Some restaurants offer gluten-free pasta, but ask that fresh water in a clean pot be used for cooking, not the same pot and water used for preparing wheat-based pasta. Also, the colander used to drain gluten-free pasta should not be the same one used to drain wheat-based pasta.

• Pizza
- Gluten-free pizza crusts may be prepared on-site or may come pre-made from an outside vendor and manufactured in a dedicated gluten-free facility. Avoid crusts that are made in-house due to a high risk for cross-contamination. Request that a pre-made pizza crust be placed and baked on a clean pan or on foil. Also request that clean utensils (not those in use along the regular preparation line) be used for dipping into fresh sauce and scooping toppings for gluten-free pizzas.

- **Vegetables**
  - Avoid battered vegetables or those prepared in sauces, which usually are thickened with wheat flour. Some vegetables may be sautéed or stir-fried with seasonings or soy sauce that contain wheat.
  - Vegetables may be heated in a colander placed in a pot of boiling pasta water.

- **Bread and Rolls**
  - Gluten-free bread toasted in a regular toaster will be cross-contaminated with crumbs from gluten-containing breads. Ask that it be toasted on a foil-lined pan in the oven.
  - Request that hands are washed and gloves changed before using a clean knife to slice gluten-free bagels, breads and rolls.

- **Desserts**
  - Ask that sorbets, ice cream and crème brûlée not be served with a cookie or wafer on top. If this occurs, ask for a new dessert. Keep the first dessert at your table until the new order arrives so the server does not merely remove the cookie or wafer and bring back the same gluten-contaminated dessert.
  - Some versions of crème brûlée are made from a mix containing flour. Either version (gluten free or not) may be poured into a dish dusted with wheat flour to prevent sticking.
  - "Flourless" cake traditionally is gluten free; however, some recipes actually do contain wheat flour.

Food Preparation Equipment

- Ask what precautions are taken to prevent cross-contamination. Are hands washed and gloves changed before or in between preparing gluten-containing foods? Will gluten-free food be prepared in an area separate from the regular flow of the kitchen or in the same area but on clean surfaces? Are gluten-free foods cooked on the same grill or pan or in the same deep fat fryer used for cooking gluten-containing items?

- Request that your food be prepared on a clean grill or in a clean pan and with clean utensils. If this is a problem, suggest cooking it on clean aluminum foil. Cooking methods such as steaming, poaching or baking are often the safest choices.

Confirm Your Order before Eating

- When your food arrives, directly ask: "Is this the special gluten-free meal I ordered?" Do not hesitate to ask further questions and/or send the meal back if it is unacceptable. If you are not satisfied with the server's responses, ask to speak to the manager.

Thank the Food Server, Chef and Manager

- After you've enjoyed a tasty and safe gluten-free meal, thank the server and leave a generous tip for good service. Also speak to the manager and chef to let them know about your positive dining experience. Assure them that you plan to patronize the establishment again, and to tell others about it.

Information about "eating away from home" was adapted from:

Restaurant Dining: Seven Tips for Staying Gluten-Free
by the Gluten Intolerance Group, Seattle, WA   www.gluten.org

Starting the Conversation on Celiac-Friendly Dining
by TheCeliacScene™   www.theceliacscene.com

Social Events

Call Ahead

- Call the host or the catering staff before the event. If the host is not aware of your food restrictions, explain that you are on a gluten-free diet. When attending a banquet, contact the catering department and/or chef several days ahead of time to explain your dietary requirements.

- Briefly explain your dietary restrictions and the need for safe foods. Ask if it is possible for your portions of the planned menu items to be prepared without marinades, sauces and/or other gluten-unsafe ingredients (e.g., request plain steak, chicken, fish, salad, vegetables, fruit), or whether a safe substitute could be made available.

- Most people are willing to accommodate special requests if they are contacted well in advance. This eliminates their having to scramble at the last minute to make changes to the menu or food preparation methods or, worse yet, to feel awkward about not having something safe for you to eat. Friends or other individuals who know you well may be able to take your needs into account either by making changes for you individually or by preparing a gluten-safe meal that is suitable for all the guests.

- Some people find preparing a gluten-free meal an interesting challenge, while others may feel very uneasy or not confident about "getting it right." If your host expresses the latter concerns or if you feel s/he may not be able to prepare items that are safe, offer to bring a gluten-free dish and be sure to serve yourself first! Another suggestion is to offer to arrive early to assist with food preparation.

- When invited to an event where you either are unable to determine the menu ahead of time or anticipate not feeling comfortable consuming what is served, to be on the safe side you may want to eat something before you leave home and/or take something with you.

Always Say "Thank You"

- A thank-you note, telephone call or email to a host or catering department that has accommodated your special dietary needs is always greatly appreciated, and paves the way for future positive encounters.

Traveling

The savvy gluten-free traveler plans the food aspect of a trip well in advance of embarking on a journey. Mode of transportation, length of trip, destination location, accommodations and language barriers are just a few of the factors that should be taken under consideration ahead of time so that meals and snacks are a safe and enjoyable part of your trip.

- Research what options for meals and snacks are available at the destination location(s). Prior to traveling, contact your hotel, airline, cruise line, family and/or friends to ensure that they will be able to accommodate your diet needs and requests.

- Check the most recent restaurant or hotel reviews on websites specializing in travel.

- Create a list of restaurants that cater to gluten free in the destination area. Additionally, make a reservation ahead of time to ensure a table is available at peak meal times.

- If traveling internationally, check out the national celiac association websites (see pp. 289, 290) as well as dining cards in international languages (p. 301).

- Always carry food with you when traveling. There may be times when you encounter unexpected delays on your journey or may not be able to find suitable options, so take along non-perishable travel-friendly items such as gluten-free snack bars, crackers, muffins; tuna or other fish in cans or vacuum-sealed pouches; single-serve packages of nut or seed butters; dried fruits, nuts, seeds; individual servings of puddings and canned fruit; granola, instant gluten-free oatmeal; gluten-free meat or poultry jerky; and gluten-free dehydrated soups. If traveling by car, bring along a cooler or cooler bag (with an ice pack) filled with individually wrapped sliced cheeses, meats or poultry; yogurt, fruits; vegetables and dip.

- When staying in a hotel or resort, request a room with a mini-kitchen or small fridge. If these are not available, ask if a small fridge can be brought to your room for medical reasons.

- Check to see if there are any grocery, health food or convenience stores nearby to purchase items to bring back to your accommodation and/or for ongoing travel. Another option is to determine if there is any delivery service(s) to bring the items directly to the accommodations.

- Take reusable toaster bags (see p. 136) with you when traveling. Gluten-free bread can be put in these bags and dropped into toasters at a hotel breakfast buffet or at friends' homes.

Gluten-Free Cooking and Baking

13

Cooking and baking gluten free at home allows for great variety and flavor, as well as the opportunity to incorporate nutritious ingredients into the diet. Whether a novice or an experienced cook, preparing gluten-free recipes does not need to be complicated. Using a few simple ingredients or substituting a gluten-free alternative in a "familiar" recipe may be all that is needed. A veggie omelet, a fruit smoothie, a green salad with chickpeas, spaghetti sauce over gluten-free pasta, a chicken stir-fry with gluten-free soy sauce and rice, lentil soup using gluten-free broth: the possibilities truly are endless!

Most of the many gluten-free cookbooks available provide a wide array of recipes using basic staple gluten-free ingredients and gluten-free substitutions appropriate in "mainline" (non-gluten-free) recipes. For a list of some popular gluten-free cookbooks and other helpful culinary resources, see pages 297–300. And on pages 157–204, there is a wide selection of tasty recipes.

Although rice and corn are the most commonly used gluten-free alternatives, cooking and baking with other grains and legumes will improve the nutritional quality of the diet. This section provides practical information about cooking and storing grains and legumes; using gluten-free flours, gums and starches; substitutions for wheat flour; and specific baking tips.

Gluten-Free Grains

Cooking Gluten-Free Grains

For stovetop cooking, bring the liquid (either water or gluten-free broth) to a rapid boil in a heavy-bottomed pot. Add the grain, stir and return to a boil. Reduce heat to low. Cover with a tight-fitting lid and simmer for the suggested cooking time (see table 13.1 on p. 144) until the liquid is absorbed. Note, though, that some of the quantities and cooking times are approximate. In general, a grain is cooked once it is tender. However, cooking times may vary depending on the desired tenderness and intended use of the grain. For example, the grain cooked for a salad or side dish should be firm in comparison to the softer-textured grain in a cooked breakfast cereal. To further soften/tenderize a cooked grain, add extra liquid and increase cooking time. Or, if the grain is cooked to desired consistency before all the liquid is absorbed, simply strain off the excess. If cooked grains are sticking to the bottom of the pot at the end of cooking time, turn off the heat, add a small amount of broth or water, put the lid back on the pot and let sit for a few minutes. Experience will be your best guide! Some packaged grains will carry cooking instructions provided by the manufacturer.

Table 13.1   Stovetop cooking instructions for gluten-free grains

Grain (1 cup raw)	Liquid (cups)	Cooking Time (minutes)	Yield (cups)
Amaranth	2	20 – 25	2 – 2½
Buckwheat (groats)	2	15 – 20	2 – 2½
Buckwheat (kasha)	2	20 – 30	2 – 2½
Corn grits (polenta)	4	10 – 15	2½
Kañiwa	2	10 – 15	2
Millet (grits)	3	10 – 15	2
Millet (whole grain)	2	20 – 25	2½ – 3
Oats (groats)*	3	50 – 60	3
Oats (old-fashioned)*	2	5 – 8	3
Oats (quick-cooking)*	2	3 – 5	3
Oats (steel-cut)*	3	20 – 25	3
Quinoa	2	15 – 20	3
Rice, brown	2½	45 – 55	3
Rice, white**	2	20 – 30	3
Sorghum (pearled)***†	3	45 – 55	3½
Sorghum (whole grain)†	3½	80	3
Sorghum (whole grain – soaked)****†	2½ – 3	45 – 55	3
Teff	3	15 – 20	3
Wild rice	4	45 – 55	3½

*   Gluten-free oats.
**   Refined grain.
***   A portion of the outer bran layer has been removed.
**** Soaking in water overnight can reduce the cooking time. Drain, rinse and cook as directed. Can be prepared without soaking but takes longer to cook.
†   Significant differences among varieties of sorghum can mean a wide range of cooking times, water requirements and final textures (chewy to soft).

Storing Gluten-Free Grains

The shelf life of uncooked grains varies depending on the type of grain and storage method (pantry versus refrigerator or freezer) as well as length of time on store shelf prior to purchase. Buckwheat and millet should be used within two months of purchase, or four months if stored in freezer. Others can be stored longer (4–6 months in the pantry or 8–12 months in the freezer).

Cook grains in large batches to save both time and energy. Leftover cooked grains can be kept covered in the refrigerator for up to 3–4 days. Most cooked grains (except buckwheat and corn grits) also can be frozen for 2–3 months, provided they have not been cooked to a porridge-like consistency. Therefore, if you're planning to freeze cooked grains, prepare with a little bit less water and cook the grain to the point where it can be fluffed with a fork. Then, to prevent clumping or mushiness, spread fluffed grain on a cookie sheet lined with plastic wrap and cool completely before freezing. Place desired-sized portions into small containers or freezer bags. Be sure to label with the name of the grain and the date it was prepared.

Frozen grains can be thawed in the microwave by transferring the grain into a microwave-safe container and defrosting on medium (50%) in one-minute intervals until thawed (3–8 minutes, depending on the grain). Alternately, frozen grains can thaw overnight on the refrigerator shelf.

Once thawed, the cooked grain can be reheated in a heavy-bottomed saucepan or non-stick skillet on medium-low heat with 1–2 tablespoons of water or broth for 3–5 minutes. Another method is to place the grain in a microwave-safe dish with the liquid, and heat on high for 30–60 seconds. Reheated grains can be added to a soup, chili or stew near the end of the cooking time.

Some of the above information is adapted with permission from the Whole Grains Council (**www.wholegrainscouncil.org**), as well as referenced from Bob's Red Mill *Everyday Gluten-Free Cookbook: 281 Delicious Whole-Grain Recipes* by Camilla V. Saulsbury.

Pulses and Soybeans

Preparing Dried Pulses and Soybeans

Beans, chickpeas, whole peas and soybeans must be soaked prior to cooking, whereas lentils and split peas can be cooked without soaking. Before rinsing and soaking, all dry pulses and soybeans should be checked and any twigs, pebbles, broken or shriveled skins and "foreign" grains (potentially gluten-containing) removed. Rinse the sorted pulses or soybeans in a strainer under cold running water.

For every 1 cup of pulses or soybeans, soak using 3–4 cups of cold water. Prior to cooking, whole peas should be soaked for 1–2 hours. Chickpeas, beans and soybeans need to be soaked for a minimum of 4 hours, and preferably 8 hours or overnight. There also are two quick-soak methods. For the first, combine pulses or soybeans and cold water in a large heavy-bottomed saucepan and bring to boil on the stovetop. Boil gently for 1–3 minutes then remove from heat; cover and let stand at room temperature for 1 hour before proceeding with recipe. Pulses and soybeans also can be soaked in the microwave. Combine water and pulses or soybeans in a large microwaveable dish, cover and microwave on high for 10–15 minutes. Remove from microwave and let stand for one hour before proceeding with recipe.

When soaking is complete, strain the pulses or soybeans, discard the soaking water and rinse well with cool water. This process reduces the amount of gas-producing compounds in the pulses and soybeans.

Cooking Dried Pulses and Soybeans

Pulses and soybeans will double or triple in volume during cooking, so choose a heavy-bottomed saucepan accordingly. Combine soaked drained pulses or soybeans and water or gluten-free broth. Add 1 teaspoon of oil to the cooking water to prevent foaming. Bring to a boil, reduce heat, cover, then simmer until desired tenderness. If the liquid is almost gone before that point, simply add more water or broth and cook longer as necessary. Table 13.2 on page 146 specifies cooking instructions for various pulses and soybeans.

When soybeans are boiling, the outer hulls will separate and float to the top. Skim these off using a large slotted spoon, and discard. Repeat as necessary.

Onions, spices and/or herbs can be added during cooking for extra flavor. Do not add vinegar, tomatoes or other acidic ingredients until pulses or soybeans are tender because these will slow the cooking process and harden the skins.

Table 13.2 Cooking pulses and soybeans

Pulse (1 cup raw)	Liquid (cups)	Cooking Time	Yield (cups)
Beans	2½ – 3	1 – 1½ hrs.	2½
Chickpeas (whole)	2½ – 3	1½ – 2 hrs.	2½
Chickpeas (split)	2	30 – 60 min.	2
Lentils (whole)	2½ – 3	10 – 30 min.	2½
Lentils (split)	2	5 – 15 min.	2
Peas (whole)	2½ – 3	1½ – 2 hrs.	2½
Peas (split)	2	45 min.	2
Soybeans (whole dried yellow)	3	2 – 3 hrs.	2½ – 3

Cooking Edamame (fresh green soybeans)

To cook fresh edamame in pods, drop into a pot of boiling water and boil for approximately five minutes. Pour off the cooking water, rinse under cold water and drain thoroughly. Remove beans from pods by squeezing gently.

Frozen edamame (in pods or shelled) can be steamed, boiled or microwaved. Follow cooking directions on the package.

Preparing Canned Pulses and Soybeans

Canned pulses and soybeans are already cooked; however, they need to be drained and rinsed well before using. Empty the can's contents into a strainer, rinse with cool water for 30–60 seconds then drain. This reduces the sodium content by up to 40%, and also decreases the amount of gas-causing compounds.

Puréeing Pulses and Soybeans

Cooked pulses and soybeans can be puréed and used in a variety of recipes such as in dips, soups and baked goods. Refrigerate or freeze unused purée.

Step 1:
Canned: Follow the above instructions for preparing canned pulses and soybeans.

Uncooked, dried: Cook according to table 13.2 until soft; drain and discard cooking water.

Step 2:
Using a food processor or an immersion (hand) blender, purée 1 cup prepared pulses or soybeans with ¼ cup hot water for about three minutes or until mixture is smooth (like canned pumpkin). If necessary, add more hot water one tablespoon at a time.

Storing Pulses and Soybeans

Dry uncooked pulses and soybeans can be stored in a sealed container in a cool, dry place for up to a year. Store cooked versions in the refrigerator (up to five days) or freezer (up to six months). To freeze cooked pulses and soybeans, pack desired-size portions in small containers or freezer bags and label with name and date.

Some of the above information regarding working with legumes is adapted from *Pulses and the Gluten-Free Diet: Cooking with Beans, Peas, Lentils and Chickpeas* by Pulse Canada. **www.pulsecanada.com**

Gluten-Free Baking

Gluten is the protein component in wheat flour that provides the structure for baked goods. When baking gluten free, in order to compensate for the lack of gluten it is essential to learn how to use different types and combinations of flours, starches and other ingredients, as well as specific baking techniques. This can require time, patience, perseverance and even a sense of humor! But do not be intimidated or get discouraged! There are many excellent gluten-free cookbooks, magazines and magazine articles, newsletters, websites and cooking classes that provide detailed information about gluten-free baking (see pp. 294–300).

Gluten-free pancakes, muffins and cookies are a good place to start because they are relatively easy to prepare. Once those recipes are mastered, move on to more challenging baked goods (e.g., breads, rolls, cakes). Before baking, read about the unique taste and texture properties of each flour and starch highlighted below. An important point is that a combination of gluten-free flours and starches results in a better product than one made with a single gluten-free flour. Flours with stronger or more distinct flavors such as amaranth, buckwheat, bean, mesquite, millet, quinoa and teff are used in smaller quantities relative to those of more neutral-flavored flours (e.g., almond, corn, oat, potato, rice, sorghum).

Examples of gluten-free flour blends that can be made at home and used in many different recipes are included on page 152. A list of substitutions and general baking hints are found on pages 153–156. Also, a variety of prepackaged gluten-free all-purpose baking mixes (see pp. 231–237) are available from various gluten-free companies.

Gluten-Free Flours, Starches and Gums

All gluten-free flours, starches and gums should be stored in airtight wide-topped plastic or glass containers and labeled with name and date. Some can be kept in a cool dry place; however, if you live in a hot and/or humid climate, refrigerator or freezer storage is best. Also, regardless of the environment, for optimum freshness the following are best stored in the refrigerator or freezer: amaranth flour, brown rice flour, corn bran, ground flax, millet flour, nut flours (almond, cashew, chestnut, hazelnut, pecan, walnut), potato flour, rice bran, rice polish and soy flour.

Almond flour, made from blanched (skin removed) ground almonds, is available in packages or alternatively can be made at home by grinding blanched slivered almonds in a food processor or clean coffee or spice grinder. High in fiber, protein and fat, almond flour adds a rich texture and nutty flavor to baked products. It also can be used as a coating for chicken or fish.

Almond meal, made from whole ground almonds with the skins intact, has a coarser texture and contains more fiber than does almond flour.

Amaranth flour, ground from the entire tiny grain-like amaranth seed, is high in fiber, protein, calcium, iron and other nutrients. It has a somewhat strong, nutty, slightly sweet toasted flavor and is best combined with other gluten-free flours, comprising no more than 15%–20% of the total flour blend. Baked goods made with amaranth flour tend to brown quickly. This flour is very good in dark-colored baked goods such as chocolate cake, brownies and items containing spices (e.g., pumpkin bread or muffins, spice cake). It can yield lighter-colored, mild-flavored baked goods when combined with almond flour, and also can be used for thickening gravies, soups and stews.

Arrowroot starch, also known as arrowroot flour or arrowroot starch flour, is ground from the root of the tropical Maranta arundinacea plant. This neutral-flavored, white-colored finely powdered starch can be blended with different flours to improve the texture of baked products. An excellent thickener for fruit and other sauces, arrowroot also can be used for breading as it produces a golden brown crust. Arrowroot starch can be substituted for cornstarch.

Bean flours can be made from various ground dried beans such as black, cranberry/Romano, fava, garbanzo (chickpea), navy, pinto and white. In order to reduce as much of the flatulent effect of the beans as possible, some companies specially process the beans before milling. Bean flours are high in fiber, protein, calcium, iron and B vitamins, especially folate. By combining bean flours with other gluten-free flours to partially or totally replace white rice flour, the nutritional quality and texture of baked products can be greatly improved. Because bean flours have a strong distinct flavor, they work well in recipes such as gingerbread and chocolate cakes where the strong taste can be offset by molasses, chocolate, brown sugar and/or spices. Introduce bean flours gradually into the diet and choose those that have been "treated" for better tolerance.

Buckwheat flour (neither a wheat nor related to wheat) is made from ground unroasted buckwheat groats and is available in light, medium and dark grades. The medium and dark flours are gray in color and have a robust flavor due to added finely milled black buckwheat hulls. The light flour, which usually does not contain added buckwheat hulls, has a milder, mellow flavor and is preferred for bread, cookie and muffin recipes. Because not everyone enjoys buckwheat's strong and distinctive flavor, its flour is best combined with other gluten-free flours. As well, chocolate, coffee, molasses or spices can offset the unique taste. Make sure you are purchasing 100% pure buckwheat flour, as some brands actually are a combination of buckwheat flour and wheat flour.

Chestnut flour, made from ground chestnuts, is higher in starch and lower in protein and fat compared to other nut flours. This light beige silky-textured flour adds a nutty flavor to baked products. It is best combined with other flours in baked products such as breads, cakes, cookies, muffins and pancakes.

Chickpea flour, ground from chickpeas / garbanzo beans, is also known as garbanzo, besan, gram or channa flour. This popular tan-colored bean flour is best combined with other flours, especially for use in breads and wraps. For more information see **Bean flours** above.

Coconut flour is made from ground dried defatted coconut meat and is high in protein and fiber. Because this flour absorbs a significant amount of liquid in a recipe, it is recommended to limit it to 10%–15% of the total flour blend in baked products. Recipes using coconut flour usually require a lot more liquid and/or eggs than equivalent recipes using other gluten-free flours. Coconut flour also can be used for breading fish, seafood and chicken.

Corn bran, made from the outer layer of the whole-grain corn kernel, is extremely high in fiber. Light in color and with a mild flavor, it can be added in small amounts to baked products such as muffins, breads and loaves.

Corn flour, milled from finely ground dried corn kernels, is very light in texture and imparts a mild nutty flavor to baked goods. It is best used in combination with other flours in recipes for breads, cakes, muffins, pancakes and tortillas.

Cornmeal is made from dried kernels of yellow, white, blue or red corn. It is not as finely ground as is corn flour, and can be used as a breading or in cornbread, corn muffins and polenta. Cornmeal can be finely ground in a coffee grinder to replace corn flour in recipes.

Cornstarch is produced from the starchy endosperm of the corn kernel and is highly refined, resulting in little nutritive value. This white flavorless powder is blended with various flours and/or other starches to lighten the texture of gluten-free baked goods. It also is an excellent thickener, especially for fruit sauces, puddings and pie fillings.

Flaxseed meal, also known as milled flaxseed or ground flaxseed, is high in fiber, omega-3 fatty acids, protein, B vitamins, calcium and other minerals. This dark brown meal adds a nutty flavor and a crunchy texture, and improves the nutritional profile of baked products. Due to its high fat content, baked products made with flax brown quickly so temperature and baking time may need to be reduced. Flaxseeds can be purchased already ground in vacuum-sealed packages or, alternatively, can be ground in a small food processor or clean coffee or spice grinder to the consistency of finely ground coffee.

Garbanzo and **fava bean flour blends** available from other companies may or may not be specially processed similar to Garfava™ flour. For more information see **Bean flours**.

Garfava™ flour, developed by Authentic Foods, is the trademark name for a blend of garbanzo bean and fava bean flours that is specially processed to create baked goods with an excellent volume and good moisture content. For more information see **Bean flours**.

Guar gum, extracted from guar beans, is a fine white powder that improves the texture and prevents crumbling of gluten-free baked goods. It is used in small amounts and, because in its pure form it will not mix with liquids, needs first to be combined with dry ingredients. This high-fiber legume has a laxative effect when used in larger quantities.

Hazelnut flour is made from ground hazelnuts, also known as filberts, and adds a rich texture and nutty flavor to gluten-free baked goods. It is high in protein, fiber and other nutrients.

Kañiwa flour, made from ground kañiwa seeds, is a light brown nutrient-rich flour high in protein, fiber, minerals and vitamins. Kañiwa is closely related to quinoa and often is referred to as "baby quinoa."

Lentil flour, ground from whole or dehulled green or red lentils, is very high in fiber, protein, B vitamins and minerals. It can be used in breads, pizza crust and tortillas or as a coating for chicken, meat or fish.

Masa harina flour is made from finely ground hominy (dried whole corn kernels that have been soaked in an alkaline liquid and then cooked). This flour traditionally is used to make corn tortillas.

Mesquite flour, made by grinding the bean pods of the mesquite tree, is available as either a light tan coarse meal or a fine flour. This very high-fiber flour has a cinnamon-mocha aroma and slightly sweet chocolate, molasses-like flavor with a hint of caramel. It is best combined with other flours to make pancakes, muffins, breads, cakes and cookies.

Millet flour, finely ground from the tiny millet seed, is light yellow and has a mild and slightly sweet, corn-like, nutty flavor. Used in a wide variety of baked goods, it yields a light dry crumb and a thin smooth crust. It should be combined with other gluten-free flours, comprising no more than 20%–25% of the total flour blend.

Nut flours, made by grinding almonds, cashews, chestnuts, hazelnuts, pecans or walnuts, can be coarsely or finely ground and may also be called "meal." Most nut flours are high in protein, fiber and fat. They add a moist, rich texture and nutty flavor to cakes, cookies, pastry crusts, muffins and other baked products. Nut flours are available packaged or can be made by grinding nuts to desired texture in a food processor. However, over-grinding will result in nut butter rather than flour.

Oat flour (gluten free) is finely milled from whole-grain oat groats. It also can be made at home by grinding rolled oats in a blender or food processor to the consistency of flour. This slightly sweet, mild-flavored flour is high in protein, iron, fiber and other nutrients. Oat flour can be used in large quantities in breads, cakes, cookies, crusts, muffins, pancakes and tortillas. For more information about the safety of oats in the gluten-free diet, see pages 9, 10, 27–30, 100 and 101.

Pea flour is made from whole or dehulled yellow or green peas and is very high in fiber, protein, B vitamins and other nutrients. Green pea flour retains its light green color so is best used in soups and dark-colored baked products. The light yellow pea flour can be added to breads, cakes, muffins, soups and tortillas and in recipes can be used interchangeably with chickpea / garbanzo bean flour. For the maximum amount of fiber, choose whole pea flour rather than split pea flour.

Peanut flour is produced from peanuts that have been roasted and processed to remove varying quantities of naturally occurring fat. Available in light, medium and dark roasts, it is very high in protein and fiber, and a good source of many vitamins and minerals. This flour can be used in a wide variety of foods ranging from baked goods, sauces and smoothies to coatings for chicken and seafood. Peanut butter can be made by combining peanut flour and water.

Potato flour, made from ground dried whole potatoes, is a relatively heavy beige flour with a slight potato flavor. Due to its heavy texture, it should be used in small amounts and combined with other flours. It adds crispness and density to baked products. Potato flour is not the same as potato starch and they cannot be substituted for one another in recipes.

Potato starch is made from only the starch portion of the potato. This bland-flavored fine white powder is used as a thickener and for coatings, as well as for improving the texture of gluten-free baked products. Because potato starch clumps easily, sift or whisk before measuring.

Quinoa flour, finely milled from quinoa seeds, is high in protein, iron and other nutrients. It has a slight nutty but strong flavor that can be overpowering in baked goods; therefore, it is best limited to 25% of the total flour mixture. This tan-colored flour works well in highly spiced or flavored sweet and savory baked goods.

Rice bran is the outer layer of the whole-grain brown rice kernel and often is combined with the germ. It is high in fiber and can be added in small amounts to baked goods to add a nutty flavor.

Rice flour (brown) is finely ground whole-grain brown rice that imparts a nutty flavor to baked goods and is best in combination with other flours and starches. This slightly tan-colored flour is higher in fiber and other nutrients than is white rice flour.

Rice flour (sweet), also known as sticky, sushi or glutinous rice flour, is different from regular white rice flour, although they look alike. Despite its name, glutinous sweet rice and its flour do not contain gluten. The flour is ground from sticky short-grain white rice that is higher in starch content than either brown or white rice. Sweet rice flour makes an excellent thickener for sauces, gravies and puddings as it keeps liquids from separating when they are chilled or frozen. In baked products, especially pie crusts, the flour can comprise up to 25% of the total flour.

Rice flour (white), made from ground white rice, contains no bran and is low in fiber and nutrients. Due to its gritty texture and nutrient profile, use in small amounts in combination with other gluten-free flours in baked products.

Rice polish contains a portion of bran and germ from the brown rice kernel. Lighter in color than pure rice bran, it is a good source of fiber and in recipes can be substituted for rice bran.

Sorghum flour (pearled) is ground from the whole-grain sorghum kernel with some of the whole bran layer removed, so thus is lower in fiber than is whole-grain sorghum flour.

Sorghum flour (whole grain) is milled from food-grade white or black sorghum varieties. These mild-flavored flours that taste similar to wheat can be used in proportions of up to 50% of a total flour blend. While the white flour is very versatile and works well in a wide range of baked goods, the black variety is reddish-brown in color so is best used in, e.g., brownies or chocolate cake.

Soy flour is made from ground dried soybeans and is available in full-fat (contains all of the fat in the soybeans), low-fat (contains about one-third the amount of fat as full-fat) and defatted (most of the fat removed) varieties. This yellow, slightly nutty and "beany-tasting" flour is best combined with other flours, especially sorghum and rice, in baked products containing fruits, nuts, spices and/or chocolate. Soy flour is very high in protein, fiber, B vitamins, iron and calcium.

Sweet potato flour is made from dried and milled orange sweet potatoes. It has a mild sweet flavor and is high in fiber, vitamin A and potassium. Due to its color, the yellowy-orange flour is best used in darker baked goods (e.g., chocolate cake; pumpkin muffins or loaf).

Tapioca starch, also known as tapioca flour or tapioca starch flour, is made from the root of the tropical cassava/manioc plant and is very low in nutrients. This pure-white fine powder can be used to make up to 25%–30% of the total flour blend in baked goods. Tapioca starch adds a light texture and chewiness to baked goods and as well thickens soups, sauces, gravies and stir-fries. It also works well for breading because it browns quickly and produces a crispy coating.

Teff flour is made by finely grinding whole-grain ivory or brown teff seeds. This nutty, molasses-tasting flour can comprise 25%–30% of the total flour blend. It works well in dark and strongly flavored baked goods (e.g., chocolate cake, brownies, pumpernickel bread, gingerbread, spice cake) and also can be added to pancakes. Teff flour is high in protein, fiber and minerals such as iron and calcium. Because of their tiny size, teff grains cannot be ground in a coffee grinder or food processor to make flour. When purchasing teff flour, make sure it is 100% teff and not in combination with wheat or barley flour. Injera, an Ethiopian flatbread, usually is made from pure teff flour; however, it sometimes is made from combined teff and wheat or barley flours, so in that case would not be gluten free.

Xanthan gum is produced by fermenting glucose (a naturally occurring simple sugar) with a plant-derived bacteria called *Xanthomonas campestris*. The resulting fine white dry powder is added to gluten-free baked goods to help with rising and prevent crumbling. It is used in small amounts and must first be combined with dry ingredients, as it does not mix with water.

For more information and recipes using some of these flours and starches, see chapter 9 (pp. 97–114) and chapter 14 (pp. 157–204). A listing of companies that sell these ingredients can be found on pages 237–241.

Gluten-Free Flour Blends

Many gluten-free recipes call for combinations of various flours and starches. Rather than measuring then combining different flours each time a recipe is prepared, to save time you can purchase premixed flour blends (see pp. 231–237) or make them at home. Following are a few examples of different gluten-free flour blend recipes. Store these mixes in plastic self-seal bags or wide-mouthed containers, in a dark, dry, cool place or in the refrigerator. Before using in a recipe, take out the amount of flour blend needed, warm to room temperature (if refrigerated) and then whisk.

Carol Fenster's Gluten-Free Sorghum Flour Blend

Makes 4 cups

1½ cups	sorghum flour
1½ cups	potato starch OR cornstarch
1 cup	tapioca flour

• Measure ingredients and whisk together.

Reprinted with permission from *Carol Fenster Cooks* at *Carolfenstercooks.com*

Beth Hillson's Gluten-Free Flour Blend

Makes 4 cups

2 cups	gluten-free oat flour
1 cup	almond flour
1 cup	arrowroot starch

• Measure ingredients and whisk together.

Reprinted with permission from Beth Hillson, Food Editor, *Living Without's Gluten Free & More*

Beth Hillson's High-Protein Flour Blend

Makes 5 cups

1 cup	sorghum OR chickpea flour
1 cup	millet, sorghum OR amaranth flour
1 cup	brown OR white rice flour
1 cup	potato starch (not potato flour) OR cornstarch
1 cup	tapioca starch

• Measure ingredients and whisk together.

Reprinted with permission from *The Complete Guide to Living Well Gluten Free* by Beth Hillson

General Baking Hints

Baking Tips

- Flours and starches that have been stored in the refrigerator or freezer should be removed and let stand until they reach room temperature before measuring.

- Because the heavier flours sink to the bottom of the mix, whisk flour blends before using.

- Measure flours and starches carefully. Inaccurate or approximate measurements can greatly affect the quality of gluten-free baked goods because each flour and starch has very unique properties. It is important to use flat-rim measuring cups designed for dry ingredients, not spouted measuring cups designed for measuring liquids.

- Loosely spoon the flour or starch into the measuring cup, leveling the top with the flat side of a knife. Never pack down the flour.

- Gluten-free bread dough tends to be heavier, softer, stickier and more batter-like than traditional wheat-based dough. If the dough is overly heavy and dry, the bread may be very crumbly.

- Forming the dough into shapes (e.g., breadsticks, buns, loaves) works best using very wet hands or an oiled spatula or spoon.

- Baking is affected by temperature and altitude. Slightly reduce the amount of liquid in the recipe if baking at a high altitude or on a very humid day. For baking at very low altitudes, slightly increase the amount of liquid.

- Gluten-free products baked in shiny light-colored metal pans (gray, not black) bake and brown more evenly than they do in dark pans, which can leave edges crisp and over-browned.

- When making a gluten-free chocolate cake or brownies, grease the pan then "flour" it with cocoa.

- If using glass baking pans or non-stick metal baking pans (gray, not black), reduce oven temperature by 25°F.

- Most gluten-free breads and pie crusts are better when baked at lower temperatures for longer periods of time because the dough is denser. After the first 10–15 minutes of baking, loosely tent the bread with foil to prevent over-browning.

- Insert a baking thermometer to the center of the bread loaf to test for doneness. The temperature should reach approximately 200°F or higher.

Texture Tips

- Because it is the gluten in wheat flour that produces an elastic and high-rising dough, gluten-free baked goods often require more leavening agents (e.g., baking powder, baking soda, eggs) than do products made with wheat flour in order to achieve a similar end product.

- To prevent crumbling, most gluten-free baked products require the addition of a very small amount of xanthan or guar gum. Add the xanthan or guar gum to the dry ingredients, as these gums will not mix with water. For every cup of gluten-free flour, use 1 teaspoon of gum for breads and 1/2–3/4 teaspoon for other baked goods.

- Substituting buttermilk for milk or water in recipes results in a lighter, more finely textured product. Carbonated beverages (not diet soft drinks) in place of water or milk also can yield a lighter-textured product (e.g., pancakes, cakes).

- Allowing gluten-free cake and muffin dough to rest for 10–15 minutes at room temperature prior to baking results in a better-textured product. Also, let pancake batter rest for 10–15 minutes before frying.

Flavor Tips

- To enhance the flavor of gluten-free baked products, use more herbs, spices and flavorings (approximately one to two times more than usual).

- Adding chocolate chips, dried fruits (e.g., apricots, cranberries, raisins); fruits and vegetables (e.g., applesauce, bananas, pumpkin, grated carrots or zucchini) and nuts to gluten-free baked goods will improve the flavor.

- Brown sugar, honey or molasses provide more flavor than does white sugar. The amount of liquid in the recipe needs to be reduced if substituting honey or molasses for sugar. For every 1 cup of sugar, use 3/4 cup honey or molasses and reduce liquid by 1/4 cup.

- Most gluten-free breads taste better when warm or toasted.

Storage Tips

- Because baked products made with gluten-free flours have no preservatives, they become stale quickly and are quite perishable (mold easily). Wrap cooled baked items tightly in plastic wrap and store in airtight plastic containers or self-seal plastic bags. If the product will not be eaten within one or two days, freeze to ensure minimal loss of moisture and flavor. For breads, it is best to thoroughly cool the loaf, slice it, then separate slices with wax paper before reassembling, bagging and freezing.

- Packaging baked products such as muffins in plastic bags when still slightly warm can preserve moisture.

- Thaw frozen baked goods at room temperature instead of microwaving at full power; microwaving causes them to become rubbery and tough.

Thickening Agents in Gluten-Free Cooking

Gluten-free flours, starches and other ingredients can be used as thickening agents in foods such as soups, stews, gravies, puddings and sauces. Due to their unique properties, some work better than others for thickening. Liquids thickened with cooked starches tend to be clear and shiny, whereas those thickened with cooked flours are more cloudy and opaque in appearance.

Table 13.3   Substitutions for 1 Tablespoon of wheat flour for thickening

Starches	Amount (Approximate)	Cooking Instructions and Traits	Suggested Use
Arrowroot Starch	1½ tsp.	Mix to a thin smooth paste with a small amount of cold liquid then add during last five minutes of cooking. Heat at a low temperature while stirring occasionally. Do not boil or overcook. Will give thickened liquid a smooth, clear, shiny appearance; semi-soft when cooled.	Fruit and savory sauces, glazes, pie fillings, stir-fries Do not use with dairy-based sauces (creates a slimy texture)
Cornstarch	1½ tsp.	Mix with a cold liquid to create a smooth slurry before adding to other liquid. Bring to a gentle boil for a few minutes while stirring constantly. Thickened liquid becomes translucent and shiny when cooked; thickens further when cooled.	Fruit and savory sauces, fruit pies and cobblers, puddings, stir-fries
Potato Starch	1½ tsp.	Mix with a small amount of cold liquid then stir constantly (lumps easily) while adding to other liquid. Do not boil or overcook. Yields a translucent thickened liquid.	Gravies, sauces, soups, stews
Tapioca Starch	1 Tbsp.	Mix with a small amount of cold liquid and add to other liquid during last five minutes of cooking, stirring constantly. Imparts a transparent and glossy appearance; produces a thick soft gel when cooled.	Pie fillings, puddings, stir-fries

Flours	Amount (Approximate)	Cooking Instructions and Traits	Suggested Use
Chickpea / Garbanzo Bean Flour	1½ Tbsp.	Make a roux for thickening sauces and gravies by combining flour with butter or oil; add roux to soup or stew at end of cooking time. Will thicken completely after 2–3 minutes of boiling. Is yellow-tan in color and produces a cloudy appearance, smooth texture and slight bean-like taste.	Gravies, savory sauces, soups, stews
Rice Flour (Brown)	1 Tbsp.	Mix with a small amount of cold liquid before using. Will thicken liquid after 5 or more minutes of boiling. Imparts a cloudy appearance and grainy texture.	Gravies, soups, stews
Rice Flour (Sweet)	1 Tbsp.	Make a roux for thickening sauces and gravies by combining flour with butter or oil; add roux to soup or stew at end of cooking time. Will thicken after 5 or more minutes of boiling. Yields an opaque and shiny appearance.	Gravies, sweet and savory sauces, puddings, soups, stews
Sorghum Flour	1 Tbsp.	Make a roux for thickening sauces and gravies by combining flour with butter or oil; add roux to soup or stew at end of cooking time. Will thicken after 2–3 minutes of boiling.	Gravies, sauces, soups, stews

Others	Amount (Approximate)	Cooking Instructions and Traits	Suggested Use
Gelatin (unflavored)	1½ tsp.	Soften in small amount of cold water then heat until liquid is clear before using. Thickness/firmness of final dish will range from semi-soft to extra firm depending on amount of gelatin used.	Cheesecakes, puddings, jellied salads
Quick-Cooking Tapioca	1½ tsp.	For fruit pies or cobblers/crisps, add dry tapioca granules to fruit and let stand for 10–20 minutes before baking.	Fruit cobblers/crisps, pies, tapioca pudding

Thank you to the following gluten-free culinary experts for some of the background information on gluten-free flours, starches and substitutions, as well as many of the baking tips:

Carol Fenster, PhD., President and Founder of Savory Palate, LLC. (a gluten-free publishing and consulting firm) and cookbook author (see pp. 297, 298).
www.carolfenstercooks.com

Heather Butt, P.H.Ec. and **Donna Washburn, P.H.Ec.**, partners in Quality Professional Services (specializing in recipe development and bread machine baking) and cookbook authors (see p. 298).
www.bestbreadrecipes.com

Beth Hilson, Food Editor, *Living Without's Gluten Free & More* and author (see p. 299).

Recipes

Brown Rice Bread 158

Wholesome Flax Bread 160

Cornbread.. 161

Teff Polenta 162

Oatmeal Bread 163

Injera (Ethiopian Flatbread) 164

Flax & Peanut Focaccia................................... 165

Apple Date Bread 166

Banana Seed Bread.. 167

Pumpkin Bread 168

Shelley's Orange Cranberry Muffins............... 169

Blueberry Almond Muffins............................. 170

Mighty Tasty Muffins 171

Carrot Cake Pancakes..................................... 172

Teff Banana Pancakes 173

Spiced Apple Cranberry Buckwheat Cereal..... 174

Sweet Sorghum Banana Date
    Breakfast Cookies...................................... 175

Carrot Apple Energy Bars 176

Fruit n' Nut Bars 177

Coconut & Banana Lentil Bites....................... 178

Sorghum Peanut Butter Cookies.................... 179

Cranberry Pistachio Biscotti 180

Chocolate Banana Rum Cake 181

Cajun Lentil Trail Mix with Dark Chocolate 182

Lentil Vegetable Soup..................................... 183

French Canadian Pea Soup 184

Moroccan Salad.. 185

Brown Rice Chickpea Kale Salad..................... 186

Quinoa Salad.. 187

Wild Rice Salad... 188

Fresh Rolls with Peanut Dipping Sauce 189

Wondergrain Sorghum Stuffing 190

Multi-Grain Pilaf 191

Moroccan Millet 192

Spicy Sweet Potato Bean Burgers 193

Hoisin Lentil Lettuce Wraps 194

Wild Rice, Chicken & Vegetable Casserole 195

Vegetable & Beef Lasagna 196

Black Bean Chili.. 197

Sahara Stew over Superblend Grains.............. 198

Turkey Meatballs with Lemon Sauce............... 199

Tabbouleh with Shrimp on Mixed Greens 200

Oven-Fried Chicken 201

Lentil Pizza Squares 202

Pepperoni Pizza 203

Thai Hot-and-Sour Sauce................................ 204

Brown Rice Bread

with variations for using teff, amaranth, quinoa and buckwheat

Yield: 1 loaf / 12 slices

So far, this is the best gluten-free bread we have tried. Adapted from a recipe adapted by Barbara Emch, a fellow celiac.

Notes:

Humidity: If humidity is high, reduce the amount of water in the recipe to avoid over-rising. Many gluten-free bakers experience the frustrating situation whereby a beautiful loaf of bread deflates once removed from the oven. You will need to experiment a little to get just the right amount of water in your bread, depending on the humidity in the air. If in doubt, use less water than the recipe calls for.

Rapid-Rise Yeast: You may use either rapid-rise yeast or regular yeast. If using rapid-rise yeast, eliminate the cold oven / pan of hot water rise method and instead follow yeast package directions for rise time.

3	large eggs (for egg-free, see substitution below*)
1/4 cup	vegetable oil
1 tsp.	lemon juice
2 cups	tapioca starch flour
2 cups	fine brown rice flour
2/3 cup	instant non-fat dry milk powder (for dairy-free, see substitution below**)
2 tsp.	xanthan gum
1 tsp.	salt
1 1/2 Tbsp.	active dry yeast
4 Tbsp.	sugar
1 1/4 cups	warm water (105°–115°F)

✦ Bring all refrigerated ingredients to room temperature. Grease a 5 x 9-inch loaf pan.

✦ In the bowl of a stand mixer, combine eggs, oil and lemon juice.

✦ In a medium bowl, combine tapioca starch flour, brown rice flour, dry milk powder, xanthan gum, salt, yeast and sugar. Add about 1 cup of the water to the egg mixture, then slowly add dry ingredients a little at a time until completely incorporated. If mixture is too dry, add remaining water (see Humidity note). Mix batter on high speed for 3 1/2 minutes, then pour into prepared pan.

✦ Cover loaf pan with foil and place in a cold oven. Set a pan of hot water on a shelf underneath the bread. Leave for 10 minutes with oven door closed. (This will cause the bread to rise quickly.) Remove bread from oven (do not uncover) and place in a warm place in the kitchen. Preheat oven to 400°F. Bread will continue to rise as oven preheats.

✦ Uncover bread and bake for 10 minutes to brown the top. Cover again with foil and continue to bake for 30 minutes. Turn bread out onto a cooling rack. When completely cooled, wrap tightly to maintain freshness for as long as possible.

* Egg-Free Substitution, Flaxseed:
Flaxseed has many healthy components such as high-quality protein, fiber, B and C vitamins, iron and zinc, anti-cancer properties and omega-3 fatty acids. To use as an egg substitute: Grind 3 tablespoons flaxseed and add 1/2 cup + 1 tablespoon boiling water, let sit for 15 minutes, then whisk with a fork – this mixture will replace 3 eggs in a recipe. A clean coffee grinder works well to grind the small flaxseed.

** Dairy-Free Substitution, Ground Almonds:
Use 2/3 cup ground almonds to replace 2/3 cup dry milk powder.

Brown Rice Bread
(continued)

Variations:

Teff Bread, Quinoa Bread, Amaranth Bread or Buckwheat Bread

Substitute the following combination of flours for the 2 cups brown rice flour and 2 cups tapioca flour in the original recipe:

1½ cups	tapioca starch flour
1½ cups	brown rice flour
1 cup	teff flour, quinoa flour, amaranth flour OR light buckwheat flour

Light buckwheat flour is preferred to dark buckwheat flour because the dark flour gives a purple cast to the bread.

Reprinted with permission from:
Cooking Gluten-Free!
A Food Lover's Collection
of Chef and Family Recipes
without Gluten or Wheat by
Karen Robertson
Celiac Publishing, 2002
www.cookingglutenfree.com

Nutritional Analysis

1 serving = 1 slice

	Original	Amaranth	Buckwheat	Quinoa	Teff	Dairy-Free & Egg-Free	Dairy Free	Egg Free
Calories	253	255	242	248	252	263	267	248
Carbohydrates (g)	47	45	42	44	45	47	46	48
Dietary Fiber (g)	2	3	3	2	2	3	3	3
Fat (g)	7	7	7	7	7	9	9	7
Protein (g)	6	7	6	6	6	4	5	5
Iron (mg)	1.0	1.8	1.2	1.8	1.6	1.1	1.2	1.0
Calcium (mg)	66	83	66	71	86	24	24	67
Sodium (mg)	257	258	256	258	258	217	234	240

Wholesome Flax Bread

Yield: 12–18 slices

This ultimate sandwich bread is free of soy, peanuts, nuts and nightshades. Feel free to experiment with different flour combinations.

1½ cups	PLUS 1 Tbsp. warm water
2 Tbsp.	pure maple syrup OR agave nectar
2½ tsp.	active dry yeast
¼ cup	PLUS 3 Tbsp. ground flaxseeds
¾ cup	PLUS 2 Tbsp. sorghum flour
½ cup	arrowroot starch OR potato starch
	(*for nightshade-free, use arrowroot starch)
½ cup	quinoa flour
¼ cup	garfava OR bean flour
¼ cup	tapioca flour
2½ tsp.	xanthan gum
1 tsp.	sea salt
2 Tbsp.	canola oil
2 tsp.	cider vinegar

✦ Lightly oil an 8½ x 4½-inch loaf pan.

✦ Put 1 cup of the water in a large measuring cup. Stir in maple syrup and yeast. Let stand for about 5 minutes, until yeast has bubbled and foamed about ½ inch.

✦ Put remaining ½ cup plus 1 tablespoon of water in a heavy-duty stand mixer or a large bowl. Stir in 3 tablespoons of the ground flaxseeds. Let stand until thickened, about 5 minutes.

✦ Put remaining ¼ cup of flaxseeds, sorghum flour, arrowroot starch, quinoa flour, garfava flour, tapioca flour, xanthan gum and salt in a medium bowl. Stir with a dry whisk until combined.

✦ Add oil and vinegar to the thickened flaxseed mixture. Using the stand mixer or a hand mixer, beat on medium speed for about 30 seconds, until well combined. Turn mixer to low speed and gradually add proofed yeast mixture and flour mixture to make a dough. Turn off mixer and scrape down sides of bowl with a rubber spatula. Resume mixing on medium-high speed for 5 minutes. The dough will be very sticky, similar to thick muffin batter.

✦ Scrape dough into prepared pan using a rubber spatula. Smooth the top. Let rise uncovered in a warm, draft-free place for about 70 minutes, just until dough reaches top of pan.

✦ About 10 minutes before dough is done rising, preheat oven to 350°F. (If dough is rising in the oven, be sure to remove it first.)

✦ Bake for 40–45 minutes, until top of the loaf is browned and a toothpick inserted into center of loaf comes out clean. Carefully remove loaf from pan and put it on a cooling rack. Let cool completely before slicing.

Reprinted with permission from:
The Allergy-Free Cook Bakes Bread by **Laurie Sadowski**,
Book Publishing Company, 2011
www.bookpubco.com
www.lauriesadowski.com

Nutritional Analysis	
1 serving = 1 slice	
Calories (kcal)	117
Carbohydrates (g)	18
Dietary Fiber (g)	3
Fat (g)	4
Protein (g)	3
Iron (mg)	1.3
Calcium (mg)	20
Sodium (mg)	145

Cornbread

Yield: 9 slices

A traditional favorite using cornmeal, brown rice flour and white bean flour for added fiber and protein.

1 cup	gluten-free cornmeal
1/2 cup	white bean flour
1/3 cup	brown rice flour blend (see below)
1/3 cup	sugar
2 tsp.	baking powder
1 tsp.	xanthan gum
1/2 tsp.	table salt
1/8 tsp.	baking soda
2	large eggs, room temperature
1 cup	milk of choice, room temperature
1/2 cup	unsalted butter OR buttery spread, melted

✦ Place rack in middle of oven. Preheat oven to 350°F.

✦ Generously grease an 8-inch-square non-stick metal pan.

✦ In a medium mixing bowl, whisk together cornmeal, white bean flour, rice flour blend, sugar, baking powder, xanthan gum, salt and baking soda until well blended. Using an electric mixer on low speed, beat in eggs, milk and butter until batter thickens slightly, about 30 seconds.

✦ Spread batter evenly in pan. Let stand 10 minutes.

✦ Bake until the top is golden brown and a toothpick inserted into the center of bread comes out clean, about 25–30 minutes.

✦ Cool bread in pan on a wire rack for 10 minutes, then remove from pan and cool another 15 minutes on wire rack.

✦ Cut into 9 squares and serve slightly warm.

Reprinted with permission from:
Pulses and the Gluten-Free Diet: Cooking with Beans, Peas, Lentils and Chickpeas by **Pulse Canada**
1212–220 Portage Ave.
Winnipeg, MB, Canada R3C 0A5
204-925-4455
www.pulsecanada.com

Brown Rice Flour Blend
1 1/2 cups brown rice flour
1 1/2 cups potato starch
1 cup tapioca flour (also called tapioca starch)

✦ Blend thoroughly. Store, tightly closed, in dark, dry place.

Nutritional Analysis	
1 serving = 1 slice (98 g)	
Calories (kcal)	258
Carbohydrates (g)	31
Dietary Fiber (g)	3
Fat (g)	13
Protein (g)	6
Iron (mg)	1
Calcium (mg)	94
Sodium (mg)	247

Teff Polenta

Yield: 4 servings

Flavored with sweet juicy tomatoes, fresh basil and garlic and decorated with bright green peppers, this is a variation on a traditional polenta. Serve garnished with grated fontina, Parmesan, manchego or sliced rounds of chèvre.

2 cups	water
2 Tbsp.	extra-virgin olive oil
8	cloves garlic, thickly sliced
1 cup	coarsely chopped onions
1 cup	coarsely chopped green pepper
⅔ cup	teff grain
½ tsp.	sea salt
2 cups	coarsely chopped plum tomatoes
1 cup	coarsely chopped fresh basil

✦ Bring water to a boil in a teakettle.

✦ Place oil in a 10-inch skillet and warm over medium heat. Add garlic and onions and sauté, stirring occasionally, for 5 minutes or until fragrant. Add peppers and sauté for 2 minutes, or until bright green. Stir in the teff.

✦ Turn off the heat to prevent splattering and add the boiling water and salt. Turn the heat on and let simmer for 2 minutes. Add tomatoes and basil.

✦ Cover and simmer for 10–15 minutes, stirring occasionally, until the water is absorbed. There may be some extra liquid from the tomatoes, but as long as the teff is no longer crunchy, the polenta is done.

✦ Taste and adjust seasonings, if desired.

✦ Transfer polenta to an unoiled 9-inch pie plate. Let cool for about 30 minutes. Slice and serve.

Reprinted with permission from:
The Teff Company
P.O. Box A
Caldwell, ID, U.S. 83606
www.teffco.com
888-822-2221

Leslie Cerier
58 Schoolhouse Rd.
Amherst, MA, U.S. 01002
413-259-1695
www.lesliecerier.com

Nutritional Analysis	
1 serving = 1 slice	
Calories (kcal)	223
Carbohydrates (g)	33
Dietary Fiber (g)	5
Fat (g)	8
Protein (g)	6
Iron (mg)	2.9
Calcium (mg)	107
Sodium (mg)	306

Oatmeal Bread
with sunflower and pumpkin seeds

Yield: 16–18 slices	

A chewy, crusty bread that is dairy-free.

Note:

Leaving the bread to cool in the oven creates a wonderfully crusty exterior. If you prefer a softer crust, remove the baked bread and turn out onto a wire rack to cool on the counter. I don't recommend making this in a bread machine.

Reprinted with permission from:
Gluten-Free Makeovers by
Beth Hillson
Da Capo Lifelong, an imprint of
The Perseus Books Group, 2011
www.dacapopress.com

Nutritional Analysis

1 serving = 1 slice	
Calories (kcal)	163
Carbohydrates (g)	24
Dietary Fiber (g)	2
Fat (g)	6
Protein (g)	4
Iron (mg)	1.1
Calcium (mg)	32
Sodium (mg)	169

2³/₄ cups	bread flour (see below)
³/₄ cup	gluten-free oat flour
¹/₂ tsp.	cream of tartar
1 Tbsp.	instant active OR active dry yeast
1 cup	PLUS 6 Tbsp. warm water (105°–110°F)
3	large eggs
3 Tbsp.	vegetable oil
3 Tbsp.	dark molasses
3 Tbsp.	raw pumpkin seeds
2 Tbsp.	raw sunflower seeds

✦ Coat an 8¹/₂ x 4¹/₂-inch loaf pan with vegetable spray or oil.

✦ In the bowl of a stand mixer, combine bread flour, oat flour and cream of tartar. Whisk to combine. Add yeast and blend. In a separate bowl, combine water, eggs, oil and molasses. Add liquid ingredients to dry ingredients and blend on medium speed for 1 minute. Scrape down sides of bowl and the beater. Beat on medium-high speed for 3–5 minutes or until mixture is smooth. Fold pumpkin and sunflower seeds into the batter.

✦ Scrape dough into the prepared loaf pan. Coat a sheet of plastic wrap with vegetable spray. Smooth top of bread and cover with plastic wrap. Set in a draft-free area and let rise until dough comes up to top of pan.

✦ Preheat oven to 350°F. Remove plastic wrap and bake 50–55 minutes, until internal temperature on an instant-read thermometer registers 190°–200°F. Remove bread from pan and set on a rack in middle of oven. Turn off oven and leave bread in until it cools completely. Remove and slice.

Tips

– This recipe makes terrific rolls, too. Just scoop the dough into oiled muffin-top pans or muffin cups, let rise for 40 minutes then bake for 25–30 minutes, until the internal temperature on an instant-read thermometer registers 190°–200°F. For a professional look, brush with egg wash or milk of choice and sprinkle with oat flakes or pumpkin seeds before baking.

– The bread also can be made using a hand-held mixer. Just be sure it's a heavy-duty mixer (200–250 watts). Krups and KitchenAid both make them.

– Don't have oat flour? Process gluten-free oats in a spice mill until finely ground. Measure out ³/₄ cup.

Bread Flour (high-protein blend with chickpea flour)

2¹/₄ cups	chickpea flour, quinoa flour OR another bean flour
2 cups	cornstarch OR potato starch
2 cups	PLUS 2 Tbsp. tapioca starch/flour
2 cups	brown rice flour
¹/₂ cup	packed light brown sugar
2 Tbsp.	PLUS 2 tsp. xantham gum
1 Tbsp.	salt

Injera (Ethiopian Flatbread)

Yield: 24 pieces

This flat, thin, porous injera is a traditional Ethiopian bread. Injera is served with "wot," a sauce or stew made with chicken, beef or lamb or spicy ground lentils and peas.

Note:

Authentic injera is made from pure teff flour; however, many North American restaurants often use a combination of teff flour and wheat flour or barley flour.

2 Tbsp.   yeast (2 packages)
6½ cups warm water
1½ lbs.   teff flour (about 4½ cups)

✦ Dissolve yeast in ½ cup water.

✦ Combine teff flour, yeast and 6¼ cups water in a large bowl. Mix well. Ensure that no clumps are left at the bottom or sides of bowl.

✦ Cover dough with plastic wrap and let it ferment for 2 to 3 days at room temperature. (Those with sensitive stomachs may consider cooking the injera the same day rather than waiting for 2–3 days. It will have a slightly "sweet" taste but that is considered normal.)

✦ Drain off any water that has risen to the top of the dough.

✦ Gradually add fresh warm water to the dough, just enough to make a thin smooth batter (like thin crêpe batter); mix well. Cover batter and let it stand until it rises, approximately 10–25 minutes.

✦ Heat a 10-inch skillet or frying pan until a drop of water bounces on the pan's surface.

✦ Scoop about ⅓ cup of batter and pour it into the pan quickly. Swirl pan so that the entire bottom is evenly coated. Cover pan quickly and let the injera cook for 1–2 minutes. (Injera does not easily stick or burn.) Remove cover and wait for a few seconds. It is cooked through when bubbles or "eyes" appear all over the top. If your first try is undercooked, cook the next one a little longer or use a smaller amount (¼ cup) of batter. Do not turn the injera over in the pan. Use a spatula to remove cooked injera and place it on a clean tea towel.

✦ Let the injera cool then stack on a serving tray. Do not stack hot as they will stick together.

✦ Continue making the injera until batter is finished.

✦ Injera should be soft and pliable, able to be rolled or folded like a crêpe or tortilla. Properly cooked, injera will be thinner than a pancake but thicker than a crêpe.

Courtesy of:
Girma and Ethiopia Sahlu
Regina, SK, Canada

Nutritional Analysis	
1 serving = 1 piece	
Calories (kcal)	105
Carbohydrates (g)	21
Dietary Fiber (g)	2
Fat (g)	1
Protein (g)	4
Iron (mg)	2
Calcium (mg)	54
Sodium (mg)	7

Flax & Peanut Focaccia

This gluten-free, golden yellow flatbread has a spectacular flavor and stays moist. Exceptionally nutritious, it's high in fiber, protein and antioxidants. To use for sandwiches, cut into large squares and slice horizontally.

Flour Mix

1/2 cup	golden flaxseeds, ground to make 3/4 cup meal
1/2 cup	almond meal
2 Tbsp.	sorghum flour
1 1/2 tsp.	baking powder
1/2 tsp.	xanthan gum
1/2 tsp.	fine sea salt
	Whole brown flaxseeds for top of bread (optional)

Liquid Ingredients

6 Tbsp.	peanut butter
2	large eggs
3/4 cup	water

✦ Heat oven to 350°F. Grease sides of an 8-inch-square baking pan with butter or non-stick cooking spray and line the bottom and two sides with parchment paper.

✦ Combine dry ingredients (except optional whole flaxseeds) in a large bowl and stir with a whisk to break up any clumps. In a food processor, blend peanut butter and eggs until creamy. Add water and process to mix. Pour over dry ingredients and stir until smooth. Batter will be very moist.

✦ Pour batter into pan, spread out evenly and smooth the surface. Sprinkle lightly with whole flaxseeds, if using. Bake for 20–25 minutes, until risen and springy to a light finger touch. Let cool in pan for 5 minutes. Loosen unlined sides with a knife tip, and lift out onto a wire rack. Peel off paper and let cool completely, right side up. Cut into portions. Refrigerate or freeze any extras.

Courtesy of:
Jacqueline Mallorca
Gluten-Free Culinary Expert

Nutritional Analysis	
1 serving	
Calories (kcal)	157
Carbohydrates (g)	8
Dietary Fiber (g)	4
Fat (g)	11
Protein (g)	8
Iron (mg)	1.2
Calcium (mg)	47
Sodium (mg)	220

Apple Date Bread

Apple juice, applesauce and dates make this bread moist and flavorful.

Note:

This recipe provides options for both bread machine and mixer.

Reprinted with permission from:
Delicious Gluten-Free Wheat Free Breads: Easy to Bake Breads Everyone will Love to Eat for the Bread Machine or Oven by **LynnRae Ries** and **Bruce Gross**
What No Wheat Publishing, 2003
www.whatnowheat.com

Nutritional Analysis	
1 serving = 1 slice (1/2" thick)	
Calories (kcal)	187
Carbohydrates (g)	39
Dietary Fiber (g)	2
Fat (g)	2
Protein (g)	4
Iron (mg)	0.7
Calcium (mg)	51
Sodium (mg)	208

3	eggs
1/2 cup	chunky applesauce
3/4 cup	apple juice or water
1 tsp.	apple cider vinegar
1 tsp.	vanilla extract
1 Tbsp.	vegetable oil
2 cups	white rice flour
1/2 cup	tapioca starch flour
1/2 cup	cornstarch

OR use 3 cups of your own favorite GF flour mix instead of the above flours

1/2 cup	non-fat dry milk
1 tsp.	salt
1 Tbsp.	sugar
2 tsp.	cinnamon
1 Tbsp.	xanthan gum
2 1/4 tsp.	yeast
3/4 cup	finely chopped GF pitted dates
1 tsp.	orange zest

Mixer

✦ In a medium-sized bowl, mix all the liquid ingredients together and set aside.

✦ Place all the dry ingredients, including the yeast, into the mixer bowl and blend flours together on slow speed.

✦ Slowly add the liquid ingredients to the dry while the mixer is on low.

✦ Beat on high for 3–4 minutes. Mixture should look silky. If the dough is too dry, add additional liquid (apple juice or water) 1 tablespoon at a time.

✦ Add the dates and orange zest after the dough has been thoroughly mixed.

✦ Place the dough into a 9 x 5-inch loaf pan that has been greased and dusted with rice flour.

✦ Bake in a preheated 350°F oven for 60–70 minutes. Start checking for the bread being done at 55 minutes.

✦ When done, remove bread from pan and place on cooling rack. Do not cut or package until the bread cools, approximately 2–3 hours.

Bread Machine

✦ Place ingredients into the bread machine according to the manual directions.

✦ Program the machine to knead (mix) the ingredients. Add the dates and orange zest at the "add in time." Allow the bread to rise once, then change to bake for 60–70 minutes. Rising time should be 50 minutes, or until the dough doubles in size.

✦ When done, remove the bread from the machine and place on a wire rack to cool. Remember to remove the bread machine paddles if they are stuck in the bread.

Banana Seed Bread
bread machine recipe

Yield: 12 slices

The combination of sorghum and bean flours really enhances the banana flavor of this loaf. Serve it for dessert or with a slice of old cheddar for lunch or a snack.

1 cup	whole bean flour
1 cup	sorghum flour
1/4 cup	tapioca starch
1/4 cup	packed brown sugar
2 1/2 tsp.	xanthan gum
1 Tbsp.	bread machine yeast OR instant yeast
1 1/4 tsp.	salt
1/2 cup	sunflower seeds*
3/4 cup	water
1 cup	mashed banana
1 tsp.	vinegar
1/4 cup	vegetable oil
2	eggs

Bread Machine

✦ In a large bowl or plastic bag, combine whole bean flour, sorghum flour, tapioca starch, brown sugar, xanthan gum, yeast, salt and sunflower seeds. Mix well and set aside.

✦ Pour water, banana, vinegar and oil into the bread machine baking pan. Add eggs.

✦ Select the Rapid 2-Hour Basic Cycle. Allow the liquids to mix until combined. Gradually add the dry ingredients as the bread machine is mixing. Scrape with a rubber spatula while adding the dry ingredients. Try to incorporate all the dry ingredients within 1 to 2 minutes. When mixing and kneading are complete, leaving the bread pan in the bread machine, remove the kneading blade. Allow the bread machine to complete the cycle.

* Use raw, unroasted, unsalted sunflower seeds. For a nuttier flavor, toast the sunflower seeds. Pumpkin seeds or chopped pecans can replace the sunflower seeds.

Reprinted with permission from:
125 Best Gluten-Free Recipes by **Donna Washburn** and **Heather Butt**
Robert Rose Inc., 2003
www.bestbreadrecipes.com

Nutritional Analysis	
1 serving = 1 slice	
Calories (kcal)	222
Carbohydrates (g)	30
Dietary Fiber (g)	4
Fat (g)	10
Protein (g)	7
Iron (mg)	2.0
Calcium (mg)	29
Sodium (mg)	282

Pumpkin Bread

Yield: 12 Slices

A moist and delicious quick bread that is a perfect treat for the autumn season.

¾ cup	chickpea (garbanzo) flour
¾ cup	brown rice flour blend (see below)
¾ cup	sugar
2 tsp.	baking powder
2 tsp.	pumpkin pie spice
1 tsp.	xanthan gum
¾ tsp.	salt
2	large eggs, room temperature
1 cup	milk of choice, room temperature
¾ cup	canned pumpkin purée (*not* pumpkin pie filling)
½ cup	canola oil
1 tsp.	vanilla extract
½ cup	chopped pecans (optional)

✦ Place rack in middle of oven. Preheat oven to 350°F. Generously grease 8 x 4-inch loaf pan.

✦ In a medium mixing bowl, whisk together the chickpea flour, rice flour blend, sugar, baking powder, pumpkin pie spice, xanthan gum and salt until well blended.

✦ Add eggs, milk, pumpkin, oil and vanilla and beat with an electric mixer on low speed until blended. Increase speed to medium and beat another 30 seconds. Stir in nuts (if desired). Spread batter evenly in pan and let stand for 10 minutes.

✦ Bake until loaf is browned and a toothpick inserted into the center comes out clean, about 55–60 minutes. Lay a sheet of foil over loaf after first 20–30 minutes to prevent over-browning. Cool in pan on a wire rack for 10 minutes, then remove bread from pan and cool completely on the wire rack.

Reprinted with permission from:
Pulses and the Gluten-Free Diet: Cooking with Beans, Peas, Lentils and Chickpeas by
Pulse Canada
1212–220 Portage Ave.
Winnipeg, MB, Canada R3C 0A5
204-925-4455
www.pulsecanada.com

Brown Rice Flour Blend
1½ cups   brown rice flour
1½ cups   potato starch
1 cup   tapioca flour (also called tapioca starch)

✦ Blend thoroughly. Store, tightly closed, in dark, dry place.

Nutritional Analysis	
1 serving = 1 slice	
Calories (kcal)	203
Carbohydrates (g)	23
Dietary Fiber (g)	2
Fat (g)	11
Protein (g)	3
Iron (mg)	1
Calcium (mg)	61
Sodium (mg)	232

Shelley's Orange Cranberry Muffins

Yield: 12 muffins

The flavor combination of cinnamon and orange zest makes these high-fiber muffins truly delectable.

Notes:

If you don't have oat flour on hand, make your own by grinding rolled oats in a food processor.

Substitute raisins for cranberries.

1 cup	GF oat flour
1/2 cup	GF rolled oats
1/2 cup	ground flax (flaxseed meal)
1 Tbsp.	baking powder
1 Tbsp.	cinnamon
1 tsp.	xanthan gum
2	eggs
1/2 cup	oil
1/2 cup	packed brown sugar
1/2 cup	orange juice
	Grated rind (zest) of 1 orange
1 tsp.	vanilla
3/4 cup	dried cranberries

✦ Preheat oven to 375°F.

✦ Combine oat flour, oats, ground flax, baking powder, cinnamon and xanthan gum in a large bowl and mix well.

✦ In separate bowl, whisk eggs and oil, then add brown sugar, orange juice, orange zest and vanilla and whisk again until mixed.

✦ Add liquid mixture to dry ingredients. Mix together until just combined. Fold in cranberries.

✦ Spoon batter into paper-lined muffin cups. Bake for 12–15 minutes, or until toothpick inserted into the center comes out clean.

✦ Cool on wire rack.

Courtesy of:
Shelley Case, RD
North America's Gluten-Free Nutrition Expert
Regina, SK, Canada
www.shelleycase.com

Nutritional Analysis	
1 serving = 1 muffin	
Calories (kcal)	238
Carbohydrates (g)	27
Dietary Fiber (g)	4
Fat (g)	12
Protein (g)	5
Iron (mg)	1.4
Calcium (mg)	50
Sodium (mg)	168

Blueberry Almond Muffins

Filled with wholesome almonds, blueberries and quinoa, these aren't just a super dessert but make a terrific snack any time of day.

1 cup	water
½ cup	white quinoa
2	large eggs, beaten
1 cup	unsweetened applesauce
¼ cup	lightly packed brown sugar
¼ cup	grapeseed oil OR vegetable oil
1 tsp.	pure vanilla extract
⅔ cup	almond flour
⅓ cup	quick-cooking rolled oats (gluten free)
3 Tbsp.	cornstarch
1 tsp.	baking powder
½ tsp.	baking soda
¼ tsp.	salt
1 cup	fresh or frozen blueberries

✦ Preheat the oven to 400°F. Lightly grease or spray with cooking oil a 12-cup muffin pan or line with paper liners.

✦ In a small saucepan, bring the water and quinoa to a boil. Reduce to a simmer, cover and cook for 15 minutes. Remove from the heat and leave covered for another 10 minutes. The quinoa must be fluffy.

✦ In a blender, combine the eggs, applesauce, brown sugar, oil, vanilla and ¼ cup of the quinoa. Blend until smooth. Repeat, adding ¼ cup quinoa, puréeing after each addition, until you have added 1½ cups.

✦ In a large bowl, whisk together the almond flour, oats, cornstarch, baking powder, baking soda and salt. Add the blueberries and stir to coat with flour mixture. Add the quinoa purée, using a spatula to get all the purée out. Stir until just blended. Divide batter among muffin cups.

✦ Bake for 30 minutes or until a toothpick inserted in the center comes out clean. Transfer to a rack to cool.

✦ Store in a sealed container for up to 1 week.

Reprinted with permission from:
Quinoa Revolution by
Carolyn Hemming and
Patricia Green
Penguin Canada Books, 2014
www.penguinrandomhouse.ca

Nutritional Analysis	
1 serving = 1 muffin	
Calories (kcal)	160
Carbohydrates (g)	17
Dietary Fiber (g)	2
Fat (g)	9
Protein (g)	4
Iron (mg)	1.1
Calcium (mg)	30
Sodium (mg)	160

Mighty Tasty Muffins

Yield: 12 muffins

The special flours and cereals used in these muffins complement the flavors of the brown sugar and spice mixtures.

Note:

Distilled white vinegar is also gluten-free and can be substituted for apple cider vinegar.

Reprinted with permission from:
Bob's Red Mill Natural Foods, Inc.
13521 SE Pheasant Ct.
Milwaukie, OR, U.S. 97222
800-349-2173 / 503-654-3215
www.bobsredmill.com

Recipe adapted by:
Carol Fenster, PhD, author of a variety of gluten-free cookbooks (see pp. 297, 298)
www.carolfenstercooks.com

2 Tbsp.	Bob's Red Mill™ Mighty Tasty GF Hot Cereal*
2/3 cup	low-fat (1%) milk
1 Tbsp.	apple cider vinegar
1	large egg
1/3 cup	molasses
1 tsp.	vanilla
3/4 cup	Bob's Red Mill™ GF Garbanzo and Fava Flour
1/2 cup	potato starch
1/4 cup	tapioca flour
1/3 cup	brown sugar, packed
1 tsp.	GF baking powder
1/2 tsp.	baking soda
1 tsp.	xanthan gum
1/4 tsp.	nutmeg
1/2 tsp.	cinnamon
1/4 tsp.	ground ginger
1/4 tsp.	allspice
1/2 tsp.	salt

✦ In a large bowl, combine the first 6 ingredients. Let sit for 15 minutes, while the cereal softens.

✦ In a separate bowl, combine remaining ingredients.

✦ Add dry ingredients to liquid ingredients and stir until just moistened.

✦ Spoon batter into greased muffin tins. Fill tins 2/3 full.

✦ Bake in preheated 350°F oven for approximately 20 minutes, or until tops of muffins are firm.

* **Mighty Tasty GF Hot Cereal:**
   Brown rice, corn, "sweet" white sorghum and buckwheat

Nutritional Analysis	
1 serving = 1 muffin	
Calories (kcal)	123
Carbohydrates (g)	27
Dietary Fiber (g)	2
Fat (g)	1
Protein (g)	3
Iron (mg)	1.1
Calcium (mg)	72
Sodium (mg)	213

Carrot Cake Pancakes

Serves 6

These golden pancakes are packed with carrots, raisins and pineapple, along with the goodness of quinoa. Tasty topped with maple syrup, or step it up with freshly whipped cream.

1½ cups	quinoa flour
1 Tbsp.	organic cane sugar OR white sugar
3½ tsp.	baking powder
½ tsp.	salt
1½ tsp.	cinnamon
½ tsp.	nutmeg
1 cup	1% or 2% milk, buttermilk OR soy milk
2	large eggs, beaten
¼ cup	applesauce
1 cup	shredded carrots
⅓ cup	crushed pineapple, drained well
⅓ cup	seedless raisins
¼ cup	chopped, toasted pecans*

✦ Measure the flour, sugar, baking powder, salt, cinnamon and nutmeg into a large bowl. Mix well. In a medium bowl, whisk together the milk, eggs and applesauce. Stir in the carrots, pineapple, raisins and pecans. Add the milk mixture to the flour mixture and stir just until blended.

✦ Grease a large skillet or spray with cooking oil and place on medium heat. When hot, pour scant ¼ cup portions of batter into the pan. The pancakes will be ready to flip when you first see bubbles and the underside is lightly golden brown. Watch them carefully, as they brown quickly. Flip and cook the pancakes for another 30 seconds, until the center springs back when pressed. If the pancakes buckle when you slide the spatula under them, lightly oil the pan again for the next batch.

✦ Serve with maple syrup.

* To toast nuts, preheat the oven to 350°F. Spread the nuts on a baking sheet and toast in the oven, stirring once if necessary, for 5–7 minutes, until fragrant and lightly toasted.

Reprinted with permission from:
Quinoa Revolution by
Carolyn Hemming and
Patricia Green
Copyright © Carolyn Hemming and Patricia Green, 2014
Penguin Canada Books
www.penguinrandomhouse.ca

Nutritional Analysis	
1 serving = 1 pancake	
Calories (kcal)	250
Carbohydrates (g)	38
Dietary Fiber (g)	6
Fat (g)	8
Protein (g)	9
Iron (mg)	1.8
Calcium (mg)	110
Sodium (mg)	240

Teff Banana Pancakes

Yield: 12 small pancakes

This basic pancake recipe is easy to make. Feel free to substitute maple syrup for honey, and juice for soy milk. Ground flaxseeds easily take the place of eggs in these delicious pancakes made with naturally sweet teff and bananas. The batter is light and looks like pudding.

2 Tbsp.	flaxseeds
2	bananas, ripe
1½ cups	vanilla soy milk
1 Tbsp.	vanilla
1 Tbsp.	honey
1½ tsp.	vegetable oil
1½ cups	teff flour
1 Tbsp.	baking powder
¼ tsp.	sea salt
½ tsp.	cinnamon

✦ Grind flaxseeds in a blender until powdery. Add banana, vanilla soy milk, vanilla, honey and ½ tsp. oil. Blend well.

✦ In a large mixing bowl, combine teff flour, baking powder, sea salt and cinnamon. Stir in banana soy milk mixture.

✦ Place griddle or skillet over medium heat. After a minute or two, brush on 1 tsp. of oil. Using a tablespoon, scoop up batter and pour it on hot griddle, 1 heaping tablespoon for each pancake.

✦ Cook pancakes for 3–4 minutes on the first side, or until tiny holes appear on the top of the pancakes. Flip pancakes over and cook for another minute or two.

✦ Serve pancakes plain or topped with yogurt.

Reprinted with permission from:
The Teff Company
P.O. Box A
Caldwell, ID, U.S. 83606
www.teffco.com
888-822-2221

Leslie Cerier
58 Schoolhouse Rd.
Amherst, MA, U.S. 01002
413-259-1695
www.lesliecerier.com

Nutritional Analysis

1 serving = 1 pancake	
Calories (kcal)	54
Carbohydrates (g)	9
Dietary Fiber (g)	1
Fat (g)	1
Protein (g)	2
Iron (mg)	0.7
Calcium (mg)	64
Sodium (mg)	79

Spiced Apple Cranberry Buckwheat Cereal

Yield: 2 servings

Knock out the same old breakfast routine with yummy cereal full of warm spices and fruit – indulge in the fabulous flavors of grains mixed with apples, cranberries, cinnamon, nutmeg and cloves in this quick and easy breakfast.

Note:

This cereal also can be made with ¼ cup millet, amaranth or teff in place of buckwheat.

1 cup	water
½ cup	unsweetened apple juice
¼ cup	quinoa seeds
¼ cup	buckwheat groats
3 Tbsp.	chopped, dried apple
1 Tbsp.	dried sweetened cranberries OR raisins
½ tsp.	cinnamon
pinch	nutmeg
pinch	ground cloves
2 tsp.	honey OR pure maple syrup (optional)
½ cup	milk (optional)

✦ Combine the water, juice, quinoa, buckwheat, apple, cranberries, cinnamon, nutmeg and cloves in a medium saucepan and bring to a boil. Reduce to a simmer, cover and cook for 15 minutes. Remove from the heat, stir and serve with honey and milk if desired.

Reprinted with permission from:
Grain Power by
Carolyn Hemming and
Patricia Green
Copyright © Carolyn Hemming and Patricia Green, 2014
Penguin Canada Books
www.penguinrandomhouse.ca

Nutritional Analysis	
1 serving	
Calories (kcal)	220
Carbohydrates (g)	45
Dietary Fiber (g)	4
Fat (g)	2
Protein (g)	6
Iron (mg)	1.8
Calcium (mg)	90
Sodium (mg)	35

Sweet Sorghum Banana Date Breakfast Cookies

Yield: 16–18 cookies

These scone-like cookies are a tasty alternative to traditional breakfast items.

³⁄₄ cup	sweet white sorghum flour
³⁄₄ cup	brown rice flour
¹⁄₂ cup	tapioca starch/flour
¹⁄₃ cup	packed light brown sugar
1 Tbsp.	baking powder
¹⁄₂ tsp.	baking soda
1 tsp.	xanthan gum
1 tsp.	ground cinnamon
¹⁄₂ tsp.	salt
5 Tbsp.	cold unsalted butter OR buttery non-dairy spread, cut into small pieces
2	large eggs
¹⁄₂ cup	buttermilk (OR soy milk combined with 2 tsp. cider vinegar)
2 tsp.	vanilla extract
³⁄₄ cup	coarsely chopped dried banana slices
³⁄₄ cup	chopped dates
	Additional buttermilk or soy milk for brushing
	Additional brown sugar for sprinkling

✦ Preheat the oven to 375°F. Line two cookie sheets with parchment paper.

✦ Combine the sorghum flour, brown rice flour, tapioca starch/flour, brown sugar, baking powder, baking soda, xanthan gum, cinnamon and salt in a large bowl. Mix until the brown sugar is blended into the ingredients. Cut in the butter until the mixture resembles coarse meal.

✦ In a separate bowl using a mixer, beat the eggs until light yellow and thick, about 3 minutes. Add the dry ingredients and beat about 1 minute. Beat in the buttermilk and vanilla until smooth. Fold in the dried banana and dates.

✦ Using a medium scoop, scoop the dough onto the prepared cookie sheets, leaving about 1 inch between each scone. Use a sheet of plastic wrap to gently press and smooth the scones into 1-inch-thick disks. Brush with buttermilk, sprinkle with brown sugar and bake for 18–20 minutes. Serve warm.

Reprinted with permission from:
Gluten-Free Makeovers by
Beth Hillson
Da Capo Lifelong, an imprint of
The Perseus Books Group, 2011
www.dacapopress.com

Nutritional Analysis	
1 serving = 1 cookie (55g)	
Calories (kcal)	167
Carbohydrates (g)	29
Dietary Fiber (g)	2
Fat (g)	5
Protein (g)	3
Iron (mg)	1
Calcium (mg)	35
Sodium (mg)	217

Carrot Apple Energy Bars

Yield: 18 bars

For a quick, easy, on-the-move breakfast or snack, choose these moist nutritious bars.

Notes:

For the dried fruit mix, we used ¼ cup dried cranberries, ¼ cup raisins, 2 Tbsp. chopped dried mangoes, 1 Tbsp. dried blueberries and 1 Tbsp. chopped dried apricots.

For a lactose-free bar, omit the milk powder.

Try substituting grated zucchini for all or half of the carrots.

Substitute cardamom for the cinnamon.

Reprinted with permission from:
The Best Gluten-Free Family Cookbook by
Donna Washburn and **Heather Butt**
Robert Rose Inc., 2005
www.bestbreadrecipes.com

1¼ cups	sorghum flour
½ cup	amaranth flour
⅓ cup	rice bran
¼ cup	ground flaxseed
¼ cup	non-fat (skim) milk powder
1½ tsp.	xanthan gum
1 Tbsp.	GF baking powder
¼ tsp.	salt
2 tsp.	ground cinnamon
2	eggs
1 cup	unsweetened applesauce
⅓ cup	packed brown sugar
1½ cups	grated carrots
¾ cup	dried fruit mix (see Notes)
½ cup	chopped walnuts

✦ Line a 13 x 9-inch baking pan with foil and grease lightly.

✦ In a large bowl or plastic bag, combine sorghum flour, amaranth flour, rice bran, ground flaxseed, milk powder, xanthan gum, baking powder, salt and cinnamon. Mix well and set aside.

✦ In a separate bowl, using an electric mixer, beat eggs, applesauce and brown sugar until combined.

✦ Add flour mixture and mix just until combined. Stir in carrots, dried fruit and nuts. Spoon the batter into the prepared pan; spread to edges with a moist rubber spatula and allow to stand for 30 minutes.

✦ Bake in a preheated 325°F oven for 30–35 minutes, or until a cake tester inserted in the center comes out clean.

✦ Let cool in pan on a cooling rack and cut into bars.

✦ Store in an airtight container at room temperature for up to 1 week or individually wrapped and frozen for up to 1 month.

Nutritional Analysis	
1 serving = 1 bar	
Calories (kcal)	144
Carbohydrates (g)	24
Dietary Fiber (g)	3
Fat (g)	4
Protein (g)	5
Iron (mg)	1.7
Calcium (mg)	99
Sodium (mg)	139

Fruit n' Nut Bars

Great for hiking trips, after a workout or anytime you need an energy boost!

1 cup	whole almonds
1 cup	whole peanuts or cashews
1½ cups	Only Oats™ Rolled Oats
¼ cup	ground flaxseed
¼ cup	hemp hearts
3 Tbsp.	chia seeds
1 cup	dried cranberries
⅔ cup	honey
¼ cup	canola oil

✦ Line a 9 x 9-inch baking pan with parchment paper, leaving extra for lifting bars out of the pan once they are baked.

✦ In a large bowl, combine almonds, peanuts, Only Oats™ Rolled Oats, flax, hemp, chia seeds and cranberries. Stir to combine.

✦ In a saucepan, heat honey and canola oil. Whisk to combine. Bring to a gentle boil, then remove from heat and pour over dry ingredients. Stir to distribute evenly.

✦ Bake at 325°F for 35–40 minutes, or until lightly browned.

✦ Let cool for 15 minutes then lift from pan and cool on rack.

✦ Cut bars into rectangles or crumble and use as a trail mix.

Reprinted with permission from:
Avena Foods, Ltd.
316 1st Ave. E
Regina, SK, Canada S4N 5H2
866-461-3663 / 306-757-3663
www.avenafoods.com

Nutritional Analysis	
1 serving = 1 bar (39 g)	
Calories (kcal)	188
Carbohydrates (g)	20
Dietary Fiber (g)	3
Fat (g)	10
Protein (g)	4
Iron (mg)	1.5
Calcium (mg)	33
Sodium (mg)	2

Coconut & Banana Lentil Bites

Yield: 30 bites

These treats are so delicious, you may be tempted to eat them all immediately!

Notes:

Almond flour can be used in place of coconut flour. Stir in enough almond flour as needed to easily roll the dough into balls.

Transform these bites into vegan snacks by using vegan chocolate chips, or omitting chips altogether.

1 cup	coconut flakes, unsweetened
1/4 cup	unroasted, unsalted sunflower seeds
1/2 tsp.	ground cinnamon
1/2 cup	mashed ripe banana (approx. 1 whole)
1/2 cup	cooked green lentils
3 Tbsp.	honey
1/4 cup	mini chocolate chips, or chopped chocolate
1 Tbsp.	coconut oil, melted (not hot)
1/2 cup	coconut flour

✦ Place coconut flakes, sunflower seeds, cinnamon, banana, lentils and honey into a food processor. Pulse until smooth, scrape down the sides and pulse again. Transfer to a bowl using a spatula.

✦ Stir in chocolate chips and oil until fully incorporated. Stir in the coconut flour until fully combined.

✦ Roll into bite-size balls, about 1 Tbsp. in size. Cover and refrigerate or freeze for 5–10 minutes so balls can solidify. Store in an airtight container in the fridge to snack on during the week, or freeze until you are ready to nibble.

Adapted and reprinted with permission from:
Canadian Lentils
207–116 Research Dr.
Saskatoon, SK, Canada S7N 3R3
306-668-3668
www.lentils.ca

Nutritional Analysis	
1 serving = 1 bite (1 Tbsp.)	
Calories (kcal)	60
Carbohydrates (g)	6
Dietary Fiber (g)	2
Fat (g)	4
Protein (g)	1
Iron (mg)	0.7
Calcium (mg)	10
Sodium (mg)	5

Sorghum Peanut Butter Cookies

Yield: 72 cookies

Peanut butter and brown sugar are a wonderful flavor combo, and sorghum and garbanzo flours add interesting texture to a favorite cookie recipe.

1½ cups	creamy peanut butter
1 cup	shortening OR margarine
2⅓ cups	firmly packed brown sugar
6 Tbsp.	low-fat (1%) milk
2 tsp.	vanilla
2	eggs
3 cups	sorghum flour
½ cup	garbanzo bean (chickpea) flour
½ cup	sweet rice flour
4 tsp.	xanthan gum
1 tsp.	salt
1½ tsp.	baking soda

✦ Combine peanut butter, shortening, brown sugar, milk and vanilla in a large bowl. With an electric mixer, beat on medium speed until well blended.

✦ Add eggs and beat just until blended.

✦ Combine the flours, xanthan gum, salt and baking soda. Add to creamed mixture at low speed. Mix just until blended.

✦ Using a mini ice cream scoop, drop dough portions 2 inches apart on baking sheets lined with parchment paper. Flatten slightly in a criss-cross pattern with the tines of a fork.

✦ Bake in a preheated 375°F oven for 8–10 minutes, or until set and just beginning to brown.

✦ Cool cookies for 2 minutes on baking sheets, then remove from pan and cool completely.

Courtesy of:
Barbara Kliment, Executive Director, Nebraska Grain Sorghum Board
301 Centennial Mall S
P. O. Box 94982
Lincoln, NE, U.S. 68509
402-471-4276
www.sorghum.state.ne.us

Nutritional Analysis	
1 serving = 1 cookie	
Calories (kcal)	113
Carbohydrates (g)	14
Dietary Fiber (g)	1
Fat (g)	6
Protein (g)	2
Iron (mg)	0.6
Calcium (mg)	11
Sodium (mg)	71

Cranberry Pistachio Biscotti

These have the appearance and texture of traditional twice-baked biscotti, but are much easier and faster to make. We like to dip them in a sweet Italian dessert wine or in coffee.

Notes:

Biscotti will be medium-firm and crunchy; for softer biscotti, bake for only 10 minutes in Step 5; for very firm biscotti, bake for 20 minutes.

Store in an airtight container at room temperature for up to 3 weeks, or freeze for up to 2 months.

If you prefer, you can use a 13 x 9-inch baking pan instead of the two 8-inch pans.

Try orange-flavored cranberries and substitute orange zest for the lemon zest.

Substitute pecans or hazelnuts for the pistachios.

Reprinted with permission from:
The Best Gluten-Free Family Cookbook by
Donna Washburn and
Heather Butt
Robert Rose Inc., 2005
www.bestbreadrecipes.com

Nutritional Analysis	
1 serving = 1 cookie	
Calories (kcal)	62
Carbohydrates (g)	10
Dietary Fiber (g)	1
Fat (g)	2
Protein (g)	2
Iron (mg)	0.5
Calcium (mg)	15
Sodium (mg)	17

1½ cups	amaranth flour
½ cup	soy flour
⅓ cup	potato starch
¼ cup	tapioca starch
1½ tsp.	xanthan gum
1 tsp.	GF baking powder
pinch	salt
4	eggs
1¼ cups	sugar
1 Tbsp.	grated lemon zest
1 tsp.	vanilla
1½ cups	coarsely chopped pistachios
1 cup	dried cranberries

✦ Line two 8-inch square baking pans with foil and grease lightly. For the second baking, use ungreased baking sheets.

✦ In a large bowl or plastic bag, combine amaranth flour, soy flour, potato starch, tapioca starch, xanthan gum, baking powder and salt. Mix well and set aside.

✦ In a separate bowl, using an electric mixer, beat eggs, sugar, lemon zest and vanilla until combined.

✦ Slowly beat dry ingredients into the egg mixture and mix just until combined. Stir in pistachios and cranberries. Spoon into the prepared pans. Using a moistened rubber spatula, spread the batter to the edges and smooth the tops.

✦ Bake in a preheated 325°F oven for 30–35 minutes, or until firm or tops are just turning golden. Let cool in the pans for 5 minutes.

✦ Remove biscotti from the pans, remove foil and let cool on a cutting board for 5 minutes.

✦ Cut biscotti into quarters, then cut each quarter into 8 slices. Arrange slices upright (cut sides exposed) at least ½ inch apart on baking sheets. Bake for an additional 15 minutes, until dry and crisp. Transfer to a cooling rack immediately.

Chocolate Banana Rum Cake

A luscious and moist chocolate cake made with high-fibre almond flour and black beans.

Note:

For an extra touch of sweetness with more rum flavor, combine 3 Tbsp. brown sugar with 2 Tbsp. dark rum; drizzle over cake while cooling.

2⅓ cups	slivered almonds
	OR 2½ cups almond flour
1 cup	brown sugar
6 Tbsp.	cocoa
½ cup	canned black beans, drained and rinsed thoroughly
2	medium bananas, very ripe
4	eggs
⅓ cup	canola oil
1 Tbsp.	rum extract

◆ Preheat oven to 350°F.

◆ If using slivered almonds, place into a food processor or coffee bean grinder. Pulse until finely ground; be careful not to over grind or it will turn to almond butter.

◆ Combine finely ground almonds or almond flour, brown sugar and cocoa in a large mixing bowl.

◆ In food processor or blender, purée beans and bananas until smooth.

◆ Add eggs, oil and rum extract to bean and banana mixture. Mix well.

◆ Add liquid mixture to dry ingredients. Mix until well blended.

◆ Pour batter into a greased 8-inch round cake pan.

◆ Bake for 30–40 minutes. After 30 minutes check for doneness: toothpick inserted into center of cake should come out clean.

◆ Cool in pan on a wire rack.

Courtesy of:
Shelley Case, RD
North America's Gluten-Free
Nutrition Expert
Regina, SK, Canada

Jessica Ethier, RD
Gluten-Free Nutrition Expert
Regina, SK, Canada

Nutritional Analysis	
1 serving	
Calories (kcal)	227
Carbohydrates (g)	23
Dietary Fiber (g)	3
Fat (g)	14
Protein (g)	6
Iron (mg)	1.3
Calcium (mg)	70
Sodium (mg)	26

Cajun Lentil Trail Mix with Dark Chocolate

Yield: 10 servings

An interesting way to incorporate lentils into your diet. This spicy, slightly sweet trail mix is an excellent high-fiber snack for when you are on-the-go.

Notes:

If you prefer more "heat," add an extra ¼ teaspoon of cayenne pepper to the recipe.

For even more crunch, use 1¼ cup uncooked lentils.

Use mini chocolate chips so that every bite has some chocolate flavor.

1 cup	uncooked split red lentils
1 cup	whole blanched almonds
1 cup	halved pecans
½ cup	shelled unroasted pumpkin seeds
½ cup	shelled unroasted sunflower seeds
1 Tbsp.	PLUS 1 tsp. canola oil
3 Tbsp.	honey
1¼ tsp.	chili powder
½ tsp.	onion powder
¼ tsp.	garlic powder
⅛ tsp.	ground black pepper
¼ tsp.	kosher salt
¼ tsp.	cayenne pepper
⅔ cup	finely chopped dried dates
⅔ cup	dark chocolate chips

✦ Rinse lentils thoroughly under cold water. Soak in cool water for 1 hour. Preheat oven to 350°F.

✦ Drain lentils and pat dry with a clean towel. Spread out on a parchment-lined tray and bake for 10 minutes. Stir, then bake another 10–15 minutes or until lentils are dry and slightly crunchy.

✦ Mix cooked lentils with almonds, pecans, pumpkin seeds, sunflower seeds, canola oil, honey, chili powder, onion powder, garlic, pepper, salt and cayenne. Spread out on lined baking tray and bake for 10 minutes at 350°F, stir, then bake for another 10–15 minutes or until golden brown. Toss into a large bowl to cool. The mixture will become crunchy as it cools.

✦ Once the mix has cooled, toss in dates and chocolate. Store in an airtight container.

Reprinted with permission from:
Canadian Lentils
207–116 Research Dr.
Saskatoon, SK, Canada S7N 3R3
306-668-3668
www.lentils.ca

Nutritional Analysis	
1 serving = ½ cup	
Calories (kcal)	310
Carbohydrates (g)	26
Dietary Fiber (g)	6
Fat (g)	20
Protein (g)	9
Iron (mg)	4.1
Calcium (mg)	70
Sodium (mg)	260

Lentil Vegetable Soup

Courtesy of:
Jessica Ethier, RD
Gluten-Free Nutrition Expert
Regina, SK, Canada

Yield: 10 servings

This wholesome soup has a slightly sweet flavor from the addition of creamed corn.

1 Tbsp.	canola oil
1	yellow onion, diced
2	garlic cloves, minced
4	carrots, sliced
1 cup	diced celery (stalk and leaves)
3	medium potatoes, cubed
1	zucchini, diced
2	(33 oz.) cartons low-sodium vegetable broth
1 cup	uncooked split red lentils
1	(28 oz.) can diced tomatoes
3 Tbsp.	tomato paste
1½ tsp.	Italian seasoning
2	bay leaves
1 tsp.	coarse ground black pepper
2	(14 oz.) cans creamed corn

- ✦ Heat oil on medium-high in a large pot.
- ✦ Add onions and garlic and cook for about 4 minutes, until onions are slightly soft and transparent.
- ✦ Add carrots and celery. Continue to cook until tender, about 10 minutes, stirring often.
- ✦ Add potatoes, zucchini, vegetable broth, lentils, diced tomatoes, tomato paste, Italian seasoning, bay leaf and pepper. Stir to combine.
- ✦ Reduce heat to medium-low. Allow soup to simmer, covered, for about 35–40 minutes.
- ✦ Mix in creamed corn and turn off heat. Remove bay leaves before serving.

Nutritional Analysis	
1 serving	
Calories (kcal)	192
Carbohydrates (g)	36
Dietary Fiber (g)	6
Fat (g)	2
Protein (g)	7
Iron (mg)	1.8
Calcium (mg)	70
Sodium (mg)	347

French Canadian Pea Soup

Yield: 6 servings

A traditional and fiber-rich soup that combines whole yellow peas and bacon to create a satisfying meal.

Note:

Soak whole yellow peas in cold water for 8 to 10 hours to shorten cooking time by 1 hour or more.

2¼ cups	Best Cooking Pulses whole yellow peas
8 cups	water
1	bay leaf
2	medium carrots, grated
¼ cup	chopped fresh sage (or 1 Tbsp. dry)
¼ cup	chopped fresh parsley
6	strips bacon
2	medium onions, chopped
1	large celery stalk, chopped
4	cloves garlic, minced
	Salt and pepper to taste

✦ Rinse and drain the peas. Place in soup pot with water and bay leaf, and bring to a boil.

✦ Boil gently for 2½–3 hours until peas purée, adding more water if required. Cooking time to the purée stage can be reduced by soaking (see Note).

✦ Add carrot, sage and parsley and continue simmering.

✦ In a skillet, slowly brown bacon strips. Remove when crisp.

✦ Add onion, celery and garlic to the rendered bacon fat and sauté over low heat until transparent. Transfer to soup pot. Salt and pepper to taste.

✦ Cook slowly for an additional ½ hour, garnish with crisp bacon strips and serve.

Reprinted with Permission from:
Best Cooking Pulses, Inc.
110 10th St., NE
Portage la Prairie, MB,
Canada R1N 1B5
204-857-4451
www.bestcookingpulses.com

Nutritional Analysis	
1 serving	
Calories (kcal)	391
Carbohydrates (g)	54
Dietary Fiber (g)	11
Fat (g)	10
Protein (g)	22
Iron (mg)	4.1
Calcium (mg)	100
Sodium (mg)	189

Moroccan Salad

Yield: 10 servings

This heart-healthy salad is packed with fiber and is sure to be a hit with everyone!

3 cups — cooked quinoa – OR can use rice, millet or a combination of millet and quinoa
1/2 — EACH, red, yellow and orange pepper, 1/4-inch diced
1 — medium red onion, 1/4-inch diced
1/2 cup — chopped GF pitted dates
1/2 cup — diced dried apricots
1/2 cup — dried cherries OR cranberries
— Grated zest and juice of 1 orange and 1 lemon
2-3 Tbsp. — extra-virgin olive oil
1/8 tsp. — turmeric
— Salt and freshly ground black pepper to taste
1/3 cup — toasted, slivered almonds
2 Tbsp. — sunflower seeds
2 Tbsp. — chopped parsley OR cilantro

To Prepare Quinoa

✦ Wash the dry quinoa, changing water at least 5 times. Rub grains with your hands and then let them settle to the bottom of the bowl each time before pouring off the water and then adding more fresh cold water.

✦ Bring a pot of lightly salted water to a boil.

✦ Add the quinoa and cook for 10 minutes.

✦ Drain quinoa into a sieve. Rinse under cold water.

✦ Set sieve over a saucepan of boiling water. Do not allow water to touch quinoa. Cover with a kitchen towel and lid. Steam until the quinoa is fluffy and dry, about 10 minutes. Check the water level in the pan, adding more if necessary.

To Make the Salad

✦ Toss everything together except almonds, sunflower seeds and parsley.

✦ Taste for seasoning.

✦ Just before serving, stir in almonds then sprinkle sunflower seeds and parsley over the salad. Serve.

Courtesy of:
Rebecca Reilly, culinary expert and author of *Gluten-Free Baking: More Than 125 Recipes for Delectable Sweet and Savory Baked Goods, Including Cakes, Pies, Quick Breads, Muffins, Cookies, and Other Delights*

Nutritional Analysis	
1 serving	
Calories (kcal)	219
Carbohydrates (g)	32
Dietary Fiber (g)	5
Fat (g)	8
Protein (g)	6
Iron (mg)	0.9
Calcium (mg)	41
Sodium (mg)	123

Brown Rice Chickpea Kale Salad
with Ginger Tahini Dressing

A meal in one dish – this salad contains a healthy dose of plant-based proteins, nutrient-rich greens and healthy fats. The lemony and gingery tahini dressing offers the perfect bold flavors to enliven the taste. It's delicious served warm or cold and holds up well for a couple of days, making it a perfect lunch to take to work or party dish for a potluck.

Salad

2 cups	cooked brown rice (short or long grain, depending on preference), cooled
1	(15 oz.) can chickpeas (garbanzo beans), rinsed, drained
5 cups	finely chopped kale
½ cup	dried cranberries

Dressing

1	lemon, juice and zest
1½ Tbsp.	red wine vinegar
3 Tbsp.	tahini (sesame seed paste)
1 tsp.	freshly grated ginger
½ tsp.	smoked red paprika
	Sea salt and black pepper (as desired)

✦ Mix together rice, chickpeas, kale and dried cranberries in a large bowl.

✦ In a small bowl, mix together lemon juice and zest, red wine vinegar, tahini, ginger, paprika and sea salt and black pepper as desired.

✦ Pour dressing over salad and combine very well to distribute all ingredients.

Courtesy of:
Sharon Palmer
The Plant-Powered Dietitian™
www.sharonpalmer.com

Nutritional Analysis	
1 serving	
Calories (kcal)	240
Carbohydrates (g)	44
Dietary Fiber (g)	7
Fat (g)	5
Protein (g)	7
Iron (mg)	3
Calcium (mg)	329
Sodium (mg)	32

Quinoa Salad

Yield: 6 servings

Nuts and seeds add crunch to this flavorful salad that can be served on its own for lunch or as a side dish at dinner.

Note:

For additional flavor, cook the quinoa in a low-sodium vegetable broth.

Lemon Garlic Dressing

4	garlic cloves, minced
1/4 cup	red wine vinegar
1/4 cup	canola oil
1/4 cup	water
1	lemon, juiced
1 tsp.	basil
1/2 tsp.	salt
	Pepper to taste

Salad Ingredients

4 cups	cooked NorQuin quinoa, cooled
1 cup	grated carrots
1/2 cup	sliced green onions
1/2 cup	chopped celery
1/4 cup	sunflower seeds
1/4 cup	slivered almonds
3 Tbsp.	sesame seeds

✦ In a small bowl, combine dressing ingredients and let stand for at least 10 minutes.

✦ Combine salad ingredients in a large bowl.

✦ Toss salad ingredients with dressing and serve.

Courtesy of:
Northern Quinoa Corporation
3002 Millar Ave.
Saskatoon, SK, Canada S7K 5X9
866-368-9304 / 306-933-9525
www.quinoa.com

Nutritional Analysis	
1 serving = 1 cup	
Calories (kcal)	358
Carbohydrates (g)	33
Dietary Fiber (g)	5
Fat (g)	19
Protein (g)	9
Iron (mg)	3.2
Calcium (mg)	100
Sodium (mg)	228

Wild Rice Salad

Yield: 4–6 servings

Wild rice isn't really rice at all, but the seed of a grass. Hearty and chewy, its nutty flavor and dark color complement the green snow peas, dried apricots and citrusy flavors in this salad. It is perfect as a buffet dish, warm or cold.

Note:

To reduce the sodium content, choose a sodium-reduced vegetable broth.

3 cups	homemade gluten-free vegetable broth OR GF store-bought vegetable broth
1 cup	wild rice, rinsed 3 times and drained
1/2 tsp.	sea salt
1 cup	fresh snow peas
4	green onions, chopped
1/2 cup	chopped dried apricots
1/4 cup	chopped toasted walnuts
2 Tbsp.	fresh parsley, plus extra for garnish
1/4 cup	freshly-squeezed orange juice
2 Tbsp.	sherry vinegar
2 tsp.	grated orange zest
1	medium garlic clove, minced
1/4 tsp.	sea salt
1/8 tsp.	freshly ground black pepper
1 tsp.	extra-virgin olive oil

✦ In a large saucepan, bring the broth to a boil over high heat. Add the wild rice and salt. Return to a boil, reduce the heat to low and simmer, covered, until done, about 45 minutes. Drain any remaining liquid, then transfer the wild rice to a serving bowl.

✦ While the wild rice cooks, bring a small pan of water to a boil. Add the snow peas and cook 1 minute, then drain and immerse in cold water to stop cooking. Add them to the serving bowl, along with the green onions, apricots, walnuts and parsley.

✦ In small bowl, whisk together the orange juice, vinegar, orange zest, garlic, salt and pepper until well blended. Whisk in the oil until slightly thickened. Drizzle it over the salad and toss to coat well.

✦ Serve at room temperature, garnished with parsley. Or chill it for 4 hours, let stand at room temperature for 20 minutes and then serve.

Reprinted with permission from:
125 Gluten-Free Vegetarian Recipes, by
Carol Fenster, PhD
Avery/Penguin Group, 2011.

Nutritional Analysis	
1 serving = 1/6th recipe	
Calories (kcal)	191
Carbohydrates (g)	36
Dietary Fiber (g)	4
Fat (g)	5
Protein (g)	5
Iron (mg)	1.3
Calcium (mg)	45
Sodium (mg)	501

Fresh Rolls with Peanut Dipping Sauce

These light and delicious fresh rolls are a great appetizer for any occasion. Learning the art of "wrapping and rolling" may take a little practice!

Notes:

Other fillings such as sliced mango, bean sprouts, zucchini, spinach, cabbage, shrimp or pork can be used.

Add a small amount of sweet chili sauce on top of the filling before wrapping for more flavor.

Dipping sauce also can be drizzled on chicken skewers or stir-fried dishes.

Courtesy of:
Jessica Ethier, RD
Gluten-Free Nutrition Expert
Regina, SK, Canada

Nutritional Analysis

1 serving = 2 rolls and 2 Tbsp. sauce	
Calories (kcal)	394
Carbohydrates (g)	41
Dietary Fiber (g)	5
Fat (g)	18
Protein (g)	15
Iron (mg)	2
Calcium (mg)	40
Sodium (mg)	537

Fresh Rolls

12	rice paper wraps
4 oz.	vermicelli rice noodles
4	large green leafy lettuce leaves, torn into small pieces
1	avocado, peeled and thinly sliced
1	small English cucumber, sliced lengthwise and cut into thin sticks
2	carrots, grated or cut into thin strips
1 cup	cooked and shredded chicken

Dipping Sauce

1/2 cup	unsweetened natural peanut butter
1/4 cup	warm water
2 Tbsp.	brown sugar
1 Tbsp.	rice vinegar
1 Tbsp.	GF soy OR tamari sauce
1	clove garlic, minced
1/4 tsp.	red pepper flakes

Assembling Fresh Rolls

✦ Prepare vegetables and chicken, and place on large platter or into small bowls.

✦ Place vermicelli noodles in a medium-sized bowl and cover with boiling water. Let stand for 3–5 minutes until noodles are soft. Drain; however, leave a small amount of water to prevent noodles from clumping. Toss the noodles lightly to separate.

✦ Fill a large casserole dish with about 2 inches of very hot water (not boiling).

✦ Place one rice paper disc into the hot water for no more than 10 seconds. It will feel slightly firm when removed but will soften when filled.

✦ Place wrap on a flat surface and pat slightly dry with paper towel.

✦ Toward edge of wrap closest to you, arrange small amounts of each filling into a compact row.

✦ Fold edge snugly over filling and fold sides in toward center.

✦ Continue rolling tightly away from you to far edge, then place filled wrap seam-down on serving plate.

✦ Repeat for each wrap.

✦ If not serving immediately, place a damp cloth or paper towel on top of the rolls.

Sauce

✦ Combine all ingredients in a small sauce pan and heat on medium-low.

✦ Whisk then heat for 5 minutes.

✦ Serve warm or cold with the rolls.

Wondergrain Sorghum Stuffing

Yield: 8–10 servings

This variation on a traditional stuffing recipe features the versatile grain, sorghum. Serve this delicious accompaniment with turkey, chicken or Cornish hens.

Notes:

See page 144 for instructions for cooking sorghum grain.

If you prefer a moister stuffing, add ¼–½ cup of broth before baking.

If Wondergrain is cooked ahead of time and frozen or refrigerated, reheat in the microwave or on the stovetop to loosen up the grains. Add water, broth, olive oil or butter if a bit dry. Fluff up with a fork before adding to recipe.

Reprinted with permission from:
Wondergrain, Nature2Kitchen
7209 NW 41st St.
Miami, FL, U.S. 33166
877-307-0253
www.wondergrain.com

Nutritional Analysis	
1 serving = 1 cup	
Calories (kcal)	133
Carbohydrates (g)	34
Dietary Fiber (g)	4
Fat (g)	9
Protein (g)	5
Iron (mg)	1.3
Calcium (mg)	30
Sodium (mg)	42

4 cups	cooked Wondergrain
¾ cup	toasted chopped pecans
1½	medium to large sweet potatoes, peeled and cubed
1½ cups	diced celery
1	large onion, diced
10 oz.	white mushrooms, chopped
2–3	cloves of garlic, finely minced (or use a garlic press)
2–3	sprigs of fresh rosemary, finely chopped
	Handful fresh sage, finely chopped
2 Tbsp.	olive oil
	Salt and pepper to taste
pinch	crushed red peppers (to taste, or feel free to omit)
½ cup	dried cranberries

✦ Cook Wondergrain according to directions on package, except use a vegetable or chicken broth instead of water. Start grain before chopping the vegetables. Or better yet, always keep cooked Wondergrain in the freezer and warm up as needed for salads, stir-fries, and pretty much any dish.

✦ Place raw pecans in a sealable heavy plastic bag and use a rolling pin to break them into smaller pieces. Sauté pecans in a pan/skillet over medium heat (about 1–2 minutes), continuously tossing to prevent burning, until the nuts start to color.

✦ Preheat oven to 400°F. In a large bowl, toss sweet potatoes, celery, onion, mushrooms, garlic, rosemary, sage and olive oil until evenly coated. Spread out evenly onto a baking sheet and roast for 15–20 minutes, stirring mixture once halfway through.

✦ Mix the roasted vegetables with the cooked Wondergrain. Add the toasted pecans, salt, pepper, red pepper flakes (optional) and cranberries. Mix thoroughly.

✦ Place stuffing mixture into a greased oven-safe dish.

✦ Bake uncovered at 375°F for 10 minutes, then broil on low until top becomes golden brown.

Multi-Grain Pilaf

Yield: 12 servings

A combination of rice, lentils and gluten-free steel-cut oats are used to make this hearty side dish.

Note:

To reduce the sodium content, choose a sodium-reduced chicken stock.

1	medium onion, chopped
1 Tbsp.	canola oil
½ cup	uncooked lentils
½ cup	sliced almonds
½ cup	uncooked wild rice
½ cup	uncooked brown rice OR white rice
½ cup	uncooked Only Oats™ Steel Cut Oats
4 cups	gluten-free chicken stock
1 tsp.	Italian seasoning
1 tsp.	salt
2 Tbsp.	cooking sherry

✦ In a large skillet, sauté onion in canola oil until soft. Add lentils, almonds, wild rice, rice and steel-cut oats and toast for 1 minute. Stir frequently.

✦ Add stock, seasoning, salt and sherry. Simmer until liquid has evaporated, about 45–50 minutes. Stir frequently to avoid burning.

Reprinted with permission from:
Avena Foods Ltd.
316 1st Ave. E
Regina, SK, Canada S4N 5H2
866-461-3663 / 306-757-3663
www.avenafoods.com

Nutritional Analysis	
1 serving = ½ cup (126 g)	
Calories (kcal)	145
Carbohydrates (g)	22
Dietary Fiber (g)	3
Fat (g)	4
Protein (g)	6
Iron (mg)	1
Calcium (mg)	18
Sodium (mg)	401

Moroccan Millet

Yield: 6 servings

This pilaf is great as a one-dish meal or served with a fresh green salad.

Note:

For a lower-sodium version, choose a sodium-reduced gluten-free vegetable stock or broth.

2 Tbsp.	coconut OR olive OR organic canola OR safflower oil
1	EACH large red and green bell pepper, sliced into strips
1	large onion, sliced into half-moons
2 Tbsp.	crushed garlic
2 tsp.	paprika
1/2 tsp.	salt
1 tsp.	ground cumin
1/2 tsp.	ground cinnamon
1/4 tsp.	ground turmeric
1/4 tsp.	ground ginger
1/8 tsp.	ground cayenne
1 1/2 cups	uncooked millet
3 cups	GF vegetable stock
1 3/4 cups	cooked chickpeas OR a 15 oz. can (drained)
1/4 cup	raisins OR chopped GF dates
1/4 cup	sunflower seeds, pumpkin seeds OR pine nuts (optional)
	Salt and pepper to taste

✦ Place 1 Tbsp. of the oil in a large roasting pan. Add peppers, onion, garlic, paprika and salt. Toss until everything is evenly coated with oil and well combined.

✦ Place in preheated 450°F oven to roast for 20 minutes, stirring 2 or 3 times.

✦ Remove vegetables from oven and allow to cool until safe to handle, then chop them coarsely.

✦ Meanwhile, heat the remaining tablespoon of oil in a large saucepan. Add cumin, cinnamon, turmeric, ginger and cayenne. Stir over medium-high heat until spices are uniform in color and well combined, about 30 seconds.

✦ Add millet and stir quickly to coat, about 1 minute.

✦ Immediately pour in the vegetable stock and bring to a boil. Reduce heat, cover and cook until all the liquid is absorbed, about 20 minutes.

✦ Place millet in a large bowl and fluff with a fork.

✦ Add the roasted vegetables, chickpeas, raisins and optional seeds. Season with salt and pepper to taste. Toss gently and serve.

Reprinted with permission from:
Food Allergy Survival Guide – Surviving and Thriving with Food Allergies and Sensitivities by **Vesanto Melina, MS, RD**, **Jo Stepaniak, MSEd** and **Dina Aronson, MS, RD**
Healthy Living Publications, 2004

Nutritional Analysis	
1 serving	
Calories (kcal)	364
Carbohydrates (g)	63
Dietary Fiber (g)	10
Fat (g)	8
Protein (g)	11
Iron (mg)	3.8
Calcium (mg)	59
Sodium (mg)	233

Spicy Sweet Potato Bean Burgers

These tasty vegetarian burgers are rich in fiber and hold together well.

Note:

Canned black beans can be used instead of kidney beans.

1	small sweet potato
2 Tbsp.	canola oil, divided
2	cloves garlic, minced
1/2	yellow onion, diced
1 cup	shredded carrots (about 2 medium)
1	(19 oz.) can kidney beans, drained and rinsed
1	egg
1/2 cup	gluten-free bread crumbs
1 1/2 Tbsp.	chili powder
1/2 tsp.	cumin
1/2 tsp.	paprika
1/4 tsp.	cayenne pepper

Optional toppings: lettuce, tomato, sharp cheddar cheese, avocado

✦ Peel sweet potato and cut into small cubes. Toss with 1 Tbsp. oil and place on a baking sheet. Bake at 400°F for 30 minutes, or until golden brown and soft. Stir once halfway through cooking time.

✦ Heat remaining 1 Tbsp. oil in a non-stick skillet over medium heat. Add garlic and onions and cook for 2 minutes. Add shredded carrots and cook mixture for another 6–8 minutes.

✦ Mash kidney beans in a separate mixing bowl until almost smooth. Add egg, bread crumbs, chili powder, cumin, paprika, cayenne pepper, cooked sweet potatoes and carrot mixture. Stir until well combined.

✦ Form into 6 patties and place on wax paper-lined plate; freeze for 30 minutes.

✦ In a non-stick skillet on medium heat, cook burgers for about 8 minutes per side, or until golden brown and heated through.

✦ Place burger on bun and top with favorite fixings.

Courtesy of:
Jessica Ethier, RD
Gluten-Free Nutrition Expert
Regina, SK, Canada

Nutritional Analysis	
1 serving = 1 patty	
Calories (kcal)	193
Carbohydrates (g)	27
Dietary Fiber (g)	6
Fat (g)	7
Protein (g)	7
Iron (mg)	2.7
Calcium (mg)	40
Sodium (mg)	180

Hoisin Lentil Lettuce Wraps

Yield: 6 servings

This delicious Asian-inspired recipe is bursting with flavors and definitely will become one of your favorite recipes.

Note:

Substitute tofu for the turkey to make this a vegetarian option.

2 tsp.	canola oil
1 lb.	ground turkey or diced firm tofu
1	red pepper, cored and diced
2	garlic cloves, minced
1 Tbsp.	fresh ginger, grated
1/4 cup	cilantro stems, chopped
1/4 cup	uncooked split red lentils
1/3 cup	water
2 Tbsp.	GF hoisin sauce or GF sweet chili sauce
1 Tbsp.	GF soy sauce
2–3	green onions, chopped
1 head	butter, romaine or leaf lettuce
	Peanuts, for garnish
	Fresh cilantro leaves, for garnish (optional)
	Lime, cut into wedges

✦ Heat oil over medium-high heat in a large, heavy skillet. Add ground turkey and red pepper and cook, breaking turkey up with a spoon until the meat is no longer pink.

✦ Add garlic, ginger, cilantro stems and lentils and cook, stirring, for a minute.

✦ Add water and simmer for 10 minutes or until lentils are tender, any excess moisture has evaporated and the meat has started to brown.

✦ Add hoisin sauce, soy sauce and green onions. Cook for another 1–2 minutes, stirring until well blended and heated through.

✦ Core the head of lettuce, separating the leaves, and arrange on plate or platter. Place lentil mix in bowl and let each person scoop/spoon into lettuce "wrap," garnishing as desired.

Adapted and reprinted with permission from:
Canadian Lentils
207–116 Research Dr.
Saskatoon, SK, Canada S7N 3R3
306-668-3668
www.lentils.ca

Nutritional Analysis

1 serving = 3/4 cup	
Calories (kcal)	190
Carbohydrates (g)	13
Dietary Fiber (g)	3
Fat (g)	6
Protein (g)	23
Iron (mg)	2.5
Calcium (mg)	40
Sodium (mg)	380

Wild Rice, Chicken & Vegetable Casserole

Yield: 6 servings

Wild rice has a nutty taste that pairs well with mushrooms and broccoli to create this comforting meal.

2 cups	cooked wild rice (½ cup dry)
3	large or 4 small chicken breasts, raw, cubed
3 cups	broccoli florets
2 cups	chopped white mushrooms
1	(10 oz.) can GF condensed mushroom soup
²/₃ cup	milk
1 tsp.	dry sage
⅛ tsp.	black pepper
⅛ tsp.	garlic powder
1 cup	low-fat cheddar cheese

Wild Rice Preparation

✦ Wash wild rice in a wire strainer and rinse under cold water.

✦ Combine 2 cups water and ½ cup wild rice in a heavy saucepan. Bring to a boil, cover and simmer over low heat for approximately 45 minutes, until rice kernels have burst their shells and fluffed out. Drain off excess water. Stir rice with a fork; cover and let stand for 15 minutes.

Casserole Preparation

✦ Preheat oven to 375°F.

✦ In a greased casserole dish with a lid, layer cooked rice, chicken, broccoli then mushrooms.

✦ In a separate bowl, whisk together condensed soup, milk, sage, pepper and garlic powder. Pour mixture over ingredients in casserole dish.

✦ Cover with lid and bake for 35–40 minutes, until chicken is cooked through.

✦ Remove from oven and take off lid. Top with cheddar cheese. Return to oven and broil on high for 3–5 minutes, until browned.

Courtesy of:
Jessica Ethier, RD
Gluten-Free Nutrition Expert
Regina, SK, Canada

Nutritional Analysis	
1 serving	
Calories (kcal)	243
Carbohydrates (g)	22
Dietary Fiber (g)	3
Fat (g)	4
Protein (g)	33
Iron (mg)	1.4
Calcium (mg)	140
Sodium (mg)	588

Vegetable & Beef Lasagna

Yield: 10 servings

This variation on a popular Italian dish is packed with nutrient-rich vegetables and tastes delicious.

Note:

Either cooked or dry lasagna noodles can be used in this recipe. If using dry noodles, do not drain liquid from diced tomatoes when adding to the sauce mixture as the extra liquid will be absorbed.

1 lb.	extra-lean ground beef
2	cloves garlic, minced
1 cup	grated carrots
1 cup	grated zucchini
2 cups	chopped spinach
1	(27 oz.) can diced tomatoes, liquid drained (see Note)
1	(23 oz.) can tomato sauce
2	(5 oz.) cans tomato paste
1 Tbsp.	dried oregano
½ Tbsp.	dried basil
½ tsp.	dried thyme
½ tsp.	freshly ground black pepper
2 tsp.	sugar
10	large GF lasagna noodles
1	egg
1	container (approx. 2 cups) low-fat ricotta cheese
1½ cups	shredded reduced-fat mozzarella cheese, divided
¼ cup	grated Parmesan cheese

✦ In a large sauté pan, cook beef until browned. Place beef in a colander to drain off excess fat. Rinse well with hot water to remove additional fat.

✦ Return drained beef into pan. Add garlic, carrots and zucchini and cook for 8 minutes, or until vegetables are tender.

✦ Add spinach and cook for another 3–4 minutes.

✦ Add diced tomatoes, tomato sauce, tomato paste, oregano, basil, thyme, black pepper and sugar to the beef vegetable mixture.

✦ Turn heat to medium-low and let simmer for 20 minutes, stirring occasionally.

✦ While sauce is simmering, in a large pot cook noodles according to package directions. Rinse with cold water.

✦ Preheat oven to 375°F.

✦ Combine egg and ricotta cheese.

✦ Add 2 cups sauce to the bottom of a greased 9 x 13-inch baking dish. Lay 3 lasagna noodles on top of the sauce. Add half the ricotta cheese mixture and spread evenly over noodles. Top with ½ cup mozzarella cheese and another 2 cups of sauce.

✦ Repeat layering with remaining sauce and ricotta cheese mixture, and ½ cup of mozzarella.

✦ Top lasagna with the final 4 noodles, the last ½ cup of mozzarella and ¼ cup of Parmesan cheese.

✦ Cover pan with foil and bake for 20 minutes. Remove foil and bake for another 15 minutes.

✦ Broil on high for 5 minutes until cheese is browned.

✦ Remove from oven and let stand for 10 minutes before serving.

Courtesy of:
Jessica Ethier, RD
Gluten-Free Nutrition Expert
Regina, SK, Canada

Nutritional Analysis	
1 serving	
Calories (kcal)	386
Carbohydrates (g)	43
Dietary Fiber (g)	6
Fat (g)	14
Protein (g)	26
Iron (mg)	3.8
Calcium (mg)	280
Sodium (mg)	412

Black Bean Chili

Yield: 6–8 servings (8 cups)

The goodness of chili in a flash. The range of ingredients provides a powerful phyto-chemical mix in this vegetarian chili.

Note:

For a hearty turkey, chicken or beef black bean chili, sauté 1 lb. of ground meat in a heavy skillet. Drain off all fat; place the cooked meat in a colander and rinse with very hot or boiling water. Add to sautéed onions and garlic.

2 tsp.	extra-virgin olive oil
1 cup	chopped onions
3	large cloves garlic, finely chopped
1	green bell pepper, diced
1 cup	½-inch cubes zucchini (1 medium)
1 tsp.	finely chopped jalapeño pepper
2	(19 oz.) cans black beans, rinsed and drained
1	(28 oz.) can whole tomatoes, coarsely chopped, with juice
1 cup	frozen corn kernels
1 Tbsp.	chili powder
1 tsp.	ground cumin
1 tsp.	dried oregano
	salt to taste
3 Tbsp.	chopped fresh coriander, for garnish
	Shredded light cheddar cheese, for garnish (optional)

✦ Heat the oil in a large, heavy pot over medium heat.

✦ Add the onions and garlic; sauté for 5 minutes.

✦ Add the green pepper, zucchini and jalapeño pepper; sauté another 3 minutes.

✦ Add the black beans, tomatoes with juice, corn, chili powder, cumin and oregano.

✦ Reduce heat to medium-low and simmer, uncovered and stirring occasionally, for 30 minutes.

✦ Season with salt to taste.

✦ Garnish with coriander and cheddar, if using, before serving.

Reprinted with permission from:
The Enlightened Eaters™ Whole Foods Guide – Harvest the Power of Phyto Foods by **Rosie Schwartz**
Penguin Group, 2003

Nutritional Analysis	
1 serving = 1 cup	
Calories (kcal)	143
Carbohydrates (g)	31
Dietary Fiber (g)	9
Fat (g)	2
Protein (g)	8
Iron (mg)	3.1
Calcium (mg)	92
Sodium (mg)	581

Sahara Stew over Superblend Grains

Spices of Morocco combine in this delightful gravy full of tender beef, sweet potato and chickpeas topped with a pinch of lemon zest and fresh parsley. Serve it over ancient grains and you have a fine-dining dinner on a shoestring budget.

2 cups	water
½ cup	quinoa seeds
¼ cup	millet seeds
3 Tbsp.	buckwheat groats OR kañiwa seeds
1 Tbsp.	amaranth seeds OR teff grains
2 Tbsp.	grapeseed OR vegetable oil
1¼ lb.	sirloin steak, trimmed and cut into 1-inch chunks
¼ tsp.	freshly ground black pepper
1 cup	chopped onion
1 cup	chopped celery
2 tsp.	minced garlic
1 tsp.	turmeric
½ tsp.	cinnamon
½ tsp.	salt (optional)
⅓ cup	unsalted tomato paste
4 cups	low-sodium beef broth
2 cups	sweet potato, cut into 1-inch chunks
1	bay leaf
1 cup	cooked chickpeas
1 Tbsp.	fresh chopped parsley
1 Tbsp.	freshly grated lemon zest

✦ Combine the water and quinoa, millet, buckwheat and amaranth in a medium saucepan and bring to a boil. Reduce to a simmer, cover and cook for 20 minutes. Remove from the heat and fluff with a fork. Set aside and keep warm.

✦ Heat a large, deep pan over high heat. Add the oil and place the steak into the pan, leaving 1½ inches between each piece. Season with pepper and caramelize two sides of each piece (approx. 2 minutes per side), in two batches if necessary. Set meat aside in a shallow bowl covered with foil.

✦ Reduce the heat to medium-low, stir in the onion and celery and cook, covered, for about 7 minutes or until they start to soften, adding water if pan looks dry. Stir in and heat the garlic, turmeric, cinnamon and salt (if using) for about 1 minute. Stir in the tomato paste. Add the broth, sweet potato and bay leaf. Bring to a boil, reduce to a simmer, cover and cook for 10 minutes. Remove the lid and continue to simmer for another 10 minutes. Add the chickpeas and sirloin and simmer an additional 8 minutes. Serve stew over ancient grains with parsley and lemon zest lightly sprinkled on top.

Reprinted with permission from:
Grain Power by
Carol Hemming and
Patricia Green
Penguin Canada Books, 2014

Nutritional Analysis	
1 serving	
Calories (kcal)	480
Carbohydrates (g)	42
Dietary Fiber (g)	7
Fat (g)	17
Protein (g)	38
Iron (mg)	4.3
Calcium (mg)	50
Sodium (mg)	250

Turkey Meatballs with Lemon Sauce

Yield: 4 servings

Kasha (roasted buckwheat groats) adds a distinctive nutty flavor to these tasty meatballs. This serves four as an hors d'oeuvre or two as a main dish with a marinated vegetable or tossed green salad.

Note:

The original recipe had 1 tsp. Worcestershire sauce; however, some brands of Worcestershire sauce contain malt vinegar (which is not gluten-free) and/or soy sauce (which often contains wheat).

Adapted and reprinted with permission from:
The Birkett Mills
163 Main St.
Penn Yan, NY, U.S. 14527
315-536-3311
www.thebirkettmills.com

1 cup	cooked kasha (any granulation)
1	egg, beaten
1 tsp.	grated lemon zest
1½ lbs.	99% fat-free ground raw turkey
2 Tbsp.	vegetable oil
1 cup	GF chicken OR turkey broth
¼ cup	plain yogurt
1 Tbsp.	cornstarch
1 Tbsp.	lemon juice
1	small carrot, finely shredded
1	green onion, diced

✦ Prepare the kasha according to package directions, using chicken broth (gluten-free) as the liquid.

✦ Combine the prepared kasha, egg, lemon zest and turkey in a mixing bowl; blend well.

✦ Shape the mixture into 12 balls.

✦ In a large skillet, heat the oil and brown the balls on all sides. Add the broth; cover and simmer for 20 minutes. Use a slotted spoon to transfer the balls to a serving dish.

✦ In a small bowl, combine the yogurt, cornstarch and lemon juice.

✦ In the skillet, combine yogurt mixture with pan juices and cook until the sauce is thickened and bubbly. Add the carrot and onion. Cook for a few minutes more then pour the sauce over the meatballs and serve.

Nutritional Analysis	
1 serving	
Calories (kcal)	203
Carbohydrates (g)	9
Dietary Fiber (g)	1
Fat (g)	6
Protein (g)	29
Iron (mg)	1.3
Calcium (mg)	30
Sodium (mg)	99

Tabbouleh with Shrimp on Mixed Greens

Sorghum is a popular cereal grain in many countries around the world. It resembles bulgur or wheat berries when cooked. It is a hearty, chewy solution to meeting our daily goal of 2 to 3 servings of whole grains per day.

Notes:

Brown rice or quinoa can be used instead of sorghum.

In place of the edamame, use other seasonal vegetables such as steamed green beans or broccoli.

Courtesy of:
Carol Fenster, PhD, author of a variety of gluten-free cookbooks (see pp. 297, 298)
www.carolfenstercooks.com

Nutritional Analysis	
1 serving	
Calories (kcal)	235
Carbohydrates (g)	31
Dietary Fiber (g)	7
Fat (g)	10
Protein (g)	9
Iron (mg)	3
Calcium (mg)	78
Sodium (mg)	363

To cook the sorghum

1 cup	uncooked whole grain sorghum (soaked overnight in water to cover)
3/4 tsp.	sea salt, divided
2 cups	water

Dressing

2 Tbsp.	freshly squeezed lemon juice
3 Tbsp.	extra-virgin olive oil
1 Tbsp.	sherry vinegar
1/8 tsp.	white pepper

Vegetables

1/4 cup	shelled raw pumpkin seeds OR pine nuts
1	English OR hothouse cucumber, unpeeled and chopped
3	green onions, chopped
1	small red bell pepper, chopped, OR 12 grape tomatoes, halved
1	small yellow bell pepper, chopped
1/2 cup	cooked edamame
1/2 cup	chopped seasonal fruit (figs, pears, apples, oranges or dried cranberries)
1/2 cup	chopped fresh parsley, plus extra for garnish
1/2 cup	chopped fresh cilantro
1/4 cup	chopped fresh mint
	Mixed greens
1/4 cup	crumbled feta cheese OR queso fresco (optional)
12	cooked large whole shrimp, peeled (or more to taste)

✦ Drain the soaked sorghum and discard water. In a heavy medium saucepan, combine sorghum, 1/2 tsp. of the salt, and 2 cups water. Bring to boil. Cover and reduce heat, simmering for 40–45 minutes. Transfer to a strainer and drain well. Set aside.

✦ Make the dressing: In a screw-top jar, shake the lemon juice, oil, vinegar, remaining 1/4 tsp. of sea salt and pepper until thoroughly blended and creamy. Set aside.

✦ Toast pumpkin seeds in a skillet over medium heat, stirring constantly until lightly browned, about 5 minutes. Set aside.

✦ In a large bowl, combine the sorghum and the vegetables (except mixed greens) and toss to blend. Add dressing and toss until all ingredients are well coated. Let stand for 20 minutes before serving.

✦ Arrange mixed greens on a large platter, top with tabbouleh, arrange shrimp (and optional cheese) on top and serve, garnished with fresh parsley.

Oven-Fried Chicken

Ground flaxseed and GF crackers or cornflakes are used to add crunch to this crispy chicken dish.

Note:
For a lower-fat version, omit the butter.

1	egg, beaten
3 Tbsp.	non-fat (skim) milk
1/2 cup	ground flaxseed (flaxseed meal)
1/2 cup	GF crackers OR GF cornflakes (finely crushed)
1/4 tsp.	ground black pepper
1 Tbsp.	dried parsley flakes
1 tsp.	chili powder
1 tsp.	garlic powder
1 tsp.	salt
2-3 lbs.	chicken thighs
2 Tbsp.	melted butter

✦ In a small bowl, combine egg and milk.

✦ In a shallow container, combine ground flax, GF cracker or cornflake crumbs, pepper, parsley, chili powder, garlic and salt.

✦ Remove skin from chicken thighs and rinse with warm water. Pat dry.

✦ Dip chicken thighs into egg mixture then coat with the crumb mixture.

✦ Place chicken thighs on a greased 10 x 15-inch baking pan so thighs do not touch.

✦ Drizzle chicken thighs with melted butter.

✦ Bake in a preheated 350°F oven for 45 minutes, or until chicken is tender and no longer pink. Do not turn chicken thighs while baking.

Adapted and reprinted with permission from:
Flax: Family Favorites – Recipes and Healthful Tips by **The Flax Council of Canada**
465–167 Lombard Ave.
Winnipeg, MB, Canada R3B 0T6
204-982-2115
www.flaxcouncil.ca

Saskatchewan Flax Development Commission
A5A – 116 103rd St. E
Saskatoon, SK, Canada S7N 1Y7
306-664-1901
www.saskflax.com

Nutritional Analysis	
1 serving	
Calories (kcal)	291
Carbohydrates (g)	10
Dietary Fiber (g)	3
Fat (g)	12
Protein (g)	34
Iron (mg)	3.1
Calcium (mg)	56
Sodium (mg)	564

Lentil Pizza Squares

Yield: 12 servings

Serve these pizza squares with a green salad for a main course or alone as a substantial snack.

¼ cup	canola oil
¾ cup	chopped onion
1 cup	sliced mushrooms
1	garlic clove, minced
4	eggs
1½ cups	lentil purée (see below)
1½ cups	low-fat sour cream
1	(7½ oz.) can tomato sauce
¾ cup	cornmeal
1 tsp.	crumbled dried basil
1 tsp.	crumbled dried oregano
½ tsp.	salt
1½ cups	grated low-fat cheddar cheese
1½ cups	grated low-fat mozzarella cheese
½ cup	sliced GF pepperoni OR salami
½ cup	diced sweet green pepper

✦ In a skillet, heat the oil and add the onion, mushrooms and garlic. Sauté until onion is translucent. Remove from heat and let cool.

✦ In a large mixing bowl, beat eggs then blend in lentil purée, sour cream, tomato sauce, cornmeal, basil, oregano, salt and mushroom mixture. Stir in the cheeses.

✦ Spoon the batter into a 9 x 13-inch baking dish sprayed with non-stick vegetable spray.

✦ Garnish with pepperoni and green pepper.

✦ Bake in preheated 350°F oven for 40–45 minutes, or until firm to the touch. Let stand 10 minutes before cutting into 12 squares.

Lentil Purée

¾ cup	lentils
2 cups	water

✦ Rinse the dry lentils and drain.

✦ Combine with water and bring to a boil. Reduce heat and simmer for 45–50 minutes.

✦ Drain off any excess liquid and mash lentils with a potato masher.

✦ Cool the purée before adding to recipe.

Courtesy of:
Saskatchewan Pulse Growers
207–116 Research Dr.
Saskatoon, SK, Canada S7N 3R3
306-668-5556
www.saskpulse.com

Nutritional Analysis	
1 serving = 1 square	
Calories (kcal)	292
Carbohydrates (g)	20
Dietary Fiber (g)	4
Fat (g)	17
Protein (g)	16
Iron (mg)	2.2
Calcium (mg)	226
Sodium (mg)	542

Pepperoni Pizza

Yield: 12" pizza

A combination of gluten-free flours and starches can be used to make a pizza crust. Here's an easy recipe for a weekend favorite that everyone will enjoy.

Note:

Add your favorite toppings such as green peppers, mushrooms, onions and olives.

Yeast Mixture

1 Tbsp.	active dry yeast
³/₄ cup	warm (110°F) milk of choice
1 tsp.	sugar

Dry Ingredients

²/₃ cup	brown rice flour, plus more for sprinkling
¹/₄ cup	potato starch
¹/₄ cup	arrowroot starch
1 tsp.	xanthan gum
1 tsp.	Italian seasoning
¹/₂ tsp.	salt

Liquids

2 tsp.	olive oil, plus extra for brushing the crust
2 tsp.	cider vinegar

Topping

1 cup	store-bought gluten-free pizza sauce
12	gluten-free pepperoni slices
1¹/₂ cups	shredded mozzarella cheese OR cheese alternative

✦ Place oven racks in the bottom and middle positions of the oven. Preheat oven to 400°F.

✦ Dissolve yeast and sugar in the warm milk for 5 minutes.

✦ In a food processor, blend all dry ingredients and liquids, including the yeast mixture, until the dough forms a ball. The dough will be very, very soft. (Or, blend in a medium bowl, using an electric mixer on low speed until well blended.)

✦ Place the dough in the center of a 12-inch non-stick (gray, not black) pizza pan greased with vegetable shortening, not cooking spray. Liberally sprinkle rice flour onto the dough then press the dough into the pan with your hands, continuing to dust the dough with flour to prevent sticking. Make edges thicker to contain toppings, taking care to make dough as smooth and even as possible for the prettiest crust.

✦ Bake the pizza crust 10 minutes on the bottom rack. Remove from oven and brush edges of crust with olive oil. Spread with pizza sauce. Arrange pepperoni on top and sprinkle with cheese. Return pizza to oven and bake on middle rack until nicely browned, about 15–20 minutes.

✦ Remove pizza from oven and cool on a wire rack for 5 minutes. At this point, you may either brush the crust with a little olive oil or immediately cut into 6 slices. Serve warm.

Courtesy of:
Carol Fenster, PhD, author of a variety of gluten-free cookbooks (see pp. 297, 298)
www.carolfenstercooks.com

Nutritional Analysis

1 serving = ¹/₆th pizza	
Calories (kcal)	265
Carbohydrates (g)	20
Dietary Fiber (g)	1
Fat (g)	15
Protein (g)	11
Iron (mg)	1
Calcium (mg)	265
Sodium (mg)	821

Thai Hot-and-Sour Sauce

Yield: 1⅓ cups

This delectable, spicy sauce is fabulous on tossed green salads, sliced tomatoes, steamed cabbage wedges, stir-fried vegetables and rice, and rice noodles with steamed veggies. You're bound to think of many other uses as well.

⅓ cup	sesame tahini, other seed butter OR almond butter
⅓ cup	fresh lime juice
3 Tbsp.	water
2 Tbsp.	balsamic vinegar
2 Tbsp.	dark sesame oil OR extra-virgin olive oil
2 Tbsp.	sugar
2 tsp.	dried basil
1 tsp.	dried spearmint
1 tsp.	ground ginger
1 tsp.	crushed garlic
¼ tsp.	crushed hot red pepper flakes

✦ Combine all of the ingredients in a small bowl and whisk until thick and smooth.

Reprinted with permission from:
***Food Allergy Survival Guide –
Surviving and Thriving with
Food Allergies and Sensitivities***
by
**Vesanto Melina, MS, RD
Jo Stepaniak, MSEd** and
Dina Aronson, MS, RD
Healthy Living Publications, 2004

Nutritional Analysis

1 serving = ⅓ cup

Calories (kcal)	218
Carbohydrates (g)	15
Dietary Fiber (g)	2
Fat (g)	18
Protein (g)	4
Iron (mg)	1.4
Calcium (mg)	52
Sodium (mg)	11

Gluten-Free Products

15

The gluten-free marketplace has expanded rapidly, especially over the past few years. Whereas historically only a handful of small specialty companies made gluten-free products, today many manufacturers of all sizes offer a wide range of options for the gluten-free consumer.

This chapter lists over 3700 gluten-free products from the U.S., Canada and other countries, providing an extensive selection of products in various categories. Availability of products will vary depending on your location and companies may choose to discontinue items at any time. Manufacturers do not pay to have their products listed in this book. The author includes product listings for informational purposes only. Product and manufacturer information, exhaustively researched between January and July 2016, is from sources believed to be reliable at the time of printing.

When purchasing a product, be sure to read the label every time because (1) manufacturers may change the ingredient formulation and (2) the brand may offer a gluten-free and non-gluten-free version of the same product with similar packaging. If ever in doubt about a product's gluten-free status, contact the manufacturer. A company directory for products listed in this chapter is found on pages 263–286. More gluten-free shopping tips are in chapter 11 (pp. 131–134.)

Gluten-Free Product Manufacturing Information

While many companies in this guide manufacture gluten-free foods exclusively, others produce both gluten-free and gluten-containing items. Production of gluten-free foods can occur in different types of facilities under various scenarios such as in a:

- Dedicated gluten-free facility

- Dedicated gluten-free production area within a shared facility (sometimes in a different room with a separate ventilation system) and on dedicated gluten-free equipment

- Shared facility and shared production area but processed on dedicated gluten-free equipment

- Shared facility and shared (thoroughly cleaned) equipment

Regardless of the type of facility, the manufacturer is required to have "Good Manufacturing Practices" (GMPs) that include strict quality control policies and protocols to mitigate the risk of cross-contamination from allergen and gluten sources. For many companies, one component of their food safety program is testing of equipment, ingredients and/or finished products for allergens and gluten sources (although the frequency of this testing can vary considerably). In addition, some companies require their ingredient suppliers to provide documentation of allergen and gluten testing.

Manufacturers making a gluten-free claim must ensure their products do not exceed the 20 ppm gluten threshold level and meet all other requirements established by governmental regulatory agencies in the U.S. and Canada. See pages 51–54 and 56–58 for information about the specific gluten-free labeling regulations.

Product Information Charts

Products are separated into general categories (see following page) then alphabetized by company or brand name. Some products are available in different sizes (e.g., single-serve, family, bulk, food service) and/or have other attributes (e.g., organic, kosher); however, these versions have not been identified in this guide. To learn more about the various product formats, review each company's website (see pp. 263–286).

Chart Symbols

♦ Diamond symbol indicates a company or brand that produces **only** gluten-free products (therefore names not carrying the symbol are manufacturers of both gluten-free **and** gluten-containing products). Regardless of whether or not the diamond symbol is present, the company manufactures all or some of its gluten-free products either (1) in dedicated gluten-free facilities, or (2) on dedicated equipment in segregated areas of its facilities, or (3) in shared facilities cleaned to mitigate the risk of cross-contamination for allergen and gluten sources. At any time manufacturers can change how and where they produce gluten-free foods, which is why this information is not included in the guide. To learn more about a particular company's methods in gluten-free food production, contact the brand directly.

GF When "GF" appears before the product name, it indicates that

   (1) a company manufacturers two "versions" of the same product – one is gluten free and one is not gluten free (e.g., GF cornflakes [without barley malt flavor] and regular cornflakes [made with barley malt flavor]), and/or

   (2) the company produces both gluten-free and gluten-containing items (e.g. turkey soup with rice [gluten free] and chicken noodle soup [not gluten free]).

   The "GF" is a reminder to check the product label so that you purchase the gluten-free item.

* Gluten-free products that contain oats will be followed by an asterisk (*) symbol. Also, appendix A on page 305 lists the brands that include oats in some or all of their gluten-free products.

The author assumes no liability for any errors, omissions or inaccuracies in this chapter. Products included in this book serve as a guide only and not all items may be suitable for every gluten-free consumer.

Gluten-Free Product Directory

Cereals and Granola 208

Baked Products 212
    Breads 212
    Yeast-Free Breads 213
    Baguettes, Flatbreads and Focaccia 213
    Pitas, Tortillas and Wraps 213
    Buns and Rolls 214
    Bagels, Biscuits, English Muffins
    and Scones 215
    Muffins and Loaves 215
    French Toast, Pancakes and Waffles 216
    Brownies and Squares 217
    Cakes and Cupcakes 217
    Cinnamon Buns and Doughnuts 218
    Cheesecakes, Pies, Tarts and
    Other Pastries 218
    Biscotti, Cookies, Graham Crackers
    and Wafers 218
    Dough – Bread, Cookie, Pie and Pizza 221
    Crusts – Pie, Pizza and Tart 221

Crackers, Breadsticks, Corn/Rice Cakes.... 222
    Savory Crackers and Breadsticks 222
    Corn and Rice Cakes 223

Communion Hosts/Wafers 224

Snacks 224
    Candy, Chips, Nuts, Seeds, Pretzels
    and Miscellaneous 224
    Ice Cream Cones/Cups 227
    Snack Bars 227

Baking Mixes 231

Flours 237
    Bean, Chickpea, Lentil and Pea Flours 238
    Other Flours and Miscellaneous 238

Starches and Gums 240

Coatings, Croûtons, Crumbs
and Stuffings 241

Grains 243

Side Dishes, Gnocchi and Perogies,
Entrées, Breaded Fish and Poultry
and Veggie Burgers 244
    Side Dishes 244
    Gnocchi and Perogies 245
    Entrées 246
    Breaded Fish and Poultry 249
    Veggie Burgers 250

Dry Pasta, Fresh Pasta and Pasta Meals .. 250
    Dry Pasta 250
    Fresh Pasta 253
    Pasta Meals 253

Pizza 256

Broths, Bouillons, Soups and Stocks 257

Gravy Mixes 260

Sauces 260

Soy Sauces 261

Beers 262

Cereals and Granola

- Most corn- or rice-based cereals are **NOT** gluten-free as they usually contain barley malt, barley malt extract or barley malt flavoring. However, there are gluten-free versions of these cereals available in the regular cereal aisle or natural food / special diet section of retail or online stores.

- Some cereals labeled "**wheat free**" are **NOT** gluten-free because they contain barley, rye and/or regular oats.

- Avoid regular oats due to high levels of contamination with wheat, rye and/or barley. Fortunately, many companies produce gluten-free oats and oat-based cereals (identified by the asterisk [*] symbol throughout this guide). To learn more about the safety of oats, see pages 27–30.

Cereals and Granola

Company or Brand	Product	Varieties or Flavors
Ancient Harvest♦	Ancient Grains Hot Cereal*	Apple Cinnamon; Banana & Brown Sugar; Honey Vanilla Spice; Maple Morning; Traditional
	Quinoa Hot Cereal Flakes	
Bakery On Main♦	Bunches of Crunches Grainola*	Dark Chocolate Sea Salt with Chia; Coconut Cacao
	Fiber Power Granola*	Cinnamon Raisin; Triple Berry
	Granola	Apple Raisin Walnut; Cranberry Orange Cashew; Extreme Fruit and Nut; Nutty Cranberry Maple; Rainforest Banana Nut
	Happy Oats*	Quick; Rolled; Steel Cut
	Hot Breakfast Instant Cereal	Amaranth Multigrain; Coffee; Dried Plum; Maple; Quinoa Multigrain
	Instant Oatmeal*	Apple Pie; Blueberry Scone; Carrot Cake; Maple Multigrain Muffin; Strawberry Shortcake; Traditional
Barbara's	GF Brown Rice Crisps	
	GF Corn Flakes	
	GF Honest O's Multigrain*	
	GF Puffins	Honey Rice; Multigrain*
Barkat♦	Chocolate Pillows	
	Corn Flakes	Chocolate; Frosted; Plain
	Porridge Flakes	
	Rice Crunchies	Chocolate; Plain
Bob's Red Mill	GF 8 Grain Hot Cereal*	
	GF Corn Grits	
	GF Brown Rice Farina Hot Cereal	
	GF Corn Grits	
	GF Creamy Buckwheat Hot Cereal	
	GF Granola*	Apple Blueberry; Honey Oat
	GF Mighty Tasty Hot Cereal	
	GF Millet Grits	
	GF Muesli*	
	GF Oat Bran Cereal*	
	GF Oatmeal Cup* with Flax & Chia	Apple Pieces and Cinnamon; Blueberry and Hazelnut; Brown Sugar and Maple; Classic
	GF Rolled Oats*	Extra Thick; Old Fashioned; Quick Cooking

Cereals and Granola (cont'd)

Company or Brand	Product	Varieties or Flavors
Bob's Red Mill (cont'd)	GF Scottish Oatmeal*	
	GF Steel Cut Oats*	
Canyon Oats◆	Granola*	Honey Crisp Vanilla & Cinnamon
	Oatmeal Cup*	Brown Sugar; Cherry, Cranberry & Walnut; Cinnamon Apple (No Sugar Added); Honey; Maple; Maple & Almond; Sweet Honey Cinnamon with Golden Raisins
Cream Hill Estates◆	Lara's Gluten-Free Oats*	Rolled
Cuisine Soleil◆	Buckwheat Flakes	
El Peto Products◆	Cream of Brown Rice	Apple Cinnamon; Plain
	Cream of White Rice	
EnviroKidz◆	Amazon Flakes	
	Chocolate Choco Chimps	
	Chocolate Koala Crisp	
	Cinnamon Jungle Munch	
	Gorilla Munch Corn Puffs	
	Oatmeal*	Apple Cinnamon; Brown Sugar Maple; Homestyle
	Peanut Butter & Chocolate Leaping Lemurs	
	Peanut Butter Panda Puffs	
Erewhon◆	GF Corn Flakes	
	GF Crispy Brown Rice	Cinnamon; Plain
	GF Granola*	Cranberry Chia; Simply Vanilla
	GF Harvest Medley	
	GF Honey Rice Twice	
Flax4Life◆	Flax Granola*	Apple Cinnamon; Banana Coconut; Chunky Chocolate; Cranberry Orange; Hawaiian Pineapple Coconut & Mango
Freedom Foods◆	All Round Goodness	Natural Maple Syrup
	Ancient Grain Flakes	
	Crunch Cereal	Cocoa; Maple; Pro-Teen
	Fruity Rainbow Rocks!	
	Quick Oats*	Berry Delight
	TropicO's	
GF Harvest◆	Granola*	Oatmeal Cookie Crisp
	Oat Groats*	
	Oatmeal GOPack*	Cinnamon Apple; Maple & Brown Sugar; Original; Sweet Cinnamon & Golden Raisins
	Old Fashioned Rolled Oats*	
	Quick Oats*	
	Steel-Cut Oats*	
Glutenfreeda Foods◆	Granola*	Apple Almond Honey; Cranberry Cashew Honey; Raisin Almond Honey
	Instant Oatmeal*	Apple Cinnamon with Flax; Banana Maple with Flax; Brown Sugar with Flax; Cranberry Cinnamon with Flax; Maple Raisin with Flax; Natural; Strawberries and Brown Sugar with Flax

Cereals and Granola (cont'd)

Company or Brand	Product	Varieties or Flavors
Glutenfreeda Foods♦ (cont'd)	Instant Oatmeal Cup*	Blueberries, Strawberries & Brown Sugar; Brown Sugar & Flax; Cranberry Apple with Walnuts & Cinnamon; Golden & Brown Raisins with Almonds
	Oats*	Quick Rolled; Steel Cut; Traditional Rolled
Gluten-Free Prairie♦	Granola*	Montana Mornings
	Oat Groats*	
	Oatmeal*	
GoGo Quinoa♦	4 Grain Hot Cereal	
	Crunchy Muesli	
	Quinoa Cocoa Puffed Cereal	
	Quinoa Crunchies	Chocolate; Cinnamon; Original
	Quinoa Instant Flakes	
	Quinoa Puffs	
Grain-Free JK Gourmet♦	Granola	Apple, Spice & Raisin; Black Cherry & Apple; Blueberry & Black Currant; Cranberry Cashew; Fig & Apricot; Hazelnut & Date; Nuts & Raisins
Hodgson Mill	GF Creamy Hot Cereal	Buckwheat with Milled Flax Seed
	GF Rolled Oats*	Quick Rolled; Thick Cut
	GF Steel-Cut Oats, Sorghum & Quinoa Hot Cereal*	
Kashi Canada	GF Corn Cereal	Indigo Morning; Simply Maize
	GF GOLEAN® Clusters Cereal	Vanilla Pepita
The Kashi Company	GF Corn Cereal	Indigo Morning; Simply Maize
	GF GOLEAN® Clusters Cereal	Vanilla Pepita
Kay's Naturals♦	Protein Cereal	Apple Cinnamon; French Vanilla; Honey Almond
Kellogg Canada	GF Brown Rice Krispies	
Kellogg Company (U.S.)	GF Special K	Touch of Brown Sugar
KIND♦	Healthy Grains Granola Clusters*	Banana Nut; Cinnamon Oat with Flax Seeds; Dark Chocolate Whole Grain; Maple Quinoa with Chia Seeds; Oats & Honey with Toasted Coconut; Peanut Butter Whole Grain; Raspberry with Chia Seeds; Vanilla Blueberry with Flax Seeds
Libre Naturals♦	Granola*	Blueberry Maple; Vanilla Caramel; Vanilla Cinnamon
	Oatmeal Cup*	Apple & Cinnamon; Blueberries & Cranberry; Blueberries, Apples & Sunflower Seeds; Pumpkin Seeds, Raisins & Spices
	Oat Flakes*	Quick; Rolled
Nature's Path	GF Corn Flakes	Fruit Juice Sweetened; Honey'd
	GF Crispy Rice	
	GF Granola*	Honey Almond; Fruit & Nut; Summer Berries; Vanilla Cranberry
	GF Hot Oatmeal*	Brown Sugar Maple with Ancient Grains; Homestyle; Spiced Apple with Flax
	GF Mesa Sunrise Cereal	Plain; With Raisins
	GF Oats*	Old Fashioned; Steel Cut
	GF Qi'a Chia, Buckwheat & Hemp Cereal	Apple Cinnamon; Cranberry Vanilla; Original Flavor
	GF Qi'a Hot Oatmeal*	Cinnamon Pumpkin Seed; Creamy Coconut; Super Seeds & Grains

Cereals and Granola (cont'd)

Company or Brand	Product	Varieties or Flavors
Nature's Path (cont'd)	GF Qi'a Superflakes Cereal	Cocoa Coconut; Coconut Chia; Honey Chia
	GF Sunrise Crunchy Cereal	Cinnamon; Honey; Maple; Vanilla
	GF Whole O's	
Only Oats (Avena Foods)♦	Oats*	Quick Flakes; Rolled; Steel-Cut
Orgran♦	O's Cereal	Buckwheat (Maple Flavor); Itsy Bitsy Cocoa; Multigrain Breakfast with Quinoa; Rice (Wildberry Flavor)
	Quinoa Flakes	
	Quinoa Porridge	Apple & Cinnamon; Berry; Plain
	Quinoa Puffs	
Pocono (The Birkett Mills)	Cream of Buckwheat Hot Cereal	
Premium Gold Flax♦	Super Booster Seeds and Grains	
Purely Elizabeth♦	Ancient Grain Granola*	Blueberry Hemp; Cranberry Pecan; Original; Pumpkin Fig
	Ancient Grain Granola + Puffs Cereal*	Blueberry Hemp; Cranberry Pecan; Original; Pumpkin Fig
	Ancient Grain Granola + Puffs Cereal Cup*	Blueberry Hemp; Cranberry Pecan; Original; Pumpkin Fig
	Ancient Grain Hot Cereal*	6 Grain
	Ancient Grain Muesli*	Apple Current; Cranberry Cashew; Mango Almond
	Ancient Grain Oatmeal*	Apple Cinnamon Pecan; Cranberry Pumpkin Seed; Original
	Ancient Grain Oatmeal Cup*	Apple Cinnamon Pecan; Cranberry Pumpkin Seed; Original
	Grain-Free Granola	Banana Nut Butter; Original
	Probiotic Granola*	Chocolate Sea Salt; Maple Walnut
Quaker	GF Instant Oatmeal*	Maple & Brown Sugar; Original
	GF Quick 1-Minute Oats*	
Udi's Gluten Free♦	Granola*	Au Natural; Cranberry; Original; Vanilla
	Granola Clusters*	Active Antioxidant Blueberry Cashew; Active with Omega 3 Cherry Walnut
	Steel Cut Oats*	Currants, Flax & Chia; Plain
Van's	GF Cereal*	Blissfully Berry; Cinnamon Heaven; Cocoa Sensation; Honey Crunch
	GF Soft Baked Whole Grain Granola*	Banana Nut; Blueberry Walnut; Cranberry Almond; Double Chocolate
Viki's♦	Granola*	Apple Cinnamon; Banana Walnut; Blueberry Almond; Maple Cranberry; Original
Wolff's (The Birkett Mills)	Cream of Buckwheat	

Baked Products

- **NOT** all "**wheat-free**" baked products (e.g., breads, cookies) are gluten free. Some may contain barley flour or regular oats.

- Gluten-free baked products are located in the bakery, dry goods, gluten-free or frozen section of retail outlets or online.

- Some gluten-free baked products are vacuum-packed for a shelf life of four months to one year from the date of manufacture.

- Ready-to-eat gluten-free baked products are convenient but usually quite expensive. For more economical options:

  - Use gluten-free mixes (see pp. 231–237) or various flours (see pp. 237–240) to make your own bread, muffins, pancakes, waffles and other baked items.

  - Try the bread, cookie and muffin recipes in chapter 14 (pp. 157–204) or check out the gluten-free cookbooks and other culinary resources listed on pages 297–300.

Breads

Company or Brand	Product	Varieties or Flavors
All But Gluten♦	Bread (Loaf)	Cinnamon Raisin; Italian Style 6 Grains & Seeds; Italian Style White; Sliced White; Whole Grain
Amy's	GF Sandwich Rounds	
Barkat♦	Par-Baked Bread	Country Loaf; White Sliced
	Sliced Bread	Brown; Multi-Grain; White; Whole-Meal
BFree Foods♦	Bread (Loaf)	Brown Seeded; Soft White
Canyon Bakehouse♦	Bread	Cinnamon Raisin; Deli Rye Style; Mountain White; Seven-Grain
	Focaccia	Rosemary & Thyme
Dempster's Bakery	GF Gluten Zero Bread (Loaf)	White; Whole Grain
El Peto Products♦	Bread	Gourmet; Italian Style; Millet; Potato; Raisin; Supreme Italian; Tapioca; White; Whole Grain Brown; Whole Grain Flax Seed; Whole Grain Multi-Grain
	Sandwich Bread	White Rice; Whole Grain Brown
Ener-G♦	Bread (Loaf)	Brown Rice; Brown Rice (Light); Corn; Hi-Fiber; Papa's; Raisin (Egg Free); Rice Starch; Seattle Brown; Tapioca (Light); Tapioca (Regular Sliced); Tapioca (Thin Sliced); White Rice; White Rice (Light); White Rice Flax; White Rice Flax (Light)
	Select Bread	Cinnamon Raisin; Deli-Style White; Northwest Banana; Pacific Molasses; Pretzel; Sourdough White
Food For Life	GF All Natural Bread	Bhutanese Red Rice; Brown Rice; Exotic Black Rice; Raisin Pecan; Rice Almond; Rice Millet; Rice Pecan; White Rice
	GF Sprouted For Life Bread	Almond; Cinnamon Raisin; Flax; Original 3 Seed
Glutenfree Bakehouse (Whole Foods)♦	Bread	Cinnamon Raisin; Corn; Honey Oat*; Light White*; Prairie; Sandwich; Sundried Tomato & Roasted Garlic
Glutino♦	Bread	Cinnamon Raisin; Seeded
	Sandwich Bread	Multigrain; White
Kinnikinnick♦	Soft Bread	Cinnamon Raisin; Multigrain; White; Whole Grain

Breads (cont'd)

Company or Brand	Product	Varieties or Flavors
Little Northern Bakehouse♦	Bread	Cinnamon & Raisin; Millet Chia; Seeds & Grains
O'Doughs♦	Bread	Flax; White
President's Choice	GF Bread (Loaf)	Multigrain; White
Promise Gluten Free♦	Bread	High Fiber Multigrain; Raisin
	Loaf	Chia Seed; White
Rudi's Gluten-Free Bakery♦	Bread (Fresh)	Multigrain; Original
	Bread (Frozen)	Cinnamon Raisin; Deli-Style with Caraway Seeds; Hearty Fiber; Multigrain; Original
	Toast (Heat & Serve)	Cheesy; Garlic
Schär♦	Bread	Deli-Style; Hearty Grain; Hearty White
	Bread (Artisan Baker)	Multigrain; White
Silver Hills	GF Bread	Chia Chia; Omega Flax
Three Bakers♦	Whole-Grain Bread	7 Ancient Grains; Cinnamon Raisin; Great Seed; MaxOmega; Rye Style; White
Udi's Gluten Free♦	Bread	Cinnamon Raisin; Millet-Chia; Omega Flax & Fiber; Rye Style; White Sandwich; Whole Grain

Yeast-Free Breads

Company or Brand	Product	Varieties or Flavors
El Peto Products♦	Bread	Flax Seed; Whole Grain Brown
Ener-G♦	Loaf	Brown Rice; Flax Meal; White Rice
Food For Life	GF Yeast Free Bread	Brown Rice; Multi Seed Rice Bread

Baguettes, Flatbreads and Focaccia

Company or Brand	Product	Varieties or Flavors
Barkat♦	Baguette	Home Fresh Par-Baked; Par-Baked
Ener-G♦	Focaccia Crust	
Glutenfreeda Foods♦	Artisan Flatbread and Pizza Crust	Original; Parmesan & Asiago Cheese; Roasted Garlic; Sun-Dried Tomato & Herbs
O'Doughs♦	Flatbread	Multigrain; Original
President's Choice	GF Baguette	White
	GF Demi-Baguette	Multigrain
Schär♦	Baguettes	
Udi's Gluten Free♦	French Baguettes	

Pitas, Tortillas and Wraps

Company or Brand	Product	Varieties or Flavors
BFree Foods♦	Pita Breads	
	Wraps	Multigrain; Quinoa & Chia Seed; Sweet Potato
Food For Life	GF Tortillas	Black Rice; Brown Rice

Pitas, Tortillas and Wraps (cont'd)

Company or Brand	Product	Varieties or Flavors
La Tortilla Factory	GF Ivory Teff Wraps	
	GF Sonoma Whole Grain Ivory Teff Wraps	
	GF Traditional Corn Tortillas	Yellow; White
Rudi's Gluten-Free Bakery◆	Tortillas	Fiesta; Plain; Spinach
Toufayan Bakeries	GF Wraps	Garden Vegetable; Original; Savory Tomato; Spinach
Udi's Gluten Free◆	Tortillas	Plain

Buns and Rolls

Company or Brand	Product	Varieties or Flavors
All But Gluten◆	Hamburger Buns	
	Hot Dog Buns	
Barkat◆	Rolls	Home Fresh; Par Baked
BFree Foods◆	Hot Dog Buns	Brown Seeded; Plain
	Rolls	Brown Seeded; Soft White
Canyon Bakehouse◆	Hamburger Buns	
	Hot Dog Buns	
El Peto Products◆	Dinner Rolls	Italian; Multi-Grain
	Hamburger Buns	Italian; Potato
	Hot Dog Buns	Italian; Potato
	Mini Subs	Gourmet
	Rolls	Gourmet
Ener-G◆	Dinner Rolls	Select; Tapioca
	Hamburger Buns	Brown Rice; Seattle; Select; Tapioca
	Hot Dog Buns	Seattle; Select; Tapioca
Flax4Life◆	Flax Toaster Buns	Cinnamon Raisin; Everything*; Original
Glutenfree Bakehouse (Whole Foods)◆	Hamburger Buns	
Kinnikinnick◆	Soft Dinner Rolls	
	Soft Hamburger Buns	
	Soft Hot Dog Buns	
Little Northern Bakehouse◆	Buns	Millet & Chia
Manini's◆	Dinner Rolls	
	Hamburger Buns	
	Sandwich Buns	
O'Doughs◆	Buns	Flax; White
	Hamburger Buns	Deluxe
	Hot Dog Buns	Original
	Sandwich Thins	Multigrain; Original
	Sub Thins	Multigrain; Original
President's Choice	GF Dinner Rolls	
	GF Hamburger Buns	
	GF Hot Dog Buns	

Buns and Rolls (cont'd)

Company or Brand	Product	Varieties or Flavors
Promise Gluten Free◆	Hamburger Buns	
	Hot Dog Rolls	
	Sandwich Rolls	Seeded Wholegrain; Supersoft White
Rudi's Gluten-Free Bakery◆	Ciabatta Rolls	Plain
	Hamburger Buns	Multigrain
	Hot Dog Rolls	Multigrain
Schär◆	Ciabatta	Multigrain; Plain
	Hamburger Buns	
	Hot Dog Rolls	
	Sandwich Rolls	
Smart Flour Foods◆	Hamburger Buns	
Three Bakers◆	Hamburger Buns	Whole Grain
	Hot Dog Buns	Whole Grain
	Hoagie Rolls	Whole Grain
Udi's Gluten Free◆	Dinner Rolls	Classic French; Seeded Whole Grain
	Hamburger Buns	Classic; Whole Grain
	Hot Dog Buns	Classic

Bagels, Biscuits, English Muffins and Scones

Company or Brand	Product	Varieties or Flavors
BFree Foods◆	Bagels	Multiseed; Plain
Canyon Bakehouse◆	Bagels	Everything; Plain
El Peto Products◆	English Muffins	
Ener-G◆	English Muffins	
Food For Life	English Muffins	Brown Rice; Multi Seed
Foods By George◆	English Muffins	Cinnamon Current; No-Rye Rye; Plain
Glutenfree Bakehouse (Whole Foods)◆	Biscuits	Cheddar; Cream
	Scones	Almond; Cranberry Orange
Glutino◆	English Muffins	Multigrain; Premium
Kinnikinnick◆	English Muffins	
	Soft Bagels	Blueberry; Cinnamon Raisin; Plain
Mikey's◆	English Muffins	Cinnamon Raisin; Original; Toasted Onion
O'Doughs◆	Bagel Thins	Apple Cranberry; Original; Sprouted Whole Grain Flax
Promise Gluten Free◆	Bagels	Cinnamon Raisin; Plain
	English Muffins	
Udi's Gluten Free◆	Bagels	Cinnamon Raisin; Everything Inside; Mighty; Plain; Whole Grain

Muffins and Loaves

Company or Brand	Product	Varieties or Flavors
All But Gluten◆	Loaf	Lemon Poppy Seed
	Muffins	Blueberry; Chocolate Chip; Double Chocolate

Muffins and Loaves (cont'd)

Company or Brand	Product	Varieties or Flavors
El Peto Products♦	Muffins	Blueberry; Chocolate Chip; Cranberry; Lemon Poppy Seed; Tropical Delight; ; Whole Grain Banana; Whole Grain Carrot
Flax4Life♦	Flax Mini Muffins	Cappuccino Brownie; Chocolate Brownie; Dark Cherry Brownie; Toasted Coconut Brownie
	Flax Muffins*	Apple Cinnamon; Carrot Raisin; Chunky Chocolate Chip; Cranberry Orange; Hawaiian Pineapple & Coconut with Ginger; Wild Blueberry
Foods By George♦	Muffins	Blueberry; Corn
Garden Lites	GF Muffins	Banana Chocolate Chip*; Blueberry Oat*; Chocolate; Chocolate Krabby Square; Ninja Power
Glutenfree Bakehouse (Whole Foods)♦	Muffins	Apple Cinnamon; Blueberry; Lemon Poppyseed; Morning Glory
Kinnikinnick♦	Muffins	Blueberry; Carrot; Chocolate Chip
O'Doughs♦	Muffins	Banana Chocolate Chip; Double Chocolate; Wild Blueberry
President's Choice	GF Loaf Cake	Banana; Lemon Poppy Seed
	GF Muffins	Blueberry; Double Chocolate
Promise Gluten Free♦	Muffins	Double Chocolate; Lemon
Udi's Gluten Free♦	Muffins	Blueberry; Double Chocolate; Double Vanilla; Harvest Crunch; Lemon Streusel
	Muffin Tops	Blueberry Oat*; Chocolate Chia

French Toast, Pancakes and Waffles

Company or Brand	Product	Varieties or Flavors
Barkat♦	Waffles	
El Peto Products♦	Belgian Waffles	Corn and Milk Free; Regular
Ian's	GF French Toast Sticks	Cinnamon
	GF Pancrepes	Sausage
The Kashi Company	GF Waffles	Cinnamon; Original
Kellogg Company (U.S.)	GF Eggo Waffles*	Original
Kinnikinnick♦	Homestyle Waffles	Cinnamon & Brown Sugar; Original
Nature's Path	GF Waffles	Buckwheat Wildberry; Chia Plus; Dark Chocolate Chip; Homestyle; Pumpkin Spice
President's Choice	GF Waffles	Blueberry; Original
Promise Gluten Free♦	Pancakes	
Qrunch Foods♦	Breakfast Toastables	Blueberry Lemon; Cinnamon Vanilla; Original; Rich Maple
Van's	GF French Toast Sticks	Cinnamon
	GF Pancakes	Totally Original
	GF Waffles	Ancient Grains Original; Apple Cinnamon; Blueberry; Totally Original

Brownies and Squares

Company or Brand	Product	Varieties or Flavors
All But Gluten♦	Mini Brownies	
Amy's	GF Brownies*	
Canyon Bakehouse♦	Brownie Bites	
El Peto Products♦	Mini Brownies	Pure Bliss
Ener-G♦	Select Brownies	
Foods By George♦	Brownies	
	Mini Brownies	
Lucy's♦	Brownie Crisps*	Mint Chocolate; Savory Seed; Triple Chocolate
1-2-3 Gluten Free♦	Gourmet Brownie Chips	Caramel; Chocolate Chip; Rainbow
PatsyPie♦	Brownies	Double Chocolate
	Mini Brownies	Double Chocolate
President's Choice	GF Mini Brownies	
Pure Genius Provisions♦	Blondie*	Chocolate Chunk
	Brownie*	Deep Chocolate
Udi's Gluten Free♦	Brownie Bites	Dark Chocolate
WOW Baking Company♦	Brownies	Peppermint

Cakes and Cupcakes

Company or Brand	Product	Varieties or Flavors
Ener-G♦	Select Poundcake	
Flax4Life♦	Cake	Birthday Sprinkles; Carrot; Chocolate Shavings
Foods By George♦	Crumb Cake	
	Pound Cake	
Glutenfree Bakehouse (Whole Foods)♦	Cakes	Angel Food; Chocolate Confetti; Coconut Raspberry; Peppermint Mousse; Salted Caramel; Shmoo; Vanilla Confetti
	Cupcakes	Chocolate; Vanilla
Kinnikinnick♦	Fruit Cake	
O'Doughs♦	Cakes	Banana Chocolate Chip; Chocolate
The Piping Gourmets♦	Whoopie Pies	Chocolate Mint; Chocolate Raspberry; Chocolate Vanilla; Classic Vanilla; Double Chocolate
President's Choice	GF Almond Torte	Chocolate Toffee; Dark Chocolate
	GF Cakes	Chocolate Layer; Strawberry Sensation
	GF Cupcakes	Chocolate; Vanilla
Promise Gluten Free♦	Cakes	Chocolate; Lemon
Schär♦	Sch'nacks Snack Cakes	Chocolate Covered

Cinnamon Buns and Doughnuts

Company or Brand	Product	Varieties or Flavors
Ener-G♦	Select Donut Holes	Plain
	Select Donuts	Plain
Kinnikinnick♦	Donuts	Chocolate Dipped; Cinnamon Sugar; Maple Glazed; Pumpkin Spice; Vanilla Glazed
	Soft Donuts with Vanilla Icing	
Udi's Gluten Free♦	Cinnamon Rolls	

Cheesecakes, Pies, Tarts and Other Pastries

Company or Brand	Product	Varieties or Flavors
Daiya Foods♦	Cheezecake	Chocolate; Key Lime; New York; Strawberry
El Peto Products♦	Pie	Apple; Blueberry; Cherry; Strawberry Rhubarb; Walnut
	Tarts	Butter; Lemon; Pecan; Raspberry
Foods By George♦	Tarts	Pecan
Glutenfree Bakehouse (Whole Foods)♦	Pie	Apple; Cherry; Pumpkin; Southern Pecan
Glutenfreeda Foods♦	Cheesecake	Chocolate Truffle; New York; Strawberry Swirl
Glutino♦	Toaster Pastries	Apple Cinnamon; Frosted Blueberry; Frosted Strawberry; Strawberry
Hail Merry♦	Mini Tarts	Blueberry Acai; Chocolate Almond Butter; Chocolate Chili Pecan; Chocolate Crème; Meyer Lemon; Strawberry Rhubarb; Sweet Potato
	Tart	Chocolate Almond Butter; Chocolate Mint; Coconut Vanilla Crème; Dark Chocolate; Meyer Lemon; Persian Lime
Schär♦	Croissants	Hazelnut Cream; Plain

Biscotti, Cookies, Graham Crackers and Wafers

Company or Brand	Product	Varieties or Flavors
Aleias♦	Cookies	Almond Horns; Chocolate Chip; Chocolate Chunk; Ginger Snap; Oatmeal Raisin*; Peanut Butter; Snickerdoodle; Vanilla Bean
	Macaroons	Chocolate; Coconut
Amy's	GF Biscotti*	Chocolate; Orange
Andean Dream♦	Quinoa Cookies	Café Mocha; Chocolate Chip; Cocoa Orange; Coconut
Annie's Homegrown	GF Bunny Cookies	Coco & Vanilla; SnickerDoodle
Barkat♦	Biscuits	Coffee; Digestive
	Chocolate Hazelnut Bar	
	Cookies	Ginger
	Cream Filled Wafers	Chocolate; Lemon; Vanilla
	Tea Cakes	Chocolate
Cybele's♦	Cookies	Chocolate Chip; Chocolate Chunk Brownie; Oatmeal Raisin*; Snickerdoodle
El Peto Products♦	Cookies	Chocolate Chip; Gingerbread

Biscotti, Cookies, Graham Crackers and Wafers (cont'd)

Company or Brand	Product	Varieties or Flavors
Ener-G♦	Cookies	Cinnamon; Ginger; Sunflower
	Select Biscotti	Chocolate; Chocolate Chip; Cranberry; Raisin
	Select Cookies	Chocolate Chip Potato; Pretzel; Vanilla
Enjoy Life♦	Crunchy Cookies	Chocolate Chip; Double Chocolate; Sugar Crisp; Vanilla Honey Graham
	Crunchy Minis	Chocolate Chip; Double Chocolate; Sugar Crisp; Vanilla Honey Graham
	Soft Baked Cookies	Chocolate Chip; Double Chocolate Brownie; Gingerbread Spice; Snickerdoodle
	Soft Baked Minis	Chocolate Chip; Double Chocolate Brownie; Snickerdoodle
Free For All Kitchen♦	Brownie Thins	Double Chocolate
Glutenfree Bakehouse (Whole Foods)♦	Bobbilicious Cookies	Chocolate Chip Walnut; Chocolatey Chocolate; Oatmeal Raisiny*
	Cookies	Chocolate Chip Walnut; Molasses Ginger; Nutmeal Raisin; Peanut Butter
Gluten-Free Prairie♦	Hunger Buster Cookie*	
Glutino♦	Animal Crackers	Graham; Original
	Cookies	Chocolate Chip; Chocolate Vanilla Crème; Double Chocolate Chip; Vanilla Crème
	Crispy Cookie Thins	Chocolate Chip; Cranberry Orange; Double Chocolate Chip
	Wafer Bites	Chocolate Covered; Hazelnut; Lemon
	Wafers	Lemon; Milk Chocolate; Vanilla
GoGo Quinoa♦	Cookies	Dark Chocolate Chip; Orange & Mango
	Kaniwa Cookies	Coconut & Vanilla
Hail Merry♦	Merry Bites	Caramel Sea Salt; Chocolate Chip Cookie Dough; Dark Chocolate; Lemon; Pure Vanilla; Salted Brownie
Homefree♦	Cookies*	Chocolate Chip
	Mini Cookies*	Chocolate Chip; Chocolate Mint; Double Chocolate Chip; Lemon Burst; Vanilla
Jovial	GF Filled Cookies	Chocolate Crème; Fig Fruit; Sour Cherry
Kay's Naturals♦	Cookie Bites	Cinnamon Almond; Honey Almond; Mocha Espresso
Kinnikinnick♦	Cookies	Gingersnap; Montana's Chocolate Chip
	KinniKritter Animal Cookies	Chocolate; Graham Style; Plain
	KinniToos Sandwich Cookies	Chocolate; Fudge; Vanilla
	S'moreables Graham Style Crackers	
	Wafers	Vanilla
Le Veneziane♦	Biscuits	Chocolate Hazelnut; Coconut; Mixed Berries
Lucy's♦	Cookies*	Chocolate Chip; Chocolate Chocolate Chunk; Chocolate Merry Mint; Cinnamon Thin; Ginger Snap; Holiday Sugars; Lemon Goodness; Oatmeal; Pumpkin Patch; Sugar
Mary's Gone Crackers♦	Cookies	Chocolate Chip; Ginger Snaps
	MiNiS Graham Bites	Cocoa; Graham; Vanilla
Milton's Craft Bakers	GF Cookies	Chocolate Chip; Double Chocolate; Snickerdoodle

Biscotti, Cookies, Graham Crackers and Wafers (cont'd)

Company or Brand	Product	Varieties or Flavors
Orgran♦	Biscotti	Amaretti; Classic Choc
	Biscuits	Vanilla; Wholefruit Wildberry
	Fruit Filled Biscuits	Apple Cinnamon; Apricot; Wild Raspberry
	Itsy Bitsy Bears Biscuits	Choc Berry; Choc Chip
	Mini Outback Animal Cookies	Chocolate; Vanilla
	Outback Animal Cookies	Chocolate; Vanilla
	Shortbread Hearts	
Pamela's♦	Biscotti	Almond Anise; Chocolate Walnut; Lemon Almond
	Cookies	Chunky Chocolate Chip; Dark Chocolate Chunk; Ginger with Sliced Almonds; Peanut Butter
	Figgies & Jammies	Blueberry & Fig; Mission Fig; Raspberry & Fig; Strawberry & Fig
	Graham Style Crackers*	Chocolate; Cinnamon; Honey
	Mini Graham Style Crackers*	Chocolate; Cinnamon; Honey
	Shortbread Cookies	Butter; Lemon; Pecan
	SimpleBites Mini Cookies	Chocolate Chip; Extreme Chocolate; Ginger Snapz; Snickerdoodle
PatsyPie♦	Biscotti	Almond; Chocolate Chip; Cranberry Orange; Pecan
	Cookies	Candy with M&M's; Chocolate Chip; Double Chocolate; Lemon Shortbread; Peanut Butter; Raisin; Snappy Ginger; White Chocolate & Macadamia Nut
President's Choice	GF Cookies	Chocolate Chip; Coconut
Schär♦	Biscuits*	Oat
	Chocolate Hazelnut Bars	
	Cookies	Butter; Chocolate Dipped; Shortbread
	Honeygrams	
	Ladyfingers	
	Sandwich Crèmes	Chocolate; Vanilla
	Thins	Chocolate
	Wafers	Cocoa; Hazelnut; Lemon; Vanilla
Simply Shari's♦	Cookies	Chocolate Chip; Fudge Brownie
	Shortbread Cookies	Almond; Lemon; Plain
Three Bakers♦	Snackers	Chocolate Chip; Chocolate Chocolate Chip; Honey Graham
Udi's Gluten Free♦	Cookies	Chocolate Chip; Ginger; Maple Pecan Chocolate Chip; Oatmeal Raisin*; Peanut Butter Coconut; Salted Caramel Cashew; Snickerdoodle
WOW Baking Company♦	Cookies	Butter Toffee; Chocolate Chip; Ginger Molasses; Key Lime White Chocolate; Lemon Burst; Maple Squares; Oregon Oatmeal*; Peanut Butter; Pumpkin Spice; Snickerdoodle; White Chocolate Cranberry

Dough – Bread, Cookie, Pie and Pizza

Company or Brand	Product	Varieties or Flavors
Cappello's◆	Cookie Dough	Chocolate Chip; Double Chocolate; Ginger Snap; Lemon Zest
Chebe◆	Breadsticks	Plain; Tomato-Basil
	Pizza Crust	
	Rolls	Cheese; Ciabatta
El Peto Products◆	Pie Dough	
The Gluten Free Bistro◆	Pizza Dough	
WOW Baking Company◆	Cookie Dough	Chocolate Chip; Ginger Molasses; Peanut Butter; Sugar

Crusts – Pie, Pizza and Tart

Company or Brand	Product	Varieties or Flavors
Barkat◆	Rice Pizza Crust	Brown; White
Cappello's◆	Naked Pizza Crust	
El Peto Products◆	Pizza Crust	Basil; White; White (Yeast Free)
	Tart Shells	Sweetened; Unsweetened
Ener-G◆	Rice Pizza Shells	Regular; Yeast Free
Foods By George◆	Pizza Crusts	
	Tart Shells	
Glutenfree Bakehouse (Whole Foods)◆	Pie Crust	
The Gluten Free Bistro◆	Pizza Crust	
Kinnikinnick◆	Pie Crusts	
	Pizza Crusts (Personal Size)	
Mikey's◆	Pizza Crusts	
PatsyPie◆	Old-Fashioned Crumble Crust	
Rustic Crust	GF Pizza Crusts	Napoli Herb
Schär◆	Pizza Crusts	
Smart Flour Foods◆	Pizza Crusts	Original
Three Bakers◆	Pizza Crusts	Traditional Thin
Udi's Gluten Free◆	Pizza Crusts	

Crackers, Breadsticks, Corn/Rice Cakes

- Most crackers and breadsticks contain wheat, rye, regular oats and/or barley.

- Some multi-grain rice cakes also may contain wheat, rye and/or barley.

- Crackers and rice cakes may contain seasonings with ingredients derived from barley or wheat.

Savory Crackers and Breadsticks

Company or Brand	Product	Varieties or Flavors
Absolutely Gluten Free◆	Crackers	Cracked Pepper; Original; Toasted Onion
	Flatbreads	Everything; Original; Toasted Onion
Barkat◆	Crackers	
	Crispbreads	
	Matzo	
Blue Diamond	GF Artisan Nut Thins	Asiago Cheese; Chia Seeds; Flax Seeds; Multi-Seeds; Sesame Seeds*
	GF Nut Thins	Almond; Cheddar Cheese; Country Ranch; Hint of Sea Salt; Pecan; Pepper Jack Cheese; Smokehouse
Breton	GF Crackers	Black Bean with Onion & Garlic; Herb and Garlic; Original with Flax; White Bean with Salt & Pepper
Crunchmaster◆	7 Ancient Grains Crackers	Hint of Sea Salt
	Multi-Grain Crackers*	Roasted Vegetable; Sea Salt; White Cheddar
	Multi-Grain Crisps	Original; Sea Salt*
	Multi-Seed Crackers	Original; Roasted Garlic; Rosemary & Olive Oil
	Rice Crackers	Artisan Four Cheese; Toasted Sesame Rice; White Cheddar
Doctor in the Kitchen◆	Flackers	Cinnamon & Currents; Dill; Rosemary; Savory; Sea Salt; Tomato & Basil
Edward & Sons	GF Brown Rice Snaps	Black Sesame; Cheddar; Onion Garlic; Plain (Unsalted); Sesame (Unsalted); Tamari Seaweed; Tamari Sesame; Toasted Onion; Vegetable
	GF Exotic Rice Toasts	Jasmine Rice & Spring Onion; Purple Rice & Black Sesame; Thai Red Rice & Flax Seeds
Ener-G◆	Crackers	Cinnamon; Flax; Seattle
Free For All Kitchen◆	Deli Crackers	Olive & Herb; Olive Oil & Sea Salt; Roasted Garlic & Rosemary
	Snack Crackers	Olive & Herb; Olive Oil & Sea Salt; Roasted Garlic & Rosemary
Glutino◆	Crackers	Cheddar; Multigrain; Original; Vegetable
	Snack Crackers	Rosemary & Olive Oil; Sea Salt
	Table Crackers	
Goldbaum's Natural Foods◆	Crisbites	French Onion; Just Salt; Nutty Sesame; Roasted Garlic
	Flatbread Crisps	French Onion; Just Salt; Nutty Sesame; Roasted Garlic
Hol•Grain	GF Brown Rice Crackers	Lightly Salted; Lightly Salted with Sesame Seeds; No Salt; Onion & Garlic; Zesty Creole
Kitchen Table Bakers◆	Parmesan Crisps	Aged; Basil Pesto; Caraway Seed; Chia Seed; Everything; Flax Seed; Garlic; Italian Herb; Jalapeño; Rosemary; Sesame
	Parmesan Mini Crisps	Aged

Savory Crackers and Breadsticks (cont'd)

Company or Brand	Product	Varieties or Flavors
Le Veneziane♦	Mini Grissini (Breadsticks)	Plain; Rosemary; Sesame & Chia
	Tockets (Corn Breadsticks)	Con Cipolla with Onion; Con Olive with Olives; Gusto Pizza Pizza Taste
Lotus Foods♦	Arare Rice Crackers	Shoyu; Sriracha; Sweet & Savory Thai
Lundberg	GF Thin Stackers	5 Grain; Brown Rice (Lightly Salted); Brown Rice (Salt-Free); Red Rice & Quinoa
Mary's Gone Crackers♦	Crackers	Black Pepper; Caraway; Herb; Jalapeño; Onion; Original; Super Seed
	Super Seed Crackers	Basil & Garlic; Chia & Hemp; Classic; Everything; Seaweed & Black Sesame
	THINS Crackers	Ancient Spice; Garlic & Onion; Italian Herb; Kale; Lightly Salted
Milton's Craft Bakers	GF Crackers	Cheddar; Crispy Sea Salt; Everything; Multi-Grain
Orgran♦	Crispbreads	Buckwheat; Chia; Corn; Essential Fibre; Quinoa; Rice
	Multi Grain Wafer Crackers	Buckwheat; Chia; Quinoa
President's Choice	GF Crackers	Blue Cheese; Sweet Chili
	GF Crisp Breads	Original; Quinoa
Saffron Road	GF Lentil Crackers	Cracked Pepper; Rosemary Herb; Sea Salt
San-J	GF Brown Rice Crackers	Tamari; Tamari Black Sesame; Tamari Brown Sesame; Teriyaki Sesame
Schär♦	Bread Sticks	Italian
	Cheese Bites	
	Crackers	Entertainment; Table
	Crispbreads	
Simple Mills♦	Almond Flour Crackers	Farmhouse Cheddar; Fine Ground Sea Salt; Rosemary & Sea Salt; Sundried Tomato & Basil
Three Bakers♦	Snackers	Cheddar Cheese
Van's	GF Crackers*	Fire Roasted Veggie; Lots of Everything!; Multigrain; Say Cheese!; The Perfect 10

Corn and Rice Cakes

Company or Brand	Product	Varieties or Flavors
Element Snacks♦	Corn Cakes	Dark Chocolate; Sweet Mint
	Corn Cakes (Minis)	Dark Chocolate
	Rice Cakes	Dark Chocolate; Milk Chocolate; Strawberry 'N' Cream; Vanilla Orange
	Rice Cakes (Minis)	Milk Chocolate
Lundberg	GF Rice Cakes	Apple Cinnamon; Brown (Lightly Salted); Brown (Salt-Free); Caramel Corn; Cinnamon Toast; Honey Nut; Kettle Corn; Koku Seaweed; Mochi Sweet; Sesame Tamari; Tamari with Seaweed; Wild
	GF Sweet Dreams Rice Cakes	Dark Chocolate; Milk Chocolate
Plum-M-Good♦	Rice Cakes	Brown Rice (Salted); Brown Rice (Unsalted); Buckwheat (Unsalted); Flax (Salted); Flax (Unsalted); Millet (Unsalted); Multigrain (Salted); Multigrain (Unsalted); Regular (Salted); Regular (Unsalted); Sesame (Salted); Sesame (Unsalted)

Corn and Rice Cakes (cont'd)		
Company or Brand	**Product**	**Varieties or Flavors**
Plum-M-Good♦ (cont'd)	Rice Thins	5 Rice Blend; Brown Rice (Sea Salt); Brown Rice (Unsalted); Brown Rice with Chia; Brown Rice with Flax; Brown Rice with Hemp; Brown Rice with Quinoa; Canadian Wild Rice; Multigrain (Unsalted); Sesame (Unsalted)
Quaker (Canada)	GF Crispy Mini's® Large Rice Cakes	Butter Popcorn; Caramel Chocolate Chip; Caramel Corn; Cracker Jack Butter Toffee; Original; Savory Tomato & Basil; White Cheddar
Quaker (U.S.)	GF Large Rice Cakes	Apple Cinnamon; Buttered Popcorn; Caramel Corn; Chocolate Crunch; Lightly Salted; Salt Free; White Cheddar
Real Foods♦	Corn Thins	Flax & Soy; Multigrain; Original; Pizza; Sesame; Sour Cream & Chives; Tasty Cheese Flavor
	Rice Thins	Whole Grain Brown Rice
Woodstock Mini Me's♦	Rice Bites	Dark Chocolate; Milk Chocolate; Strawberry Yogurt

Communion Hosts/Wafers

- Communion hosts/wafers usually contain wheat flour; however, there are rice-based and low-gluten products available. For information about low-gluten hosts/wafers made with specially processed wheat starch, see pages 19 and 40.

Communion Hosts/Wafers		
Altar Breads (Benedictine Sisters of Perpetual Adoration) (see p. 19)	Low-Gluten Hosts	People's; Presider's
Ener-G♦	Communion Wafers	

Snacks

- Many snack foods (e.g., plain and flavored potato chips; tortilla chips, nuts) contain wheat, barley, rye and/or regular oats.

- Some snack foods contain seasonings with ingredients derived from wheat or barley.

- Licorice contains wheat flour; however, there are some gluten-free versions made without wheat flour.

Candy, Chips, Nuts, Seeds, Pretzels and Miscellaneous		
Company or Brand	**Product**	**Varieties or Flavors**
Absolutely Gluten Free♦	Superseed Crunch	Toasted Coconut
Bakery On Main♦	Nut Crunch Snack*	Blueberry Cobbler; Chocolate; Chocolate Orange; Chocolate Peppermint; Maple Vanilla; Original
Barkat♦	Pretzels	
	Pretzel Sticks	

Candy, Chips, Nuts, Seeds, Pretzels and Miscellaneous (cont'd)

Company or Brand	Product	Varieties or Flavors
Beanfields◆	Bean & Rice Chips	Barbecue; Black Bean with Sea Salt; Jalapeño Nacho; Nacho; Pico De Gallo; Ranch; Salt & Pepper; Sea Salt; Simply Unsalted; White Bean with Sea Salt
Beanitos◆	Black & White Bean Skinny Dippers	
	Black Bean Chips	Honey Chipotle BBQ; The Original
	Pinto Beans Chips	Better Cheddar & Sour Cream; Simply Pinto
	White Bean Chips	Garden Fresh Salsa; Hint of Lime; Nacho Cheese; Restaurant Style; Sweet Chili & Sour Cream
	White Bean Crunch	Mac n' Cheese
Breton	GF Popped! Beans (Chickpea & Red Bean)	Sea Salt & Pepper; Sweet Chili Cheddar
CheeCha	GF Potato Puffs	Fiesta Salsa; Luscious Lime; Original; Sea Salt & Spiced Pepper; Sea Salt & Vinegar; Sea Salted Caramel
chic-a-peas◆	Baked Crunchy Chickpeas	Falafel; Fresh Salsa; Sea Salt; Sweet BBQ
Crunchmaster◆	Popped Edamame Chips	Sea Salt; Wasabi Soy
Eden Foods	GF Mochi	Brown Rice & Black Soybean; Sprouted Brown Rice; Sweet Brown Rice
Ener-G◆	Pretzels	Garlic; Original; Sesame
Enjoy Life◆	not nuts! Seed and Fruit Mix	Beach Bash; Mountain Mambo
	Plentils	Dill & Sour Cream; Garlic & Parmesan; Original Sea Salt; Margherita Pizza
	ProBurst Bites	Cinnamon Spice Chocolate; Cocoa & Roasted SunSeed Butter; Cranberry Pomegranate; Mango Habanero
The GFB: Gluten Free Bar◆	Bites	Chocolate Cherry Almond; Coconut Cashew Crunch; Dark Chocolate Coconut; Dark Chocolate Hazelnut; Dark Chocolate Peanut Butter; PB + J
Glutino◆	Bagel Chips	Cinnamon & Sugar; Original; Parmesan Garlic
	Big Pretzels	
	Pretzel Chips	
	Pretzels	Buffalo Style; Chocolate Covered; Honey Mustard; Peppermint Yogurt Covered; Salted Caramel Covered; Sesame Rings; Yogurt Covered
	Pretzel Sticks	
	Pretzel Twists	
Goldbaum's Natural Foods◆	Kale Chips	Cracked Pepper; Piedmont BBQ; Salt & Vinegar; Touch of Salt
	Quinoa Crisps	Barbeque; Onion & Garlic; Sea Salt
The Good Bean◆	Bean Chips with Sweet Potato & Quinoa	BBQ Bacon; Cheesy Nacho; Jalapeño Cheddar; Sea Salt; Sweet Chili
	Roasted Chickpea Snacks	Chocolate; Cracked Pepper; Mesquite BBQ; Sea Salt; Smoky Chili & Lime; Sweet Cinnamon; Thai Coconut
GoPicnic	GF Black Bean Dip & Plantain Chips	
	GF Edamame Kale Dip & Plantain Chips*	
	GF Sunflower Butter & Multigrain Crackers*	
	GF Traditional Hummus & Multiseed Crackers	
	GF Turkey Pepperoni & Asiago Cheese*	
	GF Turkey Stick & BBQ Chips	

Company or Brand	Product	Varieties or Flavors
Gorilly Goods♦	Fruit & Nut Clusters	Forest (Dark Chocolate); Jungle (Original)
	Nut & Seed Snacks	Baja (Pumpkin Seed, Hemp & Cilantro); Coast (Sweet Curry Cashew & Fruit); Hillside (Pumpkin Seed & Kale); Trail (Nut, Goji & Cacao Nib)
Grain-Free JK Gourmet♦	GG Bites	Chocolate; Cranberry; Crushed Chilli and Cayenne; Hemp Seeds; Pepper; Ginger and Black Pepper; Original
Kay's Naturals♦	Pretzel Sticks	Cinnamon Toast; Jalapeño Honey Mustard; Original
	Protein Chips	Chili Nacho Cheese; Crispy Parmesan; Lemon Herb
	Protein Kruncheeze	White Cheddar Cheese
	Protein Puffs	Almond Delight; Mac & Cheese; Veggie Pizza
	Snack Mix	Sweet BBQ
Mary's Gone Crackers♦	Pretzels	Everything; Sea Salt
Orgran♦	Molasses Licorice	
Nourish Snacks♦	Fruit and Nut Snack	Cinnamon-Spiced Apples & Almonds
	Granola Bites*	Blueberry-Apple; Chocolate-Banana; Coconut-Vanilla
	Half-Popped Corn Kernels	Dark Chocolate; Plain
	Roasted Chickpeas & Virginia Peanuts	BBQ
	Roasted Corn	Mild Chili; Spicy Habanero
President's Choice	GF Pretzel Bites	
	GF Pretzels	
Quaker (Canada)	GF Crispy Mini's® Rice Chips	BBQ; Butter Popcorn; Caramel Kettle Corn; Cheddar; Crunchy Dill; Ketchup; Salt & Vinegar; Sea Salt & Lime; Sour Cream & Onion; Smoky Chipotle; Sweet Chili; Tortilla Style Cheesy Nacho; Tortilla Style Creamy Ranch
Quaker (U.S.)	GF Popped Rice Crisps	Apple Cinnamon; BBQ; Caramel Corn; Cheddar Cheese; Chocolate; Kettle Corn; Ranch; Sea Salt & Cracked Black Pepper; Sour Cream & Onion; Sweet Chili
Quinn Foods♦	GF Pretzels	Sea Salt; Touch of Honey
Saffron Road	GF Baked Lentil Chips	Cucumber Dill; Garlic Parmesan; Moroccan Barbecue; Rosemary; Sea Salt
	GF Bean Stalks	Barbecue; Cheddar; Sea Salt
	GF Crunchy Chickpeas	Bombay Spice; Chipotle; Falafel; Korean BBQ; Sea Salt; Wasabi
SimplyProtein♦	Protein Chips	BBQ Tomato; Herb; Sea Salt & Cracked Pepper; Spicy Chili
	Protein Crunch	Banana, Caramel and Cashew Nuts; Lemon, Cranberry and Pumpkin Seeds; Raspberry and Coconut
Tonya's Gluten Free Kitchen♦	Soft Pretzel Pieces	Original
	Soft Pretzels	Cinnamon Sugar; Original
Udi's Gluten Free♦	Ancient Grain Crisps	Aged Cheddar; Jalapeño Cheddar; Simply Sea Salt
Van's	Multigrain Chips	BBQ!; Nacho Nacho Man!
Watusee Foods♦	Chickpeatos	Cinnamon Toast; Rosemary; Spicy Cayenne; Tomato Basil

Ice Cream Cones/Cups

Company or Brand	Product	Varieties or Flavors
Barkat♦	Ice Cream Cones	Regular; Waffle
Goldbaum's Natural Foods♦	Cones	Cup; Regular; Sugar; Sugar Cocoa
	Dessert Cups	
Let's Do…	GF Ice Cream Cones	Regular; Sugar
Let's Do…Organic	GF Ice Cream Cones	Regular; Sugar

Snack Bars

Company or Brand	Product	Varieties or Flavors
Ancient Harvest♦	Ancient Grains Nutrition Bar	Garden Vegetable; Garlic & Herb; Roasted Jalapeño
Annie's Homegrown	GF Granola Bar*	Double Chocolate Chip; Oatmeal Cookie
Bakery on Main♦	Granola Bar*	Double Chocolate; Oat & Honey; Peanut Butter & Chocolate; Peanut Butter & Jelly
	True Bar	Apricot Almond Chai; Coconut Cashew; Fruit & Nut; Hazelnut Chocolate Cherry; Raspberry Chocolate Almond; Walnut Cappuccino
Bobo's Oat Bars♦	Bobo's Bites*	Apple Pie; Coconut; Lemon Poppyseed; Maple Pecan; Original; Peanut Butter & Jelly
	Oat Bar*	Almond; Apple Pie; Apricot; Banana; Chocolate; Chocolate Almond; Cinnamon Raisin; Coconut; Cranberry Orange; Lemon Poppyseed; Maple Pecan; Original; Peach; Peanut Butter; Peanut Butter & Jelly; Strawberry
BumbleBar♦	Juno Bar	Apple Crisp; Brownie Batter; Peanut Butter Cookie
	Sesame Bar	Amazing Almond; Chai Almond; Chocolate Crisp; Chocolate Mint; Chocolate Peanut Butter; Classic Cashew; Harvest Hazelnut; Luscious Lemon; Mixed Nut Medley; Original Peanut
	Sesame Bar (Junior)	Amazing Almond; Chocolate Crisp; Original Peanut
Ener-G♦	Snack Bar	Chocolate Chip
Enjoy Life♦	Chewy Bar	Caramel Apple; Coco Loco; Mixed Berry; SunSeed Crunch
	Decadent Bars	Cherry Cobbler; Chocolate SunSeed Crunch; Cinnamon Bun; S'mores
EnviroKidz♦	Crispy Rice Bar	Berry Blast; Chocolate; Peanut Butter; Peanut Choco Drizzle
	Granola Bar*	Chocolate Chip; Strawberry
Freedom Foods♦	Chewy Crunchola Granola Bar*	Oats, Apple & Cinnamon; Oats, Apricot, Coconut & Chia
	Chewy Oats & Seeds Muesli Bar*	Cranberries & Mixed Seeds
	Crafted Blend with Superfoods Snack Bar	Cranberry, Pomegranate & Goji Berry; Maca, Chickpea & Raisin; Pumpkin Seed, Spinach & Chickpea
The GFB: Gluten Free Bar♦	Snacks Bar	Chocolate Peanut Butter; Coconut Cashew Crunch; Cranberry Toasted Almond; Dark Chocolate Coconut; Oatmeal Raisin*; Peanut Butter
Gluten Free Café♦	Sesame Bar	Chocolate; Cinnamon; Lemon
Glutino♦	Breakfast Bar	Apple; Blueberry; Cherry; Strawberry
	Organic Bar	Chocolate & Banana; Chocolate & Peanut; Wild Berry

Snack Bars (cont'd)

Company or Brand	Product	Varieties or Flavors
GoMacro♦	Macro Bar	Almond Butter + Carob; Apples + Walnuts*; Banana + Almond Butter; Cashew Butter; Cashew Caramel; Cherries + Berries*; Coconut + Almond Butter + Chocolate Chips; Granola + Coconut*; Peanut Butter; Peanut Butter Chocolate Chip; Sesame Butter + Dates; Sunflower Butter + Chocolate
	Macro Bar (Mini)	Almond Butter + Carob; Apples + Walnuts*; Banana + Almond Butter; Cashew Butter; Cashew Caramel; Cherries + Berries*; Granola + Coconut*; Peanut Butter; Peanut Butter Chocolate Chip; Sesame Butter + Dates; Sunflower Butter + Chocolate
	Thrive Ancient Seeds Nut Bar	Almond Apricot; Blueberry Lavender; Caramel Coconut; Chocolate Nuts & Sea Salt; Chocolate Peanut Butter Chip; Ginger Lemon
The Good Bean♦	The Fruit & NO-NUT Bar	Apricot Coconut; Chocolate Berry; Fruit & Seeds Trail Mix
Goodnessknows♦	Snack Squares*	Apple, Almond & Peanut, Dark Chocolate; Cranberry, Almond, Dark Chocolate; Peach & Cherry, Almond, Dark Chocolate
Grain-Free JK Gourmet♦	Granola Bar	Roasted Nuts & Blueberries; Roasted Nuts & Cranberries; Roasted Nuts & Dates; Roasted Nuts & Raisins; Roasted Nuts & Seeds
The Kashi Company	GF GOLEAN® Plant-Powered Bar	Dark Chocolate Cashew Chia; Honey Pecan Baklava; Peanut Hemp Crunch; Salted Dark Chocolate & Nuts
	Kashi Savory Bar	Basil, White Bean & Olive Oil; Quinoa, Corn & Roasted Pepper
Kellogg Canada	Special K Nourish Snack Bar	Chocolate Chunks & Almonds; Cranberries & Almonds
Kellogg Company (U.S.)	Special K Nourish Chewy Nut Bar	Chocolate Almond; Cranberry Almond
KIND♦	Breakfast Bar*	Blueberry Almond; Dark Chocolate Cocoa; Honey Oat; Peanut Butter; Raspberry Chia
	Pressed by KIND Fruit Bar	Apricot Pear Carrot Beet; Cherry Apple Chia; Mango Apple Chia; Pineapple Banana Kale Spinach; Pineapple Coconut Chia
	Healthy Grains Snack Bar*	Caramel Macchiato; Dark Chocolate Chunk; Dark Chocolate Mocha; Maple Pumpkin Seeds with Sea Salt; Oats & Honey with Toasted Coconut; Peanut Butter Berry; Peanut Butter Dark Chocolate; Popped Dark Chocolate with Sea Salt; Popped Salted Caramel; Vanilla Blueberry
	Popped Snack Bites*	Dark Chocolate with Sea Salt; Salted Caramel

Snack Bars (cont'd)

Company or Brand	Product	Varieties or Flavors
KIND◆ (cont'd)	Snack Bar	Almond & Apricot; Almond & Coconut; Almond Cashew with Flax + Omega-3; Almond Coconut Cashew Chai; Almonds & Apricots in Yogurt; Almond Walnut Macadamia with Peanuts; Apple Cinnamon & Pecan; Black Truffle Almond & Sea Salt; Blueberry Pecan + Fiber; Blueberry Vanilla & Cashew; Caramel Almond & Sea Salt; Cashew & Ginger Spice; Cranberry Almond + Antioxidants; Dark Chocolate Almond & Coconut; Dark Chocolate Almond Mint; Dark Chocolate Cherry Cashew + Antioxidants; Dark Chocolate Chili Almond; Dark Chocolate Cinnamon Pecan; Dark Chocolate Mocha Almond; Dark Chocolate Nuts & Sea Salt; Fruit & Nut Delight; Fruit & Nuts in Yogurt; Honey Roasted Nuts & Sea Salt; Madagascar Vanilla Almond; Maple Glazed Pecan & Sea Salt; Peanut Butter & Strawberry; Peanut Butter Dark Chocolate + Protein; Pomegranate Blueberry Pistachio + Antioxidants; Raspberry Cashew & Chia; Salted Caramel & Dark Chocolate Nut
	STRONG & KIND Almond Protein Bar	Hickory Smoked; Honey Mustard; Honey Smoked BBQ; Roasted Jalapeño; Thai Sweet Chili
Larabar (Canada)◆	Fruit & Nut Energy Bar	Apple; Blueberry; Cashew; Chocolate Brownie; Chocolate Chip; Cocoa Coconut Chew; Coconut Cream; Lemon; Peanut Butter; Peanut Butter Chocolate Chip
Larabar (U.S.)◆	Fruit & Nut Bar	Apple Pie; Banana Bread; Blueberry Muffin; Cappuccino; Carrot Cake; Cashew Cookie; Cherry Pie; Chocolate Chip Brownie; Chocolate Chip Cherry Torte; Chocolate Chip Cookie Dough; Chocolate Coconut Chew; Coconut Cream Pie; Coconut Chocolate Chip; Gingerbread; Key Lime Pie; Lemon; Peanut Butter & Jelly; Peanut Butter Chocolate Chip; Peanut Butter Cookie; Pecan Pie; Pumpkin Pie; Snickerdoodle
	Snack Bar with Superfoods	Coconut Kale & Cacao; Hazelnut, Hemp & Cacao; Turmeric, Ginger & Beet
Libre Naturals◆	Granola Bar*	Apple Cinnamon; Chocolate Chip; Double Chocolate; Red Berry
Nature's Path	GF Chewy Granola Bar*	Chunky Chocolate Peanut; Dark Chocolate Chip; Trail Mixer
	GF Qi'a Snack Bar	Blueberry Cashew Pumpkin Seed; Dark Chocolate Cranberry Almond; Mocha Cocoa Hazelnut; Nuts & Seeds & Sea Salt; Roasted Peanut Dark Chocolate
NoGii◆	High Protein Bar	Chocolate Coconut; Chocolate Mint; Coca Brownie; Peanut Butter & Chocolate
	Paleo Protein Bar	Nuts About Berries; Nuts About Nuts; Nuts About Tropical Fruit
	Protein D'LITES	Chocolate Caramel Bliss; Cookies & Crème Dream
	Super Protein Bar	Chocolate Peanut Butter Caramel Crisp; Cookies & Crème; Rocky Road
Pamela's◆	Whenever Oat Bar*	Blueberry Lemon; Chocolate Chip Coconut; Cranberry Almond; Double Chocolate; Peanut Butter Chocolate Chip; Raisin Walnut Spice

Snack Bars (cont'd)

Company or Brand	Product	Varieties or Flavors
Perfect Bar♦	Perfect Bar	Almond Acai; Almond Butter; Almond Coconut; Blueberry Cashew; Carob Chip; Coconut Peanut Butter; Cranberry Crunch; Fruit & Nut; Maple Almond; Peanut Butter
Promax Nutrition Company♦	Carb Sense Protein Bar	Chocolate Mint; Honey Peanut; Salted Caramel
	Lower Sugar Protein Bar	Chocolate Fudge; Peanut Butter Chocolate; Peanut Butter Cookie Dough
	Original Protein Bar	Chocolate Chip Cookie Dough; Chocolate Peanut Crunch; Cookies n' Cream; Double Fudge Brownie; Lemon; Nutty Butter Crisp
	Pro Series Crisp Bar	Peanut Butter; Triple Chocolate
Promise Gluten Free♦	Snack Bar	Chocolate & Marshmallow Biscuit; Yogurt, Fruit & Nut Bar
PureFit♦	Nutrition Bar	Almond Crunch; Berry Almond Crunch; Chocolate Brownie; Granola Crunch*; Peanut Butter Chocolate Chip; Peanut Butter Crunch; Peanut Butter Toffee Crunch
	ProLean Protein Bar	Cookies N' Cream; Cookie Dough; Double Chocolate
Pure Organic♦	Ancient Grains Bar	Chocolate Chunk Nut; Chocolate; Triple Berry Nut; Vanilla Almond
	Fruit & Nut Bar	Banana Coconut; Cashew Coconut; Cherry Cashew; Chocolate Brownie; Dark Chocolate Berry; Peanut Butter Chocolate Chip; Wild Blueberry
Rise Bar♦	Breakfast Bar	Cranberry Apple; Crunchy Cashew Almond; Crunchy Macadamia Pineapple; Crunchy Perfect Pumpkin
	Energy Bar	Apricot Goji; Blueberry Coconut; Coconut Acai; Raspberry Pomegranate
	Protein Bar	Almond Honey; Carob Chip; Cacao Banana; Lemon Cashew; Snicker Doodle; Sunflower Cinnamon
	Protein Bar (Mini)	Almond Honey; Cacao Banana; Lemon Cashew; Snicker Doodle
Rudi's Gluten-Free Bakery♦	Bars*	Cherry Almond
SimplyProtein♦	Decadent Bar	Dark Chocolate Cherry; Dark Chocolate Salted Caramel
	Kid's Bar	Apple Maple; Banana Chocolate; Chocolate Brownie; Strawberry Vanilla
	Nut & Fruit Bar	Apricot Almond Coconut; Dark Chocolate Cherry Almond; Dark Chocolate Peanut Butter Strawberry
	Snack Bar	Chocolate Caramel; Cinnamon Pecan; Cocoa Coffee; Cocoa Raspberry; Lemon Coconut; Maple Pecan; Peanut Butter Chocolate
	Veggie Savory Bar	Sesame Chives; Smoky BBQ Peppers
	Wellness Bar	Fodmap Coconut Almond; Lemon Coconut "0" Fibre; Soothe Apricot
	Whey Bar	Apple Cinnamon; Banana Butterscotch; Chocolate Mint; Coconut
SOYJOY♦	Baked Soy & Fruit Bar	Banana; Berry; Blueberry; Cranberry; Dark Chocolate Cherry; Mango Coconut; Strawberry

Snack Bars (cont'd)

Company or Brand	Product	Varieties or Flavors
Taste of Nature♦	Protein Snack Bar	Dark Chocolate Cherry; Dark Chocolate Orange; Dark Chocolate Peanut & Sea Salt
	Snack Bar	Almond; Apple*; Blueberry; Brazil Nut; Cherry; Coconut; Cranberry; Ginger; Goji; Maple; Orange; Peanuts; Pineapple; Pomegranate
Udi's Gluten Free♦	Granola Bar*	Ancient Grains; Chocolate Chip; Cranberry Almond
Van's	GF Sandwich Bar*	Gramwich Chocolate and Graham-Style; PB + J Blueberry and Peanut Butter; PB + J Strawberry and Peanut Butter
	GF Snack Bar*	Banana Bread; Chocolate Chip; Cranberry Almond; Peanut Butter Chocolate
Zing♦	Snack Bar	Almond Blueberry; Cashew Cranberry Orange; Coconut Cashew Crisp; Dark Chocolate Coconut; Dark Chocolate Hazelnut; Dark Chocolate Mint; Dark Chocolate Mocha; Dark Chocolate Peanut Butter; Double Nut Brownie; Lemon Cashew Crunch; Oatmeal Chocolate Chip*; Peanut Butter Chocolate Chip*
	Snack Bar (Mini)	Coconut Cashew Crisp; Dark Chocolate Coconut; Dark Chocolate Mint; Oatmeal Chocolate Chip*; Peanut Butter Chocolate Chip

Baking Mixes

Baking Mixes

Company or Brand	Product	Varieties or Flavors
Allen Creek Farm♦	Pancake and Waffle Mix	Chestnut Buttermilk
Arnel's Originals♦	All Purpose Flour & Pie Crust Mix	
	Bread Mix	Buckwheat
	Cake Mix	Make-A-Cake-Your-Way
	Pancake & Waffle Mix	
Authentic Foods♦	Bread Mix	Cinnamon; Wholesome
	Brownie Mix	Double Chocolate
	Cake Mix	Devil's Food Chocolate; Lemon; Vanilla Bean
	Cookie Mix	Chocolate Chunk
	Flour Blend	Bette's Gourmet Featherlight; Bette's Gourmet Four Flour; Classical; Multi; Steve's GF Cake Flour; Steve's GF Flour
	Muffin Mix	Blueberry; Chocolate Chip
	Pancake & Baking Mix	
	Pie Crust Mix	
	Pizza Crust Mix	
Barkat♦	All Purpose Flour Mix	
	Bread Mix	
	Muffin Mix	Chocolate
	Pancake & Batter Mix	

Baking Mixes (cont'd)

Company or Brand	Product	Varieties or Flavors
Bob's Red Mill	GF Biscuit & Baking Mix	
	GF Bread Mix	Cinnamon Raisin; Cornbread; Hearty Whole Grain; Homemade Wonderful
	GF Brownie Mix	
	GF Cake Mix	Chocolate; Vanilla
	GF Cookie Mix	Chocolate Chip; Shortbread
	GF Flour Mix	1-to-1 Baking; All Purpose Baking; Paleo Baking
	GF Muffin Mix	
	GF Pancake Mix	
	GF Pie Crust Mix	
	GF Pizza Crust Mix	
Breads From Anna♦	Bread Mix	Banana; Classic Herb; Dairy & Corn Free; Original; Pumpkin; Yeast Free
	Brownie Mix	Black Bean
	Pancake & Muffin Mix	Apple; Cranberry; Maple
	Pie Crust Mix	
	Pizza Crust Mix	
Chebe♦	Bread Mix	All Purpose; Original Cheese
	Breadstick Mix	Garlic-Onion
	Cinnamon Roll Mix	
	Focaccia Mix	
	Pizza Crust Mix	
Cherrybrook Kitchen	GF Brownie Mix	Fudge
	GF Cake Mix	Carrot; Chocolate; Yellow
	GF Cookie Mix	Chocolate Chip; Sugar
	GF Pancake & Waffle Mix	
	GF Pancake Mix	Chocolate Chip
Cloud 9 Specialty Bakery♦	All-Purpose Baking Mix	
	Bread Mix	
	Brownie Mix	
	Cake and Cupcake Mix	Chocolate
	Cookie Mix	Chocolate Chip
	Granola Bar Mix*	
	Pancake & Waffle Mix	
Cuisine Soleil♦	All Purpose Mix	
	Bread Mix	Artisan; Homemade Style; Multigrain
	Pancake Mix	4 Grain
Cup4Cup♦	Brownie Mix	Chocolate
	Cake Mix	Vanilla
	Flour Mix	Multipurpose; Wholesome
	Pancake & Waffle Mix	
	Pizza Crust Mix	
Domata♦	Pizza Crust Mix	
	Recipe Ready Flour	

Baking Mixes (cont'd)

Company or Brand	Product	Varieties or Flavors
Dowd & Rogers♦	Brownie Mix	Dark Chocolate
	Cake Mix	Dark Vanilla; Dutch Chocolate; Golden Lemon
	Pancake & Baking Mix	
Duinkerken Foods♦	Biscuit Mix	
	Bread Mix	White Sandwich
	Brownie Mix	Fudge
	Cake Mix	Chocolate; Lemon; Vanilla
	Cookie Mix	Classic; Shortbread
	Muffin Mix	
	Pizza Crust Mix	
	Waffle/Pancake Mix	
El Peto Products♦	Bread Mix for Bread Maker	Brown Rice; Italian Style; White Rice
	Cake Mix	Chocolate; Lemon; White
	Cookie Mix	Sugar
	Flour Mix	All Purpose; Corn-Free All Purpose
	Muffin Mix	Corn Free; Regular
	Pancake Mix	Corn Free; Regular
Ener-G♦	Corn Mix	
	Potato Mix	
	Rice Mix	
Enjoy Life♦	All Purpose Flour Mix	
	Brownie Mix	
	Muffin Mix	
	Pancake & Waffle Mix	
	Pizza Crust	
Freedom Foods♦	Pancake Mix	Original; Quinoa
gfJules♦	All Purpose Flour Mix	
	Bread Mix	Cornbread; Regular
	Brownie Mix	
	Cookie Mix	Cut Out; Regular
	Graham Cracker / Gingerbread Mix	
	Muffin Mix	
	Pancake & Waffle Mix	
	Pizza Crust Mix	
Gluten-Free Naturals♦	All Purpose Flour	
	Bread Flour Mix	Multi-Grain; Sandwich
	Brownie Mix	Homemade
	Cake Mix	Yellow
	Cookie Blend Mix	
	Cornbread & Corn Muffin Mix	
	Pancake Mix	
	Pizza Crust Mix	Pizzeria-Style
Gluten-Free Prairie♦	Brownie Mix	Deep Dark Chocolate
	All Purpose Flour	Simply Wholesome

Baking Mixes (cont'd)

Company or Brand	Product	Varieties or Flavors
Glutino♦	All Purpose Flour Mix	
	Bread Mix	Favorite Sandwich; Yankee Cornbread
	Brownie Mix	Double Chocolate
	Cake Mix	Decadent Chocolate; Old Fashioned Yellow
	Cookie Mix	Chocolate Chip; Sugar
	Muffin Mix	
	Pancake Mix	Fluffy; Instant
	Perfect Pie Crust Mix	
	Pizza Crust Mix	
GoGo Quinoa♦	Cake Mix	Dark Chocolate
	Pancake Mix	Whole Grains
Grain-Free JK Gourmet♦	Cookie Mix	
	Muffin Mix	
	Pancake & Waffle	
	Pie & Tart Crust Mix	
Hodgson Mill	GF All Purpose Baking Flour	
	GF Bread Mix	
	GF Brownie Mix	
	GF Cake Mix	Chocolate; Yellow
	GF Cookie Mix	Chocolate Chip; Plain
	GF Cornbread Mix	Sweet Yellow
	GF Muffin Mix	Apple Cinnamon with Milled Flax Seed
	GF Multi Purpose Baking Mix	
	GF Pancake & Waffle Mix	
	GF Pizza Crust Mix	
Hol•Grain	GF Brownie Mix	Chocolate
	GF Cookie Mix	Chocolate Chip
	GF Pancake & Waffle Mix	
Jovial	GF Ancient Grain Bread Flour Mix	Regular; Whole Grain
	GF Ancient Grain Pastry Flour Mix	Regular; Whole Grain
King Arthur Flour	GF All-Purpose Baking Mix	
	GF Bread & Pizza Crust Mix	
	GF Bread Mix	Banana; Corn; Pumpkin*
	GF Brownie Mix	
	GF Cake Mix	Chocolate; Yellow
	GF Cookie Mix	Plain; Sugar*
	GF Doughnut Mix	
	GF Flours	Ancient Grains Blend; Measure For Measure; Multi-Purpose; Whole Grain Blend
	GF Gingerbread Mix	
	GF Muffin Mix	
	GF Pancake Mix	
	GF Pie Crust Mix	
	GF Scone Mix	

Baking Mixes (cont'd)

Company or Brand	Product	Varieties or Flavors
Kinnikinnick♦	All Purpose Flour Blend	
	Cake Mix	Angel Food; Chocolate; White
	Cookie Mix	Sugar
	Cornbread Mix	
	Kinni-Kwik Bread & Bun Mix	
	Pancake & Waffle Mix	
Larrowe's (The Birkett Mills)	GF Pancake Mix	Buckwheat
Manini's♦	Bread Mix	Old Fashioned
	Flour Mix	Multi-Grain; Multi-Purpose
Namaste Foods♦	Blondie Mix	
	Bread & Roll Mix	
	Brownie Mix	Dark Chocolate; Regular
	Cake Mix	Chocolate; Pure Vanilla; Spice
	Cookie Mix	
	Muffin & Scone Mix	
	Muffin Mix	Sugar-Free
	Perfect Flour Blend	
	Pizza Crust Mix	
	Pumpkin Baking Mix	
	Waffle & Pancake Mix	
Nu Life Market♦	All-Purpose Flour Mix	
	Pizza Crust Mix	
1-2-3 Gluten-Free♦	Biscuit Mix	Southern Glory
	Brownie Mix	Devilishly Decadent; Divinely Decadent
	Bundt Poundcake Mix	Delightfully Gratifying Lemon; Delightfully Gratifying Lemon (Sugar Free); Peri's Perfect Chocolate; Peri's Perfect Chocolate (Sugar Free)
	Cake Mix	Devil's Food; Yummy Yellow
	Cookie Mix	Chewy Chipless; Lindsay's Lipsmakin' Sugar
	Corn Bread Mix	Micah's Mouthwatering
	Muffins/Quickbread Mix	Meredith's Marvelous
	Multi-Purpose Fortified Flour Mix	Olivia's Outstanding
	Pan Bars Mix	Sweet Goodness
	Pancake Mix	Allie's Awesome
	Rolls Mix	Aaron's Favorite
Only Oats (Avena Foods)♦	Cookie Mix*	Grandma's Oatmeal
	Muffin Mix*	Chocolate; Cinnamon Spice
	Pancake Mix*	Whole Oat

Baking Mixes (cont'd)

Company or Brand	Product	Varieties or Flavors
Orgran♦	Bread Mix	Alternative Grain Wholemeal; Easy Bake; Multigrain with Quinoa and Chia
	Brownie Mix	Caramel Fudge; Chocolate
	Cake Mix	Banana with Caramel Icing; Chocolate; Vanilla
	Falafel Mix	
	Flour Mix	All Purpose Plain; Multigrain All Purpose Plain with Quinoa; Self Raising; Self Raising with Quinoa
	Gluten-Free Gluten (GFG) Substitute	
	Muffin Mix	Chocolate; Chocolate Caramel
	Pancake Mix	Apple Cinnamon; Buckwheat
	Pastry Mix	All Purpose
	Pizza & Pastry Multimix	
Pamela's♦	All-Purpose Flour	Artisan Blend
	Baking & Pancake Mix	
	Biscuit & Scone Mix	
	Bread Mix	Plain; Pumpkin
	Brownie Mix	Chocolate
	Cake Mix	Chocolate; Spice; Vanilla
	Cookie Mix	Chocolate Chunk; Oatmeal*; Sugar
	Cornbread & Muffin Mix	
	Grain-Free Pancake Mix	
	Nut Flour Blend	
	Pancake & Waffle Mix	
	Pizza Crust Mix	
	Sprouted Grain Pancake Mix	6 Grain; Buckwheat; Buttermilk; Non-Dairy; Protein
PatsyPie♦	Scone Mix	Classic; Cranberry
Premium Gold Flax♦	All-Purpose Flour	Flax & Ancient Grains
	Ancient Grain Baking & Pizza Flour	
	Brownie Mix	Double Chocolate Chip
	Cookie Mix	Chocolate Chip; Sugar
	Muffin Mix	
	Pancake & Waffle Mix	
President's Choice	GF All Purpose Flour Blend	
	GF Cake Mix	Chocolate; Golden; Yellow Loaf
	GF Cookie Mix	Chocolate Chip
	GF Pancake Mix	
The Really Great Food Company♦	Bread Mix	Banana; Irish Soda; Pumpkin
	Brownie Mix	
	Cake Mix	Chocolate; Classic Pound; Coffee Crumb; Devil's Food; Golden; Yellow
	Muffin Mix	Cornbread; Vanilla
	Pancake Mix	Classic
	Pizza Crust Mix	
Schär♦	Bread Mix	Classic White
	Pancake & Waffle Mix	

Baking Mixes (cont'd)

Company or Brand	Product	Varieties or Flavors
Simple Mills◆	Bread Mix	Artisan
	Cake Mix	Vanilla
	Cookie Mix	Chocolate Chip
	Muffin & Bread Mix	Banana; Pumpkin
	Muffin & Cake Mix	Chocolate
	Pancake & Waffle Mix	
	Pizza Dough Mix	
Smart Flour Foods◆	Pancake & Waffle Mix	
Whole Note Food Company◆	Crêpe Mix*	Original
	Muffin Mix*	Cappuccino and Dark Chocolate; Create-A-Muffin-Mix; Lemon Ginger
	Multipurpose Flour Blend*	
	Pancake Mix*	Buttermilk; Non-Dairy
	Pizza Crust Mix*	Original
	Pumpkin Bread and Muffin Mix*	
	Waffle Mix*	Non-Dairy; Original
Wondergrain◆	All Purpose Flour Mix	
	Cookie Mix	
WOW Baking Company◆	Cake Mix	Chocolate; Spice; Yellow
XO Baking Co.◆	All Purpose Flour Blend	
	Biscuit and Scone Mix	
	Blondie Mix	
	Bread Mix	Banana; Corn; Pumpkin; Zucchini
	Brownie Mix	Fudge
	Cake Mix	Chocolate; Pound; Vanilla
	Cookie Mix	Chocolate Chip; Double Chocolate Chip; Double Chocolate Peppermint; Gingerbread; Oatmeal*; Sugar
	Muffin Mix	All-Purpose
	Pancake and Waffle Mix	
	Pie Crust Mix	

Flours

- Avoid buying gluten-free flours from bulk bins due to a high risk of cross-contamination from gluten-containing flours.

- It should be noted that some companies not displaying the diamond symbol ◆ nonetheless produce their gluten-free grains in dedicated gluten-free facilities (e.g., Bob's Red Mill, King Arthur Flour).

- Information about a wide variety of gluten-free flours is found on pages 147–151.

Bean, Chickpea, Lentil and Pea Flours

Flour Type	Company or Brand
Black Bean Flour	Best Cooking Pulses♦
	Bob's Red Mill
Chickpea Flour / Garbanzo Bean Flour	Authentic Foods♦
	Best Cooking Pulses♦
	Bob's Red Mill
	Cuisine Soleil♦
	Namaste Foods♦
Fava Bean Flour	Bob's Red Mill
Garbanzo Bean Flour and Fava Bean Flour	Authentic Foods♦ (developed original blend called "Garfava™ Flour")
	Bob's Red Mill
Lentil Flour	Best Cooking Pulses♦
	CanMar Grain Products♦
	Cuisine Soleil♦
Navy Bean Flour	Best Cooking Pulses♦
Pea Flour	Best Cooking Pulses♦ (green; yellow)
Pinto Bean Flour	Best Cooking Pulses♦
White Bean Flour	Bob's Red Mill

Other Flours and Miscellaneous

Flour Type	Company or Brand
Almond Flour or Almond Meal Flour	Authentic Foods♦
	Bob's Red Mill
	Dowd & Rogers♦
	Grain-Free JK Gourmet♦
	Hodgson Mill
	King Arthur Flour
Amaranth Flour	Bob's Red Mill
	Cuisine Soleil♦
	King Arthur Flour
Buckwheat Flour	Bgreen Food♦
	Cuisine Soleil♦
	King Arthur Flour
	Pocono (The Birkett Mills)
Chestnut Flour	Allen Creek Farm♦
	Dowd & Rogers♦
Coconut Flour	Bob's Red Mill
	Cloud 9 Specialty Bakery♦
	Cuisine Soleil♦
	Dowd & Rogers♦
	Hodgson Mill
	King Arthur Flour
	Let's Do…Organic
Corn Flour	Bob's Red Mill
	El Peto Products♦

Other Flours and Miscellaneous (cont'd)

Flour Type	Company or Brand
Cornmeal	Bob's Red Mill
	El Peto Products♦
Green Banana Flour	Let's Do…Organic
Hazelnut Flour	Bob's Red Mill
Mesquite Flour	Casa de Mesquite♦
	Dowd & Rogers♦
Millet Flour	Authentic Foods♦
	Bgreen Food♦
	Bob's Red Mill
	Cuisine Soleil♦
	King Arthur Flour
	Namaste Foods♦
Oat Bran (Gluten Free)	Bob's Red Mill
	Only Oats (Avena Foods)♦
Oat Flour (Gluten Free)	Bob's Red Mill
	Cream Hill Estates♦
	GF Harvest♦
	Gluten-Free Prairie♦
	King Arthur Flour
	Only Oats (Avena Foods)♦
Potato Flour	Authentic Foods♦
	Bob's Red Mill
	El Peto Products♦
	Ener-G Foods♦
Quinoa Flour	Ancient Harvest♦
	Bob's Red Mill
	Cuisine Soleil♦
	Dowd & Rogers♦
	GoGo Quinoa♦
	King Arthur Flour
	Namaste Foods♦
	NorQuin♦
Rice Bran	Bob's Red Mill
Rice Flour (Black)	Bgreen Food♦
Rice Flour (Brown)	Authentic Foods♦
	Bgreen Food♦
	Bob's Red Mill
	Cloud 9 Specialty Bakery♦
	Cuisine Soleil♦
	El Peto Products♦
	Hodgson Mill
	King Arthur Flour
	Namaste Foods♦

Other Flours and Miscellaneous (cont'd)

Flour Type	Company or Brand
Rice Flour (Sweet)	Authentic Foods♦
	Bob's Red Mill
	El Peto Products♦
	Ener-G♦
	Namaste♦
Rice Flour (White)	Authentic Foods♦
	Bgreen Food♦
	Bob's Red Mill
	Club House
	Cuisine Soleil♦
	Duinkerken Foods♦
	El Peto Products♦
	Ener-G♦
	Hodgson Mill
Sorghum Bran	Nu Life Market♦ (black; burgundy; sumac)
Sorghum Flour	Authentic Foods♦
	Bgreen Food♦
	Bob's Red Mill
	Cuisine Soleil♦
	El Peto Products♦
	Namaste Foods♦
	Nu Life Market♦ (black; burgundy; white)
	Wondergrain♦
Sweet Potato Flour	Let's Do…Organic
Teff Flour	Bob's Red Mill (brown)
	Nu Life Market ♦ (brown; ivory)
	The Teff Company♦ (brown; ivory)

Starches and Gums

Starches

Starch Type	Company or Brand
Arrowroot Starch	Authentic Foods♦
	Bob's Red Mill
	El Peto Products♦
	Namaste Foods♦

Starches (cont'd)

Starch Type	Company or Brand
Potato Starch / **Potato Starch Flour** Note: This is not the same as Potato Flour.	Authentic Foods ◆
	Bob's Red Mill
	Club House
	Cuisine Soleil ◆
	Duinkerken ◆
	El Peto Products ◆
	Ener-G ◆
	Hodgson Mill
	King Arthur Flour
Tapioca Starch / **Tapioca Starch Flour /** **Tapioca Flour**	Authentic Foods ◆
	Bob's Red Mill
	Cuisine Soleil ◆
	Duinkerken ◆
	El Peto Products ◆
	Ener-G ◆
	Hodgson Mill
	King Arthur Flour
	Let's Do…Organic
	Namaste Foods ◆

Gums

Gum Type	Company or Brand
Guar Gum	Authentic Foods ◆
	Bob's Red Mill
	Duinkerken ◆
	El Peto Products ◆
Xanthan Gum	Authentic Foods ◆
	Bob's Red Mill
	Duinkerken ◆
	El Peto Products ◆
	Ener-G ◆
	Hodgson Mill
	King Arthur Flour
	Namaste ◆

Coatings, Croûtons, Crumbs and Stuffings

• These items usually contain wheat and/or may contain seasonings derived from wheat or barley.

• Make your own coatings or crumbs from gluten-free breads, chips or crackers.

• Gluten-free grains or dry bread can be used to make homemade stuffing. A recipe for stuffing made with sorghum grain is on page 190.

Coatings, Croûtons, Crumbs and Stuffings

Company or Brand	Product	Varieties or Flavors
Aleias♦	Bread Crumbs	Italian; Plain
	Coat & Crunch	Crispy Spicy; Extra Spicy
	Croutons	Classic; Parmesan
	Real Panko	Original
	Stuffing Mix	Plain; Savory
Barkat♦	Stuffing Mix	Sage & Onion
Domata♦	Seasoned Flour	
El Peto Products♦	Bread Crumbs	
	Stuffing	
Ener-G♦	Bread Crumbs	
	Croutons	Plain
Glutenfree Bakehouse (Whole Foods)♦	10 Minute Stuffing*	
	Stuffing Cubes	
Glutino♦	Bread Crumbs	Original
	Stuffing	Corn Bread
Goldbaum's Natural Foods♦	Mini Croutons	
Hilary's Eat Well♦	Holiday Stuffing	
Hodgson Mill	GF Seasoned Coating Mix	
Hol•Grain	GF Batter Mix	Onion Rings; Tempura
	GF Bread Crumbs	Brown Rice
	GF Coating Mix	Chicken
Ian's	GF Breadcrumbs	Ancient Grain with Quinoa & Amaranth; Whole Grain Brown Rice
	GF Croutons	Italian Style; Kale Garlic; Rosemary Garlic; Sea Salt & Pepper
	GF Homestyle Stuffing	Savory
	GF Panko Breadcrumbs	Italian; Original
Kikkoman	GF Panko Style Coating	
Kinnikinnick♦	Bread Crumbs	Panko Style
	Bread Cubes	
	Crumbs	Chocolate Cookie; Graham Style Cracker
Namaste Foods♦	Seasoned Coating Mix	Barbecue; Homestyle; Hot 'n Spicy; Italian Herb
Olivia's Croutons	GF Croutons	Garlic
	GF Stuffing	
Orgran♦	Bread Crumbs	All Purpose Rice; Corn Crispy; Quinoa
	Quinoa Croutons	Garlic & Herbs; Sea Salt
Plum-M-Good♦	Breading Crumbs	Brown Rice
President's Choice	GF Bread Crumbs	Plain
Schär♦	Bread Crumbs	
	Croutons	
Three Bakers♦	Whole Grain Cubed Stuffing Mix	Herb Seasoned
Watusee Foods♦	Chickpea Crumbs	Plain

Grains

- Avoid buying gluten-free grains from bulk bins due to a high risk of cross-contamination from gluten-containing grains.

- It should be noted that some companies not displaying the diamond symbol (♦) nonetheless produce their gluten-free grains in dedicated gluten-free facilities (e.g., Bob's Red Mill, King Arthur Flour).

- Learn more about the different gluten-free grains (see pp. 97–104, 143–145).

Grains	
Grain Type	**Company or Brand**
Amaranth	Bob's Red Mill
	GoGo Quinoa♦
Buckwheat (Whole Groats, Roasted Groats [Kasha], Grits)	Bob's Red Mill
	Hodgson Mill
	Pocono (The Birkett Mills)
	Wolff's (The Birkett Mills)
Millet	Bob's Red Mill
	Eden Foods
Oats (Gluten-Free Oat Groats, Steel-Cut)	Bakery On Main♦
	Bob's Red Mill
	Cream Hill Estates♦
	GF Harvest♦
	Glutenfreeda Foods♦
	Gluten-Free Prairie♦
	Libre Naturals♦
	Only Oats (Avena Foods)♦
	Udi's Gluten Free♦
Quinoa	Ancient Harvest♦
	Bob's Red Mill
	GoGo Quinoa♦
	Hodgson Mill
	Norquin♦
	TruRoots♦
Sorghum	Bob's Red Mill
	Hodgson Mill
	Nu Life Market♦
	Wondergrain♦
Teff	Bob's Red Mill (brown)
	Nu Life Market ♦ (brown, ivory)
	The Teff Company♦ (brown, ivory)

Side Dishes, Gnocchi and Perogies, Entrées, Breaded Fish and Poultry and Veggie Burgers

- Side dishes and entrées may contain seasonings that include a carrier agent such as wheat flour or wheat starch.

- Some vegetarian and vegan side dishes, entrées and meat replacement products are made with gluten-containing ingredients (e.g., wheat-based soy sauce, wheat gluten, barley) and therefore are **NOT** gluten free.

- Grain-based side dishes (e.g. couscous, pilafs) often contain ingredients not allowed (e.g., wheat berries, barley).

- Most breaded products, such as chicken and fish, typically contain wheat-based coatings and therefore are **NOT** gluten free.

Side Dishes

Company or Brand	Product	Varieties or Flavors
Ancient Harvest◆	Polenta	Basil Garlic; Green Chili & Cilantro; Heirloom Red & Black Quinoa; Sun-Dried Tomato Garlic; Traditional Italian
	Quinoa, Millet & Amaranth Blend	Butter & Parmesan; Sea Salt & Herb; Spanish Style; Spicy Curry
Annie Chun's	GF Rice Express (Sticky Rice)	Sprouted Brown; White
Cooksimple◆	Ancient Grains Salad	
	Pilaf	Sorghum; Wild Rice
	Spanish Rice	
Dr. Praeger's	GF Cakes*	Broccoli; Spinach
	GF Hash Browns	Four Potato; Root Veggie; Southwest; Sweet Potato
	GF Littles	Broccoli; Kale; Spinach; Sweet Potato
	GF Veggie Puffs	Carrot; Kale; Taro
Feel Good Foods◆	Dumplings	Chicken; Pork; Vegetable
	Egg Rolls	Chicken & Vegetable; Shrimp & Vegetable; Vegetable
	Fried Brown Rice	Vegetable
Garden Lites	GF Bake	Cheddar Broccoli
	GF Soufflé	Butternut Squash; Kale & Quinoa; Roasted Vegetable
	GF Veggie Bites	Broccoli & Brown Rice; Cornbread; Italian; Kale & Brown Rice
	GF Veggie Cakes	Superfood
GoGo Quinoa◆	Granissimo	5 Grains; Andean Mix & Pumpkin Seeds
	Paella	Vegetarian
	Pilaf	Basmati & Wild Quinoa
	Quinoa	Provençal; With Vegetables
Goldbaum's Natural Foods◆	Israeli CousCous (Tapioca and Potato)	
Grainful◆	Steel Cut Sides*	Cheesy Oats; Jambalaya; Madras Curry; Tomato Risotto
Hilary's Eat Well◆	Veggie Bites	Broccoli Casserole; Mediterranean; Original; Spicy Mesquite

Side Dishes (cont'd)

Company or Brand	Product	Varieties or Flavors
Hodgson Mill	GF Quinoa & Brown Rice	Garlic & Herb; Italian; Lemon Pepper; Mediterranean; Spicy
	GF Sorghum, Quinoa & Brown Rice	Chipotle; Parmesan; Pesto Herb; Rosemary & Garlic; Southwest
Ian's	GF Alphatots	
	GF Crispy Potato Puffs	
	GF Onion Rings	
	GF Tempura-Style Green Beans	
	GF Tempura-Style Sweet Potato Sticks	
Lotus Foods♦	Heat & Eat Rice Bowl	Brown Jasmine; Forbidden; Volcano
Lundberg	GF Brown Rice Bowl	Country Wild; Long Grain; Short Grain
	GF Crabby Rice	Chesapeake Bay Style Seasoning
	GF Sprouted Risotto	Butter & Chive; Cheddar & Peppers; Sweet Corn & Bell Pepper
	GF Sprouted Whole Grain Rice	Chili Verde; Korean BBQ; Thai Red Curry; Toasted Coconut; Vegetable Fried
	GF Traditional Risotto	Alfredo; Butternut Squash; Creamy Parmesan; Florentine; Garlic Primavera; Porcini Mushroom
	GF Whole Grain Quinoa & Rice	Basil & Bell Pepper; Rosemary Blend; Spanish Style
	GF Whole Grain Rice & Seasoning Mix	Black Beans & Rice; Jambalaya; Masala; Red Beans & Rice; Southwestern; Spanish; Tuscan; Yellow
	GF Whole Grain Rice & Wild Rice & Seasoning Mix	Garlic & Basil; Original; Wild Porcini Mushroom
President's Choice	GF Corn Couscous	
Taste Adventure	GF Black Beans & Rice	Santa Fe Fiesta
	GF Lentils & Rice	Bombay Curry
	GF Louisiana Red Bean	Jambalaya
TruRoots♦	Accents	Sprouted Lentil Trio; Sprouted Quinoa Trio; Sprouted Rice Trio
	Multigrain Pilaf	Coconut Lemon Grass; Curry Rice; Mediterranean Vegetable; New World Blend; Roasted Garlic; Savory Herb; Spanish Spice
	Sprouted Medley	Bean & Lentil; Quinoa & Ancient Grain; Rice & Quinoa

Gnocchi and Perogies

Company or Brand	Product	Varieties or Flavors
Caesar's Pasta	GF Gnocchi	Potato; Spinach
Cappello's♦	Gnocchi	
Conte's Pasta	Gnocchi with Marinara Sauce	
	GF Pierogies	Potato and Cheese with Onion; Potato and Onion
	GF Potato Gnocchi	
Gabriella's Kitchen	Gnocchi in Pomodoro Sauce	
	Sweet Potato Gnocchi in Pomodoro Sauce	
Joe's Gluten-Free Foods♦	Potato Perogies	Bacon & Cheddar; Cheddar Cheese; Jalapeño & Cream Cheese; Onion; Roasted Garlic; Sauerkraut

Gnocchi and Perogies (cont'd)

Company or Brand	Product	Varieties or Flavors
Leo's Gluten Free♦	Gnocchi	Butternut Squash; Potato; Roasted Red Pepper; Spinach
	Gnocchi (Stuffed)	Asiago; Portobello Mushroom; Spinach
Le Veneziane♦	Gnocchi	Potato

Entrées

Company or Brand	Product	Varieties or Flavors
Amy's	GF Asian Meal	Thai Green Curry; Thai Pad Thai; Thai Red Curry; Thai Stir-Fry
	GF Bowl	3 Cheese Kale Bake; Baked Ziti; Black-Eyed Peas & Veggies; Broccoli & Cheddar Bake; Brown Rice; Brown Rice & Vegetables; Brown Rice & Vegetables (Light in Sodium); Brown Rice, Black Eyed Peas and Veggies; Harvest Casserole; Mexican Casserole; Mexican Casserole (Light in Sodium); Mushroom Risotto; Santa Fe Enchilada; Sweet and Sour (Light & Lean); Teriyaki; Tortilla Casserole & Black Beans
	GF Burrito	Black Bean & Quinoa; Cheddar; Non-Dairy
	GF Chile Relleno Casserole	
	GF Chili	Black Bean; Medium; Medium (Light in Sodium); Medium with Vegetables; Spicy; Spicy (Light in Sodium)
	GF Enchiladas	Black Bean & Cheese (Light & Lean); Black Bean Vegetable; Black Bean Vegetable (Light in Sodium); Cheese; Vegan Cheeze & Black Bean
	GF Enchilada Whole Meal	Black Bean; Cheese; Verde
	GF Indian Meal	Mattar Paneer; Mattar Paneer (Light & Lean); Mattar Paneer (Light in Sodium); Mattar Tofu; Palak Paneer; Paneer Tikka; Vegetable Korma
	GF Pies	Mexican Tamale; Shepherd's
	GF Pot Pie	Vegetable
	GF Quinoa & Black Beans with Butternut Squash and Chard (Light & Lean)	
	GF Roasted Polenta (Light & Lean)	
	GF Scramble	Breakfast*; Mexican Tofu; Tofu
	GF Soft Taco Fiesta (Light & Lean)	
	GF Tamale	Roasted Vegetable
	GF Tamale Verde	Black Bean; Cheese
	GF Veggie Loaf Whole Meal*	Light in Sodium; Regular
	GF Wrap	Indian Aloo Mattar; Teriyaki; Tofu Scramble Breakfast
Apetito	GF Apple Braised Pork	
	GF Beef & Vegetable Casserole	
	GF Country Chicken With Gravy	
	GF Hawaiian Chicken	
	GF Lemon Herb Fish	
	GF Pot Roast	
	GF Turkey with Gravy	

Entrées (cont'd)

Company or Brand	Product	Varieties or Flavors
Applegate Farms	GF Breakfast Sausage Patties	Chicken & Apple; Chicken & Maple; Savory Turkey
	GF Breakfast Sausages	Chicken & Apple; Chicken & Maple; Chicken & Sage; Classic Pork; Savory Turkey
	GF Corn Dogs	Beef
Beetnik◆	Frozen Meal	Beef Chili; Beef Kheema; Beef Meatballs with Marinara; Chicken Creole; Chicken Meatballs with Marinara; Moroccan Seasoned Chicken Stew; Peruvian Seasoned Chicken Stew; Sesame Ginger Chicken; Thai Style Beef with Coconut Rice
Blue Horizon	GF Surf Burgers	Alaskan Salmon; Alaskan Salmon & Blue Cheese; Alaskan Salmon Cilantro Lime; Pacific Tuna Teriyaki
Campbell Company of Canada	GF Chunky Chili	Homestyle; Hot & Spicy
Cooksimple◆	Chili	Cowboy; White Bean
	Jambalaya	
	Sloppy Joe	
	Tamale Pie	
Evol Foods	GF Fajita Cup	Beans, Veggie & Cheddar; Grilled White Chicken with Rice; Pork & Poblano Pesto with Rice, Bell Peppers & Cheese; Southwest Veggie, Rice, Bean & Cheddar; Srircha Queso Grilled Chicken
	GF Meals for Two	Chicken Tikka Masala; Teriyaki Chicken; Thai Style Curry Chicken; Truffle Parmesan & Portabella Risotto
	GF Scramble Cup	Chicken Apple Sausage, Egg White with Potato & Cheese; Egg, Basil Pesto, Potato & Cheese; Egg, Uncured Bacon & Cheese with Bell Peppers & Potato; Egg White, Veggies & Cheese
	GF Single Serve Entrée	Chicken Enchilada Bake; Chicken Enchiladas; Chicken Tikka Masala; Coconut Lemongrass Chicken; Fire Grilled Chicken Poblano; Fire Grilled Steak; Parmesan Polenta & Veggies; Quinoa & Roasted Veggies; Sriracha Chicken; Teriyaki Chicken; Vegetable Enchiladas
	GF Street Tacos	Shredded Chicken & Caramelized Onion; Sweet Potato, Black Bean & Goat Cheese; Uncured Bacon, Potato & Poblano Pepper
	GF Veggie Cup	Balsamic Brussels with Uncured Bacon & Parmesan; Broccoli & Cheddar with Uncured Ham & Potato; Ginger Sesame Sweet Potato; Truffle Parmesan Roasted Cauliflower
Feel Good Foods◆	Broad Noodles with Chicken & Chinese Broccoli	
	General Tso's Chicken	
	Mongolian Beef with Asparagus & Scallions	
	Stir-Fry Chicken & Vegetables with Mandarin Pancakes & Dipping Sauce	
Gluten Free Café◆	Homestyle Chicken & Vegetables	
	Lemon Basil Chicken	
	Savory Chicken Pilaf	

Entrées (cont'd)

Company or Brand	Product	Varieties or Flavors
Glutenfreeda Foods♦	Burrito	Beef & Potato; Chicken & Cheese; Chipotle Chicken & Black Bean; Shredded Beef; Vegetarian Bean & Cheese; Vegetarian Dairy Free
	Pizza Wrap	Italian Sausage; Pesto Chicken; Three Cheese
	Pocket Sandwich	Bacon & Eggs with Cheddar; Hickory Smoked Ham & Cheddar; Roast Beef with Caramelized Onions & Provolone
Grainful♦	Steel Cut Meals*	Cheddar Broccoli; Porcini Mushroom Chicken; Thai Curry; Tuscan Bean & Kale; Unstuffed Pepper; Vegetarian Chili
Ian's	GF Corn Dogs	Popcorn Uncured Turkey
Neat Foods♦	Meat Replacement Mix*	Breakfast; Italian; Mexican; Original
Pacific Foods	GF Burmese Tofu	Chipotle; Italian Herb; Original
President's Choice	GF Breakfast Sausage	Loads of Cheddar Potato & Bacon; Loads of Maple Syrup, Apple & Bacon; Loads of White Cheddar & Apple
	GF Frozen Entrée	Butter Chicken; Cashew Chicken; Chicken Korma; Chicken Madras; Red Curry Chicken
	GF Frozen Entrée (Blue Menu)	Butter Chicken; Chicken Korma; Chicken Vindaloo; Quinoa Lemon & Herb Chicken; Quinoa Mediterranean Chicken; Quinoa Southwest Chicken; Sweet & Sour Chicken
Saffron Road	GF Achiote Roasted Chicken	
	GF Beef Bulgogi	
	GF Beef Chile Colorado	
	GF Bibimbop	Beef; Vegetable
	GF Bowls	Lemongrass Basil Fish; Masala Curry Fish; Sesame Ginger Salmon; Thai Red Curry Fish
	GF Chana Saag	
	GF Chicken Biryani	
	GF Chicken Enchiladas Poblano	
	GF Chicken Nuggets	Plain; Tandoori Seasoned
	GF Chicken Pad Thai	
	GF Chicken Saag	
	GF Chicken Tenders	
	GF Chicken Tikka Masala	
	GF Chicken Vindaloo	
	GF Enchiladas Al Chipotle	
	GF Gochujang Chicken	
	GF Lamb Saag	
	GF Lamb Vindaloo	
	GF Lemongrass Basil Chicken	
	GF Manchurian Dumplings	
	GF Palak Paneer	
	GF Thai Basil Chili Tofu	
	GF Vegetable Pad Thai	
Sea Fare Pacific♦	GF Curry Entrée	Red Albacore; Yellow Albacore

Entrées (cont'd)

Company or Brand	Product	Varieties or Flavors
Sol Cuisine	GF BBQ Tofu Ribs	
	GF Falafel with Tahini Sauce	
	GF Meatless Beef	Mongolian BBQ
	GF Meatless Chicken	Ginger Lime Teriyaki; Korean BBQ; Lightly Seasoned; Smoky Chipotle Tinga
Taste Adventure	GF Chili Mix	5 Bean; Black Bean; Lentil; Red Bean
Thai Kitchen	GF Curry Kit	Green; Red
The Tofurky Company	GF Ground	Beef Style; Chorizo Style
	GF Tempeh Cake	Five Grain; Soy
	GF Tempeh Strips	Coconut Curry
Udi's Gluten Free♦	Breakfast Burrito	Chicken Apple Sausage; Sausage, Spicy Southwest Veggie; Uncured Bacon
	Breakfast Sandwich	Chicken Maple Sausage; Egg White & Cheddar; Ham & Cheddar; Sausage
	Burrito	Bean & Green Chili; Chicken; Spicy Southwest Veggies; Steak

Breaded Fish and Poultry

Company or Brand	Product	Varieties or Flavors
Applegate Farms	GF Chicken Nuggets	
	GF Chicken Tenders	
Blue Horizon	GF Bites	New England Crab; Wild Alaskan Salmon
	GF Crab Cakes	Maryland Style
Dr. Praeger's	GF Crusted Fish Sticks	Rice; Southern Cornmeal; Thai
	GF Fish Fillets	Quinoa & Herb Crusted; Herb Crusted Cod; Rice Crusted
	GF Rice Crusted Fishies	
Golden Platter♦	GF Boneless Chicken Wyngz	Buffalo Style
	GF Buffalo Style Bites	
	GF Chicken Nuggets	Dinosaurs; Disney's Frozen; Disney's Star Wars; Disney's Winnie The Pooh Honey; Marvel's Avengers
	GF Chicken Patties	
	GF Chicken Tenders	
Ian's	GF Chicken Nuggets	Plain; Smokin' Sweet BBQ
	GF Chicken Nuggets Kids Meal	
	GF Chicken Patties	
	GF Chicken Patty Fritters	Sriracha Fire Sticks
	GF Chicken Tenders	Plain; Southwest
	GF Fish Filets	Herb Crusted
	GF Fish Sticks	
President's Choice	GF Chicken Breast Fillets	
	GF Chicken Breasts	Ancient Grains; Quinoa
	GF Cod Burgers	Fish & Chips; Quinoa Pacific

Veggie Burgers

Company or Brand	Product	Varieties or Flavors
Amy's	GF Veggie Burgers	Bistro; Sonoma*
Dr. Praeger's	GF Veggie Burgers	Black Bean Quinoa; GF California*; Heirloom Bean; Kale; Mushroom Risotto; Super Greens
GoGo Quinoa♦	Burger	Tex Mex
	Quinoa Burger Mix	Quinoa & Amaranth
Hilary's Eat Well♦	Burgers	Adzuki Bean; Black Rice; Curry; Hemp & Greens; Kimchi; Root Veggie; Spicy Thai; World's Best Veggie
President's Choice	Vegetarian Burger	Portobello Swiss
Qrunch Foods♦	Quinoa Burgers	Green Chile with Pinto Beans; Original; Saucy Buffalo; Spicy Italian
Sol Cuisine	GF Burgers	Chickpea Sweet Potato; Original; Portobello Mushroom; Spicy Black Bean; Sprouted Quinoa Chia; Sweet Curry
	GF Veggie Breakfast Sausages	
Sunshine Burger♦	Veggie Breakfast Patties	Hemp & Sage
	Veggie Burgers	Barbecue; Black Bean Southwest; Falafel; Garden Herb; Quarter Pound Original; Shiitake Mushroom
The Tofurky Company	GF Veggie Burgers	Hearty Hemp; Spicy Black Bean; White Quinoa

Dry Pasta, Fresh Pasta and Pasta Meals

- Some brands of buckwheat pasta contain a mixture of both buckwheat flour and wheat flour.
- There are many different types of gluten-free pastas in various shapes made with ingredients such as amaranth, buckwheat, corn, flax, millet, pulses, quinoa, rice, soy, vegetables (e.g., potato, sweet potato) and/or wild rice.
- Fresh pastas can be found in the refrigerated or frozen sections of the store.

Dry Pasta

Company or Brand	Product	Varieties or Flavors
Ancient Harvest♦	Black Bean & Quinoa Pasta	Elbows
	Corn & Quinoa Pasta	Elbows; Garden Pagotas; Linguine; Penne; Rotini; Shells; Spaghetti; Veggie Curls
	Green Lentil & Quinoa Pasta	Penne; Spaghetti
	Red Lentil & Quinoa Pasta	Rotini; Linguine
Andean Dream♦	Quinoa Pasta	Fusilli; Macaroni; Orzo; Shells; Spaghetti
Annie Chun's	GF Rice Noodles	Maifun; Maifun Brown; Pad Thai; Pad Thai Brown
Banza♦	Chickpea Pasta	Elbows; Penne; Rotini; Shells
Barilla	GF Corn and Rice Pasta	Elbows; Penne; Rotini; Spaghetti
Barkat♦	Buckwheat Pasta	Penne; Spirals
	Corn Pasta	Alphabet Shapes; Animal Shapes; Macaroni; Shells; Short Cut Tagliatelli; Spaghetti; Spirals
	Corn and Rice Pasta	Lasagne

Dry Pasta (cont'd)

Company or Brand	Product	Varieties or Flavors
Bgreen Food♦	Black Rice Pasta	Angel Hair
	Brown Rice Pasta	Angel Hair
	Buckwheat Pasta	Angel Hair
	Fensi (Pea Starch) Noodles	Vermicelli
	Millet Pasta	Angel Hair
	Ramen	Black Rice; Brown Rice; Buckwheat; Millet & Brown Rice
	White Rice Pasta	Angel Hair
Bionaturae	GF Potato, Rice and Soy Pasta	Elbows; Fusilli; Linguine; Penne Rigate; Rigatoni; Spaghetti
Cappello's♦	Almond Pasta	Fettuccine; Lasagne Sheets
Catelli	GF Corn, Quinoa, Brown and White Rice Pasta	Fusilli; Lasagna; Linguine; Macaroni; Penne; Spaghetti
Cooksimple♦	Vegetable & Bean Rotini	Beet; Carrot; Pea; Sweet Potato
DeBoles	GF Corn Pasta	Elbows Style; Spaghetti Style
	GF Multigrain Pasta	Penne; Spaghetti
	GF Quinoa + Golden Flax Pasta	Penne; Spaghetti
	GF Rice + Golden Flax Pasta	Angel Hair; Spirals
	GF Rice Pasta	Angel Hair; Fettuccini; Lasagna; Penne; Spaghetti Style; Spirals
Eden Foods	GF Bifun Rice Pasta	
	GF Kuzu Pasta	
	GF Mung Bean Pasta (Harusame)	
Explore Cuisine♦	Adzuki Bean Pasta	Spaghetti
	Black Bean Pasta	Spaghetti
	Brown Rice Noodles	Pad Thai
	Brown Rice Pasta	Fusilli; Rigatoni
	Chickpea Pasta	Fusilli; Spaghetti
	Edamame & Mung Bean Pasta	Fettuccine
	Edamame Pasta	Spaghetti
	Green Lentil Pasta	Lasagna; Penne
	Red Lentil Pasta	Penne; Spaghetti
	Red Rice Noodles	Pad Thai
	Red Rice Pasta	Elbows
	Soybean Pasta	Spaghetti
GoGo Quinoa♦	Rice & Amaranth Pasta	Penne
	Rice & Quinoa Pasta	Fusilli; Macaroni; Spaghetti; Vegetable Anelli
Goldbaum's Natural Foods♦	Brown Rice Pasta	Elbows; Fettuccini; Fusilli; Penne; Radiatore; Shells; Spaghetti; Spirals
	Chow Mein Noodles	
	Pasta Noodles	Medium Cut; Thin Cut
Hodgson Mill	GF Brown Rice Pasta with Golden Milled Flax	Angel Hair; Elbows; Lasagna; Linguine; Penne; Spaghetti
Jovial	GF Brown Rice Pasta	Capellini; Caserecce; Elbows; Farfalle; Fusilli; Lasagna; Manicotti; Penne Rigate; Spaghetti; Tagliatelle

Dry Pasta (cont'd)

Company or Brand	Product	Varieties or Flavors
Le Asolane♦	Corn Pasta	Capellini; Ditalini; Eliche; Penne Rigate; Spaghetti; Tagliatelle
	Corn Pasta with Fiber	Anellini; Bucatini; Capellini; Cellentani; Ditalini; Eliche; Farfalle; Gnocchi; Penne Rigate; Pipe Rigate; Rigatoni; Risetti; Spaghetti; Stelline; Tagliatelle; Tubetti Rigati
Le Veneziane♦	Corn Pasta	Anellini; Capellini; Ditalini; Elbows; Eliche (Fusilli); Farfalle; Fettucce; Lasagne; Penne Rigate; Pipe Rigate (Shells); Rigatoni; Spaghetti
Lotus Foods♦	Ramen Noodles	Forbidden Rice; Jade Pearl Rice; Millet & Brown Rice
Lundberg	GF Brown Rice Pasta	Elbows; Penne; Rotini; Spaghetti
Modern Table♦	Bean & Lentil Pasta	Confetti
	Lentil Pasta	Elbows; Penne; Rotini
	Mixed Lentil Pasta	Penne
Mrs. Leeper's♦	Corn Pasta	Elbows; Rotelli; Spaghetti; Vegetable Radiatore
	Rice Pasta	Spaghetti; Vegetable Twists
Orgran♦	Buckwheat Pasta	Spirals
	Corn & Vegetable Pasta	Shells; Spirals
	Corn Pasta	Spirals
	Italian Style Pasta	Spaghetti
	Quinoa Pasta	Penne; Spirals
	Rice & Corn Pasta	Farm Animal Vegetable; Lasagne Mini Sheets; Macaroni; Outback Animal Vegetable; Penne; Spaghetti; Spaghetti Noodles; Spirals; Tortelli
	Rice & Millet Pasta	Spirals
	Rice Pasta	Spirals
	Super Trio Brown Rice, Quinoa and Kale Pasta	Penne
	Super Trio Millet, Quinoa and Buckwheat	Spirals
	Vegetable Rice Pasta	Penne; Spirals
Pasta Legume♦	Whole Green Lentil Pasta	Elbows; Penne; Spirals
Pastariso♦	Brown Rice Pasta	Elbows; Penne; Rotini; Spaghetti; Vegetable Rotini
	White Rice Pasta	Elbows; Ziti
Pastato♦	Fortified Potato Pasta	Elbows; Penne; Spaghetti
President's Choice	GF Corn Pasta	Fusilli; Macaroni; Penne; Spaghetti
Rizopia♦	Brown and Wild Rice Pasta	Elbows; Fusilli; Penne; Shells; Spaghetti
	Brown Rice Pasta	Elbows; Fantasia; Fettuccine; Fusilli; Lasagne; Penne; Shells; Spaghetti; Spaghetti; Spirals
	Quinoa and Brown Rice Pasta	Fusilli; Penne; Spaghetti
	White Rice Pasta	Spaghetti
Ronzoni	GF Corn, Quinoa, Brown and White Rice Pasta	Elbow; Penne Rigate; Rotini; Spaghetti; Thin Spaghetti
Schär♦	Corn & Rice Pasta	Fusilli; Penne; Spaghetti
Thai Kitchen	GF Rice Noodles	Stir Fry; Thin

Dry Pasta (cont'd)

Company or Brand	Product	Varieties or Flavors
Tinkyada♦	Brown Rice Pasta	Elbows; Fettuccine; Fusilli; Grand Shells; Lasagne; Little Dreams; Penne; Shells; Spaghetti; Spirals
	Spinach Brown Rice Pasta	Spaghetti
	Vegetable Brown Rice Pasta	Spirals
	White Rice Pasta	Spaghetti
Tolerant Foods♦	Energy Legume Blend Black Bean & Pea Pasta	Penne; Spaghetti
	Energy Legume Blend Green Lentil & Pea Pasta	Elbows; Penne; Rotini; Spaghetti
	Energy Legume Blend Red Lentil & Pea Pasta	Penne; Rotini; Spaghetti
	Simply Legume Black Bean Pasta	Penne
	Simply Legume Green Lentil Pasta	Elbows; Penne; Shells
	Simply Legume Red Lentil Pasta	Mini Fettucini; Penne; Rotini
TruRoots♦	Ancient Grains Pasta (Brown Rice, Quinoa, Amaranth & Corn)	Elbows; Fusilli; Penne; Spaghetti

Fresh Pasta

Company or Brand	Product	Varieties or Flavors
Gabriella's Kitchen	GF Teff skinnypasta	Linguine; Macaroni; Penne
Leo's Gluten Free♦	Brown Rice Fresh Pasta	Cavatelli; Elbow Macaroni; Fettuccine; Lasagna Sheets; Penne; Rotini; Spaghetti
Manini's♦	Ancient Grains Pasta	Fettuccini; Fettuccini (Roasted Garlic); Lasagna Sheets; Linguini; Linguini (Lemon Thyme); Macaroni; Rigatoni; Spaghetti
President's Choice	GF Buckwheat, Potato and Rice Fresh Pasta	Spaghetti; Tagliatelli
RP's Pasta Company	GF Black Bean Pasta	Penne
	GF Brown Rice Pasta	Fettuccine; Fettuccini (Spinach); Fusilli; Lasagna Sheets; Linguine
	GF Chickpea Pasta	Linguini
	GF Heat & Serve Brown Rice Pasta (Frozen)	Fusilli; Macaroni; Penne; Shells; Ziti
	GF Red Lentil Pasta	Fusilli

Pasta Meals

Company or Brand	Product	Varieties or Flavors
Amy's	GF Asian Meal	Asian Noodle Stir Fry; Chinese Noodles & Veggies
	GF Chili Mac	
	GF Lasagna	Garden Vegetable; Vegetable (Dairy Free)
	GF Rice Mac & Cheeze	Dairy Free
	GF Rice Mac & Cheese	

Pasta Meals (cont'd)

Company or Brand	Product	Varieties or Flavors
Ancient Harvest♦	Corn & Quinoa Mac & Cheese	Mild Cheddar with Elbows; Mild Cheddar with Llamas; Sharp Cheddar with Shells; White Cheddar with Shells
	Lentil & Quinoa Mac & Cheese	Mild Cheddar Elbows; Sharp Cheddar Shells; White Cheddar Shells
	Lentil & Quinoa Pasta Meal	Cubanitos; Italiano
Annie's Homegrown	GF Deluxe Rice Pasta Dinner	Rice Pasta & Extra Cheesy Cheddar Sauce
	GF Mac & Cheese Microwaveable	Real Aged Cheddar
	GF Macaroni & Cheese	Rice Pasta & Cheddar; Rice Shells & Creamy White Cheddar
	GF Quinoa Rice Pasta	White Cheddar
	GF Rice Pasta & Cheddar Microwavable Cup	
	GF Rice Pasta Dinner	Vegan Elbows & Creamy Sauce
Banza♦	Chickpea Pasta Mac & Cheese	Deluxe Cheddar; White Cheddar
	Chickpea Pasta Shells and Cheese	Classic Cheddar
Barkat♦	Mac 'n' Cheese	
Beetnik♦	Pasta Meal	Beef Bolognese; Beef Stroganoff; Chicken Cacciatore
Caesar's Pasta	GF Cannelloni	Beef
	GF Gluten-Free Gourmet	3 Cheese Herb Rigatoni & Meat Sauce; Buffalo Style Chicken Mac & Cheese
	GF Lasagna	Cheese; Chicken; Vegetable
	GF Manicotti	With Cheese in Marinara Sauce
	GF Meals for Two	Mexican Mac & Cheese; Portobello Mushroom Mac & Cheese; Tofu & Kale Penne
	GF Ravioli	Beef; Cheese
	GF Stuffed Shells	With Cheese in Marinara Sauce
Conte's Pasta	GF Microwave Meal	Cheese Lasagna; Cheese Ravioli
	GF Ravioli	Butternut Squash; Cheese; Spinach & Cheese
	GF Stuffed Shells	Cheese
	GF Tortolloni	Four Cheese
Cooksimple♦	Pasta Meal / Side Dish Kit	Alfredo; Buffalo Blue; Cheesy Broccoli; Herb & Butter Noodles; Lasagna; Pasta Salad; Stroganoff
Daiya Foods♦	Cheezy Mac	Deluxe Alfredo Style; Deluxe Cheddar Style; Deluxe White Cheddar Style Veggie
DeBoles	GF Rice Pasta & Cheese	Elbow Style
Evol Foods	GF Mac & Cheese	Smoked Gouda; Uncured Bacon
Gabriella's Kitchen	GF skinnypasta Kids Meal	3 Cheese & Spinach Ravioli; Teff Macaroni and Cheese; Teff Penne in Ragu Sauce
	GF skinnypasta Meal	3-Cheese & Spinach Ravioli; Butternut Squash Ravioli; Roasted Vegetable Lasagna
Gluten Free Café♦	Asian Noodles	
	Fettuccini Alfredo	
	Pasta Primavera	
Leo's Gluten Free♦	Ravioli	Butternut Squash; Four Cheese; Portobello Mushroom; Roasted Red Pepper; Spinach & Cheese
Lundberg	GF Brown Rice Pasta & Sauce Mix	Garlic & Olive Oil; Leek & Mushroom; Roasted Red Pepper; Spinach & Rosemary

Pasta Meals (cont'd)

Company or Brand	Product	Varieties or Flavors
Manini's♦	Ancient Grains Fresh Pasta	Ravioli (4 Cheese); Ravioli (Portobello & Cheese); Ravioli (Spinach & Cheese)
Modern Table♦	Bean Pasta & Veggie Kit	Cheddar Broccoli; Creamy Mushroom; Homestyle Mac & Cheese; Italian; Mediterranean; Pesto; Southwest; Teriyaki
Mrs. Leeper's♦	Pasta Dinner	Beef Lasagna; Beef Stroganoff; Cheeseburger Mac; Chicken Alfredo; Creamy Tuna
Namaste Foods♦	Pasta Dinner	Pasta Pisavera; Say Cheez; Taco
Orgran♦	Canned Spaghetti in Tomato Sauce	
Pastariso♦	Brown Rice Mac & Cheeze	White Cheddar; Yellow Cheddar
	Mac Uncheddar	
	Microwaveable Mac & Cheese Meal Cup	Brown Rice; Brown Rice (Reduced Sodium); White Rice; White Rice (Reduced Sodium)
	White Rice Mac & Cheeze	Yellow Cheddar
Pastato♦	Fortified Potato Mac & Cheeze	White Cheddar; Yellow Cheddar
President's Choice	GF Fresh Tortellini	Four Cheese
Road's End Organics	GF Alfredo Mac & Chreese	
	GF Cheddar Penne & Chreese	
Schär♦	Cannelloni with Spinach and Ricotta	
	Caserecce Pasta with Pesto Sauce	
	Fusilli with Arrabbiata Sauce	
	Ravioli with Ricotta & Swiss Chard	
Thai Kitchen	GF Noodle Kit	Pad Thai; Thai Peanut
	GF Rice Noodle Cart	Spicy Thai Basil; Tangy Lemongrass; Pad Thai; Sweet Citrus Ginger
Udi's Gluten Free♦	Bakeable Meal	Lasagna with Meat Sauce; Mac & Cheese; Vegetable Lasagna
	Frozen Entrée	Broccoli & Kale Lasagna; Chicken Florentine; Chicken Puttanesca; Italian Sausage Lasagna; Penne & Cheese; Penne & Cheese with Bacon; Sweet Potato Ravioli; Ziti & Meatballs
	Frozen Skillet Meal	Chicken Florentine; Chicken Parm Penne; Chicken Penne Alfredo; Three Cheese Ravioli; Ziti & Meatballs
Van's	GF Pasta Side Kit	Creamy Herb & Garlic; Rotini & Red Sauce; Ultimate Cheddar Penne

Pizza

- Gluten-free pre-made fresh or frozen pizzas are convenient but costly. For a more economical option, make homemade pizza crust from a gluten-free mix (see pp. 231–237) or use various flours (see pp. 237–240) and add your favorite toppings.

Pizza

Company or Brand	Product	Varieties or Flavors
Absolutely Gluten Free♦	Cauliflower Crust Pizza	Dairy Free; Regular
Amy's	GF Rice Crust Pizza	Cheese; Pesto; Pesto (Dairy Free); Spinach; Spinach Cheese
	GF Single Serve Rice Crust Pizza	Cheese; Cheeze (Dairy Free); Margherita; Roasted Vegetable
Bold Organics	GF Pizza	Deluxe; Meat Lovers; Vegan Cheese; Veggie Lovers
Cappello's♦	Pizza	Cheese; Pepperoni; Sheep's Milk Cheese
Conte's Pasta	GF Pizza	Margherita with Roasted Garlic and Olive Oil; Mushroom Florentine
	GF Pizza (Bake in Bag)	Margherita with Roasted Garlic and Olive Oil; Mushroom Florentine; Pepperoni
Daiya Foods♦	Pizza	Cheeze Lover's; Fire-Roasted Vegetable; Margherita; Mushroom & Roasted Garlic; Spinch & Mushroom; Supreme
Foods By George♦	Pizza	Cheese
The Gluten Free Bistro♦	Bistro Bites Mini Deep Dish Pizzas	Greek Vegan; Margherita; Pepperoni
Glutino♦	Pizza	Duo Cheese; Uncured Pepperoni; Spinach & Feta
Ian's	GF French Bread Pizza	Cheesy; Pepperoni
O'Doughs♦	Pizza Kit	Flax; White
Schär♦	Pizza	Cheese; Veggie
Smart Flour Foods♦	Pizza	Chicken Sausage; Classic Cheese; Garden Margherita; Italian Sausage; Tuscan Inspired Two Meat; Uncured Pepperoni
Three Bakers♦	Pizzas	Classic Cheese; Mild Pepperoni; Sweet Italian Sausage
The Tofurky Company	GF Pizza	Barbecue Chick'n; Pepp'roni & Mushroom; Pesto Supreme
Udi's Gluten Free♦	Pizza	Margherita; Pepperoni; Spinach & Feta; Supreme; Three Cheese

Broths, Bouillons, Soups and Stocks

- Most canned soups are **NOT** gluten-free as they contain **wheat flour**, **barley**, **noodles** and/or hydrolyzed plant protein / hydrolyzed vegetable protein (HPP/HVP) made from **wheat**.

- Bouillon cubes and soup broths often contain wheat flour or hydrolyzed plant / vegetable protein (HPP or HVP) made from wheat, so therefore are **NOT** gluten free.

Broths, Bouillons, Soups and Stocks

Company or Brand	Product	Varieties or Flavors
Amy's	GF Canned Soup	Black Bean Vegetable; Cream of Tomato; Curried Lentil; Fire Roasted Southwestern Vegetable; Indian Golden Lentil; Lentil; Lentil Vegetable; Mushroom Bisque with Porcini; Quinoa, Kale & Red Lentil; Split Pea; Summer Corn & Vegetable; Thai Coconut; Tuscan Bean & Rice
	GF Canned Soup (Chunky)	Tomato Bisque; Tomato Bisque (Vegan); Vegetable
	GF Canned Soup (Hearty)	French Country Vegetable; Rustic Italian Vegetable; Spanish Rice & Red Bean
	GF Canned Soup (Light in Sodium)	Chunky Tomato Bisque; Cream of Tomato; Lentil; Lentil Vegetable; Split Pea
	GF Frozen Soup	Broccoli Cheddar; Corn & Potato Chowder
Andean Dream♦	Quinoa Vegetarian Noodle Soup	
Boulder Organic Foods♦	Fresh Soup	Butternut Squash with Sage; Carrot Ginger with Coconut; Chicken Quinoa and Kale; Chicken Vegetable Chili; Cuban Black Bean; Garden Minestrone; Golden Quinoa and Kale; Green Chili Corn Chowder; Potato Leek; Red Lentil Dahl; Roasted Tomato Basil; Summer Gazpacho; Tuscan White Bean; Vegetable Chili
Campbell Company of Canada	GF Chunky Soup	Chicken & Sausage Gumbo; Split Pea with Ham
	GF Condensed Soup	Chicken with Rice; Chicken with White & Wild Rice; Tomato with Basil and Oregano
	GF Everyday Gourmet Soup	Fire Roasted Sweet Pepper & Tomato; Red Pepper Black Bean; Roasted Potato & Spring Leek; Sweet Potato Tomatillo; Thai Tomato Coconut; Tomato Basil Bisque
	GF Healthy Request Soup	Curried Cauliflower Lentil
	GF Ready To Serve Soup	Herb Chicken with Rice; Homestyle Rustic Lentil
	GF Ready To Use Broth	Beef; Beef (30% Less Sodium); Vegetable; Vegetable (No Salt Added)
	GF Stock First	Beef
Campbell Soup Company (U.S.)	GF Campbell's Organic Soup	Chicken Tortilla; Creamy Butternut Squash; Garden Vegetable with Herbs; Lentil; Sun-Ripened Tomato & Basil Bisque
CelifibR♦	Soup Cubes	Vegetable Medley; Vegetarian Beef; Vegetarian Chicken
Cuisine Santé♦	GF Base for Soups and Sauces	White Roux
	GF Soup Mix	Sweet Corn; Tomato
	GF Stock	Beef Flavored; Beef Flavored (Low Sodium); Chicken Flavored; Chicken Flavored (Low Sodium); Vegetable
Eden Foods	GF Instant Miso Soup Pockets	White Miso Kuzu Tofu & Green Onion

Broths, Bouillons, Soups and Stocks (cont'd)

Company or Brand	Product	Varieties or Flavors
Edward & Sons	GF Bouillon Cubes	Garden Veggie; Not-Beef; Not-Chick'n; Not-Chick'n (Low Sodium); Veggie (Low Sodium); Yellow Curry
	GF Miso-Cup	Japanese Restaurant Style; Original Golden Vegetable; Reduced Sodium; Savory Seaweed; Traditional with Tofu
Explore Cuisine◆	GF Soybean Noodle Soup	Vegetable Flavor; Vegetarian Beef Flavor; Vegetarian Chicken Flavor
Gluten Free Café◆	Canned Soup	Black Bean; Chicken Noodle; Cream of Mushroom; Veggie Noodle
GoGo Quinoa◆	Dry Soup Mix	Minestrone; Mushroom and Quinoa Cream; Quinoa and Vegetables
Habitant	GF Canned Soup	Pea with Garden Vegetables
Imagine Foods	GF Broth	Beef Flavored; Free Range Chicken; Free Range Chicken (Kosher); Miso; Vegetable; Vegetarian No-Chicken
	GF Broth (Low Sodium)	Beef Flavored; Free Range Chicken; Free Range Chicken (Kosher); Vegetable; Vegetarian No-Chicken
	GF Cooking Stock	Beef Flavored; Chicken; Vegetable
	GF Cooking Stock (Low Sodium)	Beef Flavored; Chicken
	GF Heat & Serve Creamy Soup	Acorn Squash & Mango; Broccoli; Butternut Squash; Carrot Almond; Cauliflower & Potato; Celery; Golden Beet; Portobello Mushroom; Potato Leek; Pumpkin; Sweet Corn; Sweet Pea; Sweet Potato; Tomato; Tomato Basil
	GF Heat & Serve Creamy Soup (Light in Sodium)	Butternut Squash; Garden Broccoli; Garden Tomato; Harvest Corn; Red Bliss Potato & Roasted Garlic; Sweet Potato
Kitchen Basics◆	Beef Stock	Original; Unsalted
	Bone Broth	Chicken
	Bouillon Stock Cubes	Roasted Garlic & Chicken Flavor; Roasted Vegetable & Herbs
	Chicken Stock	Original; Unsalted
	Seafood Stock	Original
	Stock Cubes	Roasted Garlic & Chicken Flavor; Roasted Vegetable & Herbs
	Turkey Stock	Original
	Vegetable Stock	Original; Unsalted
Lotus Foods◆	Ramen with Miso Soup	Forbidden Rice; Jade Pearl Rice; Millet & Brown Rice
	Ramen with Vegetable Broth	Buckwheat & Mushroom; Purple Potato & Brown Rice; Wakame & Brown Rice
Mrs. Leeper's◆	Soup Mix	Minestrone; Pasta Fagioli
Namaste Foods◆	Soup Cup	Broccoli & Non-Dairy Cheddar; Chicken Flavored Noodle; Hearty Vegetable
Orgran◆	Soup Cup Mix	Tomato

Broths, Bouillons, Soups and Stocks (cont'd)

Company or Brand	Product	Varieties or Flavors
Pacific Foods	GF Broth	Beef; Free Range Chicken; Mushroom; Turkey; Vegetable
	GF Broth (Bone)	Chicken; Chicken Original; Chicken with Ginger; Chicken with Lemongrass; Turkey; Turkey with Rosemary, Sage & Thyme
	GF Broth (Low Sodium)	Beef; Free Range Chicken; Vegetable
	GF Stock	Chicken; Chicken Unsalted
	GF Stock (Bone)	Chicken Unsalted; Turkey Unsalted
	GF Stock (Simply)	Chicken Unsalted; Vegetable Unsalted
	GF Bisque	Butternut Squash; Cashew Carrot Ginger; Hearty Tomato; Roasted Red Pepper & Tomato
	GF Cream Condensed Soup	Chicken; Mushroom
	GF Creamy Soup	Butternut Squash; Tomato; Tomato Basil
	GF Creamy Soup (Low Sodium)	Butternut Squash; Tomato
	GF Soup	Cashew Carrot Ginger; Chicken & Wild Rice; Chipotle Sweet Potato; French Onion; Roasted Garlic & Potato; Roasted Red Pepper & Tomato; Rosemary Potato Chowder; Thai Sweet Potato Soup; Vegetable Quinoa
	GF Soup (Low Sodium)	Roasted Red Pepper & Tomato
	GF Soup Starters Soup Base	Chicken Pho; Tom Yum; Tortilla; Vegetarian Pho
Saffron Road	GF Broth	Artisan Roasted Chicken; Lamb; Traditional Chicken (Low Sodium); Vegetable (Low Sodium)
San-J	GF Soup Mix	Wakame Seaweed & Shiitake Mushrooms; White Miso with Tofu & Scallions
Savory Choice♦	Bag in Box Liquid Broth Concentrate for Foodservice	Beef; Chicken; Clam; Lobster; Mushroom; Seafood; Turkey; Veal; Vegan Beef; Vegan Chicken; Vegetable
	Clean & Healthy Liquid Broth Concentrate Packets for Foodservice (Reduced Sodium)	Beef; Chicken; Vegetable
	Liquid Base for Foodservice (Reduced Sodium)	Beef; Chicken; Turkey; Vegan Beef; Vegan Chicken; Vegetable
	Liquid Broth Concentrate Packets	Beef Flavor; Chicken; Turkey
	Liquid Broth Concentrates Packets (Reduced Sodium)	Chicken; Vegetable
	Pho Liquid Broth Concentrate Packets	Beef Flavor; Chicken; Veggie
	Stock Pot In-A-Pouch Liquid Broth Concentrate for Foodservice (Low Sodium)	Beef; Chicken; Vegetable
Sea Fare Pacific♦	GF Chowder	Clam; Salmon
	GF Seafood Bisque	
	GF West Coast Cioppino	
Swanson	GF Broth (Canned)	Chicken; Chicken (50% Less Sodium); Vegetable
	GF Broth (Carton)	Beef; Beef (Lower Sodium); Chicken; Vegetable
	GF Natural Goodness Broth	Chicken (canned); Chicken (carton)
	GF Stock (Carton)	Beef; Chicken; Unsalted Beef Flavor; Unsalted Chicken Flavor
Taste Adventure	GF Dried Soup	Black Bean; Curry Lentil; Golden Pea; Navy Bean; Split Pea; Sweet Corn Chowder

Broths, Bouillons, Soups and Stocks (cont'd)		
Company or Brand	**Product**	**Varieties or Flavors**
Thai Kitchen	GF Instant Rice Noodle Soup	Bangkok Curry; Garlic & Vegetable; Lemon Grass & Chili; Spring Onion; Thai Ginger
	GF Instant Rice Noodle Soup Bowl	Lemon Grass & Chili; Mushroom; Roasted Garlic; Spring Onion; Thai Ginger

Gravy Mixes

- Most gravy mixes are **NOT** gluten free as they usually contain wheat flour or wheat starch.

- Purchase a gluten-free gravy mix or prepare from gluten-free broth or stock. For tips on how to thicken gravy, see pages 155 and 156.

Gravy Mixes		
Company or Brand	**Product**	**Varieties or Flavors**
Barkat◆	Gravy Mix	Vegetable
Club House	GF Gravy Mix	Brown; Chicken; Poutine (25% Less Sodium); Pork; Turkey
Cuisine Santé◆	GF Gravy Mix	Au Jus Clear
Hol•Grain	GF All Purpose Gravy Thickener	
Imagine Foods	GF Gravy	Roasted Turkey Flavored; Savory Beef Flavored; Vegetarian Wild Mushroom
Orgran◆	Gravy Mix	Vegetable
Pacific Foods	GF Gravy	Vegan Mushroom
Road's End Organics	GF Gravy Mix	Golden; Savory Herb; Shiitake Mushroom

Sauces

- Both store-bought and homemade sauces often are made with gluten-containing ingredients such as wheat flour, wheat starch and/or soy sauce.

- Some BBQ sauces are **NOT** gluten free as they contain beer or malt vinegar.

- Certain brands of Worcestershire sauce contain malt vinegar (which is **NOT** gluten-free).

Sauces		
Company or Brand	**Product**	**Varieties or Flavors**
Cuisine Santé◆	GF Demi-Glace / Brown Sauce Mix	
Eden Foods	GF Miso Paste	Genmai (Soy & Brown Rice); Shiro (Rice & Soybeans)
Imagine Foods	GF Culinary Simmer Sauce	Latin Veracruz; Louisiana Creole; Portobello Red Wine; Thai Coconut Curry

Sauces (cont'd)

Company or Brand	Product	Varieties or Flavors
Kikkoman	GF Hoisin Sauce	
	GF Marinade & Sauce	Teriyaki; Teriyaki (50% Less Sodium)
	GF Oyster Sauce	Blue Label; Green Label
	GF Sweet Chili Sauce	
Premier Japan♦	Sauce	Hoisin; Teriyaki
Saffron Road	GF Simmer Sauce	Coconut Curry Korma Style; Harissa; Korean Stir-Fry; Lemongrass Basil; Moroccan; Thai Red Curry; Tikka Masala
San-J	GF Sauce	Asian BBQ; Hoisin; Mongolian; Orange; Sweet & Tangy; Szechuan; Teriyaki; Thai Peanut
Savory Choice♦	Demi-Glace Concentrate	Beef; Chicken
	Demi-Glace Concentrate for Foodservice	Beef; Chicken; Veal
Simply Asia	GF Stir-Fry Seasoning Mix	Beef & Broccoli; Mandarin Teriyaki Chicken; Spicy Szechwan Chicken & Green Bean; Sweet Ginger Garlic Chicken & Vegetable
Thai Kitchen	GF 10-Minute Simmer Sauce	Green Curry; Panang Curry; Red Curry; Yellow Curry
	GF Paste	Green Curry; Red Curry; Roasted Red Chili
	GF Sauce	Original Pad Thai; Peanut Satay; Pineapple & Chili; Premium Fish; Spicy Thai Mango; Spicy Thai Chili; Sweet Red Chili; Thai Chili & Ginger
The Wizard's	GF Sauce	Hot Stuff; Worcestershire

Soy Sauces

- Many brands of soy sauce are a combination of soy and wheat and therefore are **NOT** gluten-free.
- Soy sauce usually is an ingredient in teriyaki sauce and also may be present in other foods such as salad dressings.

Soy Sauces

Company or Brand	Product	Varieties or Flavors
Bgreen Food♦	Tamari Soy Sauce	Traditional
Eden Foods	GF Tamari Soy Sauce Imported	Green & White Label
	GF Tamari Soy Sauce U.S. Brewed	Red & White Label
Kikkoman	GF Soy Sauce	Full Size; Packets
	GF Sweet Soy Sauce for Rice	
	GF Tamari Soy Sauce	50% Less Sodium; Regular
San-J	GF Organic Tamari Soy Sauce	Full Size; Packets
	GF Organic Tamari Soy Sauce	Reduced Sodium
	GF Tamari Lite Soy Sauce	50% Less Sodium
	GF Tamari Soy Sauce	Reduced Sodium

Beers

- Regular beer is **NOT** gluten-free because it contains barley, wheat and/or rye.

- Gluten-reduced beer made from barley is **NOT** gluten-free (see p. 33).

- Various gluten-free beers are available made with grains such as amaranth, buckwheat, chestnuts, corn, millet, quinoa and/or rice (see below).

Beers

Company or Brand	Product	Grains
Anheuser-Busch	GF Redbridge Beer	Made with sorghum
Bard's Tale Beer Company♦	American Lager	Made with sorghum
Glutenberg♦	American Pale Ale	Made with millet, buckwheat, corn and quinoa
	Blonde Ale	Made with millet and corn
	India Pale Ale	Made with millet, buckwheat, corn and black rice
	Red Ale	Made with buckwheat, millet, chestnuts and quinoa
	White Beer	Made with buckwheat, millet, amaranth and quinoa
Lakefront Brewery	GF New Grist Pilsner	Made with sorghum and rice
La Messagère	GF Aux Fruits	Made with buckwheat
	GF Millet	Made with millet
	GF Pale Ale	Made with buckwheat
	GF Red Ale	Made with buckwheat and millet

16

Company Directory

This directory lists the manufacturers of products featured in chapter 15 on pages 205–262. It includes contact information and a short description of the types of products the manufacturer offers (products and/or spellings vary according to the manufacturer). When the diamond symbol ♦ appears in front of a brand name, it indicates that the company produces only gluten-free items. Regardless of whether or not the diamond symbol is present, the company manufactures all or some of its gluten-free products either (1) in dedicated gluten-free facilities, or (2) on dedicated equipment in segregated areas of its facilities, or (3) in shared facilities cleaned to mitigate the risk of cross-contamination for allergen and gluten sources. At any time manufacturers can change how and where they produce gluten-free foods, which is why that information is not included in the guide. To learn more about a particular company's methods in gluten-free food production, contact the company directly.

Company information, exhaustively researched between January and July 2016, is from sources believed to be reliable at the time of printing. **The author assumes no liability for any errors, omissions or inaccuracies in this section.**

A	264	J	275	S	283
B	265	K	276	T	284
C	267	L	277	U	285
D	270	M	278	V	285
E	270	N	279	W	286
F	271	O	279	X	286
G	272	P	280	Z	286
H	274	Q	282		
I	275	R	282		

A

◆ Absolutely Gluten Free
35 West St.
Spring Valley, NY, U.S. 10977
845-517-3670
www.absolutelygf.com
- Gluten-free crackers, snack bites and frozen pizzas

◆ Aleias Gluten Free Foods
4 Pin Oak Dr.
Branford, CT, U.S. 06405
203-488-5556
www.aleias.com
connect@aleias.com
- Gluten-free breads, cookies, coatings, croûtons, crumbs and stuffings

◆ All But Gluten, Weston Bakeries, Ltd.
1425 The Queensway
Toronto, ON, Canada M8Z 1T3
800-661-7246 (CAN)
www.allbutgluten.ca
- Gluten-free baked products (breads, brownies, buns, cupcakes, cookies, loaf cakes and muffins)

◆ Allen Creek Farm
P.O. Box 841, 29112 NW 41st Ave.
Ridgefield, WA, U.S. 98642
360-887-3669
www.chestnutsonline.com
info@chestnutsonline.com
- Chestnuts (fresh, dried, chips, flour) and a gluten-free pancake and waffle mix made with chestnut flour

Amy's Kitchen, Inc.
P.O. Box 449
Petaluma, CA, U.S. 94953
707-568-4500 / 707-781-7535
www.amys.com
www.amyskitchen.ca
- Burritos, chili, baked and refried beans, pasta meals, pizza, pot pies, snacks, soups, veggie burgers, pasta sauces, salsas, brownies, cakes, cookies and candy bars, as well as an extensive line of vegetarian prepared meals including Asian, Indian and Mexican cuisines
- Over 130 products are gluten free

◆ Ancient Harvest Quinoa Corporation
1722 14th St., Suite 212
Boulder, CO, U.S. 80302
310-217-8125
www.ancientharvest.com
quinoacorp@quinoa.net
- Gluten-free quinoa products including cereal flakes; hot cereals containing quinoa, gluten-free oats, millet and amaranth; flour, grain, pastas, quinoa mac & cheese; side dishes made with quinoa, millet and amaranth; cornmeal polenta and snack bars

◆ Andean Dream, LLC.
P.O. Box 411404
Los Angeles, CA, U.S. 90041
310-281-6036
www.andeandream.com
info@andeandream.com
- Quinoa-based gluten-free cookies, pastas and a soup

Anheuser-Busch
(see **Redbridge**, p. 282)

Annie Chun's, Inc.
Fullerton, CA, U.S. 92831
800-459-3445
www.anniechun.com
info@anniechun.com
- Asian meal starters, noodles (chow mein, rice, soba), pot stickers and mini-wontons, rice, sauces, soup bowls and sushi wraps
- Rice noodles and Rice Express (pre-cooked rice in microwaveable cups) are gluten free

Annie's Homegrown, Inc.
1610 Fifth St.
Berkeley, CA, U.S. 94710
800-288-1089 / 510-558-7500
www.annies.com
www.annieshomegrown.ca
- Condiments, cookies, crackers, fruit snacks, pastas, pizza, sauces, salad dressings and granola bars
- Many products are gluten free

Apetito

12 Indell Lane
Brampton, ON, Canada L6T 3Y3
800-268-8199 / 905-799-1022
www.apetito.ca

- Frozen products, in bulk and portioned formats, for home use; for hospitals, long-term care and other institutions; and for Meals-on-Wheels
- A line of gluten-free complete meals (also suitable for lactose-free and renal diets) in bulk and individual trays

Applegate Farms

750 Rt. 202 S, Suite 300
Bridgewater, NJ, U.S. 08807
866-587-5858
www.applegate.com
help@applegate.com

- Frozen entrées and meat products (breaded chicken, breakfast sausages, burgers, corn dogs, deli meats, hot dogs)
- Many products are gluten free

◆ Arnel's Originals

381 Sonoma Ct.
Ventura, CA, U.S. 93004
805-322-6900
www.arnelsoriginals.com
arnels@arnelsoriginals.com

- Gluten-free baking mixes (all purpose flour & pie crust, bread, cake, pancake & waffle)

◆ Authentic Foods

1850 W 169th St., Suite B
Gardena, CA, U.S. 90247
800-806-4737
www.authenticfoods.com
sales@authenticfoods.com

- Gluten-free baking mixes (bread, brownie, cake, cookie, flour blend, muffin, pancake & baking, pie crust, pizza crust), flours and other baking ingredients
- Mixes contain Garfava™ flour (garbanzo and fava beans) developed by founder of this company

◆ Avena Foods, Ltd. (Only Oats)

316 1st Ave. E
Regina, SK, Canada S4N 5H2
866-461-3663 / 306-757-3663
www.avenafoods.com
info@avenafoods.com

- Gluten-free oat products (bran, flour, regular and quick flakes, steel-cut) and mixes (cookie, muffin, pancake)
- Oats produced using the gluten-free purity protocol (see p. 28)

B

◆ Bakery On Main

127 Park Ave., Suite 100
East Hartford, CT, U.S. 06108
860-895-6622
www.bakeryonmain.com
info@bakeryonmain.com

- Gluten-free granolas, oats (instant oatmeal, quick, rolled, steel-cut), other hot cereals, snacks and snack bars

◆ Banza

760 Virginia Park St.
Detroit, MI, U.S. 48202
313-899-7884
www.eatbanza.com
info@eatbanza.com

- Gluten-free chickpea pasta and pasta with cheese sauce

Barbara's

500 Nickerson Rd.
Marlboro, MA, U.S. 01752
800-343-0590
www.barbaras.com
info@barbarasbakery.com

- Cereals, chips, crackers, cookies and snack bars
- Some cereals are gluten free

◆ Bard's Tale Beer Company, LLC.

P.O. Box 24835
Minneapolis, MN, U.S. 55424
877-440-2337
www.bardsbeer.com
info@bardsbeer.com

- Gluten-free beer made from sorghum

Barilla, Barilla America, Inc.
1200 Lakeside Dr.
Bannockburn, IL, U.S. 60015
800-922-7455
www.barilla.com
www.barilla.ca

* Variety of pastas
* Some pastas (made with corn and rice) are gluten free

◆ Barkat, Gluten Free Foods
Unit 270 Centennial Park
Elstree, Hertfordshire, London, U.K. WD6 3SS
44 208 953 4444
www.glutenfree-foods.co.uk
info@glutenfree-foods.co.uk

* Gluten-free baking mixes (all purpose flour, bread, muffin, pancake & batter), baguettes, breads, cereals, cookies, crackers, gravy mix, ice cream cones, pasta, pizza crusts, pretzels, rolls, stuffing mix and waffles

◆ Beanfields Snacks
11693 San Vicente Blvd., Suite 328
Los Angeles, CA, U.S. 90049
855-328-2326
www.beanfieldssnacks.com
info@beanfieldssnacks.com

* Gluten-free chips (made with beans and rice)

◆ Beanitos, Inc.
3601 South Congress, Suite B–500
Austin, TX, U.S. 78704
512-609-8017
www.beanitos.com
customers@beanitos.com

* Gluten-free snacks (made with black, pinto or white beans and rice)

◆ Beetnik Foods, LLC.
2600 E Cesar Chavez
Austin, TX, U.S. 78702
512-584-8228
www.beetnikfoods.com

* Gluten-free baked products, frozen entrées, meat products, pasta and other items

◆ Best Cooking Pulses, Inc.
110 10th St. NE
Portage la Prairie, MB, Canada R1N 1B5
204-857-4451
www.bestcookingpulses.com
retail@bestcookingpulses.com

* Gluten-free pulse flours (whole black bean, whole chickpea, whole lentil, whole navy bean, whole pinto bean, split green pea, whole yellow pea) and pea fiber

◆ BFree Foods, Ltd.
10 Clyde Rd.
Dublin 4, Ireland
3 531 779 0500
www.bfreefoods.com

◆ BFree Foods USA
5042 Wilshire Blvd., #34665
Los Angeles, CA, U.S. 90036
844-775-4647
us.bfreefoods.com
info@bfreefoods.com

* Gluten-free bagels, breads, buns, pita breads, rolls and wraps

◆ Bgreen Food, Big Green (USA), Inc.
6549 Mission Gorge Rd., Suite 351
San Diego, CA, U.S. 92120
619-825-9330
www.bgreenfood.com
info@bgreenfood.com

* Gluten-free flours, noodles, pasta, ramen, rice, soy sauce and other items

Bionaturae, LLC.
P.O. Box 98
North Franklin, CT, U.S. 06254
877-642-0644 / 860-642-6996
www.bionaturae.com
info@bionaturae.com

* Variety of Italian products (balsamic vinegar, fruit nectars and spreads, olive oil, pastas, tomatoes, tomato paste)
* Many products are gluten free, including pastas (made with potato, rice and soy flours)

The Birkett Mills
P.O. Box 440
Penn Yan, NY, U.S. 14527
315-536-3311
www.thebirkettmills.com
contact@thebirkettmills.com

* Gluten-free products sold under the brand names Pocono (cream of buckwheat, buckwheat groats, buckwheat flour, kasha), Larrowe's (instant buckwheat pancake mix) and Wolff's (cream of buckwheat, buckwheat groats, kasha)

Blue Diamond Almonds, Blue Diamond Growers
1701 C St.
Sacramento, CA, U.S. 95811
800-987-2329 / 916-442-0771
www.bluediamond.com

* Almonds, crackers and non-dairy almond beverages
* Most products are gluten free

Blue Horizon, Elevation Brands, LLC.
190 Fountain St.
Framingham, MA, U.S. 01702
800-543-6637
www.bluehorizonseafood.com
customerservice@elevationbrands.com

- Frozen fish and shellfish products (bites, burgers, crab cakes)
- Many products are gluten free

◆ Bobo's Oat Bars
6325 Gunpark Dr., Suite B
Boulder, CO, U.S. 80301
303-938-1977
www.bobosoatbars.com
info@bobosoatbars.com

- Snack bars and mini bites

Bob's Red Mill Natural Foods, Inc.
13521 SE Pheasant Ct.
Milwaukie, OR, U.S. 97222
800-349-2173 / 503-654-3215
www.bobsredmill.com

- Extensive variety of baking flours, mixes and other baking ingredients; cereals, granolas, grains, legumes, protein powders and seeds
- Over 100 gluten-free products including baking flours, mixes (1-to-1 baking, all purpose baking, biscuit & baking, bread, brownie, cake, cookie, muffin, Paleo baking, pancake, pie crust, pizza crust) and other baking ingredients; cereals, grains, legumes, protein powders and seeds

Bold Organics
2090 7th Ave., Suite 201A
New York, NY, U.S. 10027
212-666-6097
www.bold-organics.com
consumerinfo@bold-organics.com

- Frozen calzones and pizzas
- Some pizzas are gluten free

◆ Boulder Organic Foods, LLC.
6363 Horizon Lane
Niwot, CO, U.S. 80503
303-530-0470
www.boulderorganicfoods.com
info@boulderorganicfoods.com

- Gluten-free refrigerated soups

◆ Breads From Anna, Anna's Allergen Free, Inc.
3007 Sierra Ct.
Iowa City, IA, U.S. 52240
877-354-3886 / 319-354-3886
www.breadsfromanna.com
info@breadsfromanna.com

- Gluten-free mixes (bread, brownie, pancake & muffin, pie crust, pizza crust) made with a combination of flours (beans, chia, millet)

Breton, Dare Foods
2481 Kingsway Dr.
Kitchener, ON, Canada N2C 1A6
800-668-3273
www.darefoods.com

- Crackers and popped bean snacks
- Some products are gluten free

◆ BumbleBar, Inc.
3014 North Flora Rd., Bldg. 4B
Spokane Valley, WA, U.S. 99216
509-924-2080
www.bumblebar.com

- Gluten-free snack bars

C

Caesar's Pasta, LLC.
1001 Lower Landing Rd.
Blackwood, NJ, U.S. 08012
888-432-2372 / 856-227-2585
www.caesarspasta.com
www.caesarskitchenmeals.com
caesars@caesarspasta.com

- Frozen products (gnocchi, meatballs, pasta, pasta entrées)
- Some products are gluten free

Campbell Company of Canada
60 Birmingham St.
Toronto, ON, Canada M8V 2B8
800-410-7687
www.campbellsoup.ca

Campbell Soup Company
1 Campbell Pl.
Camden, NJ, U.S. 08103
800-257-8443
www.campbellsoup.com

- Broths, chili, condensed soups, juices, ready-to-serve soups, salsas, sauces and stocks
- Some products are gluten free

◆ CanMar Grain Products, Ltd.
2480 Sandra Schmirler Way
Regina, SK, Canada S4W 1B7
866-855-5553 / 306-721-1375
www.roastedflax.com

- Mill and manufacture gluten-free roasted flax products (whole seed, ground flax) and de-hulled red lentil flour
- Retail flax products sold under the name "Flax for Nutrition"

◆ Canyon Bakehouse
1510 E 11th St.
Loveland, CO, U.S. 80537
888-566-3590 / 970-461-3844
www.canyonglutenfree.com

- Gluten-free breads, bagels, brownies, buns and focaccia

◆ Canyon Oats
(see **GF Harvest**, p. 272)

◆ Cappello's
P.O. Box 11757
Denver, CO, U.S. 80211
844-353-2863
www.cappellos.com
talk@cappellosglutenfree.com

- Gluten-free almond flour-based products (cookie dough, gnocchi, pasta, pizza crust, pizzas)

◆ Casa de Mesquite
27520 Hawthorne Blvd., Suite 285
Rolling Hills Estate, CA, U.S. 90274
310-651-2364
www.casademesquite.com
info@casademesquite.com

- Gluten-free mesquite flour

Catelli, Catelli Foods Corporation
6890 Rue Notre-Dame Est.
Montreal, QC, Canada H1N 2E5
888-293-1333
www.catelli.ca

- Variety of pastas
- Some pastas (made with corn, quinoa, brown and white rice) are gluten free

◆ CelifibR, Maplegrove Gluten Free Foods, Inc.
5010 Eucalyptus Ave.
Chino, CA, U.S. 91710
909-823-8230
www.pastarisofoods.com/celifibr

- Gluten-free bouillon cubes made with vegetables

◆ Chebe
1840 Lundberg Dr.
Spirit Lake, IA, U.S. 51360
800-217-9510 / 712-336-4211
www.chebe.com

- Gluten-free baking mixes (bread, breadsticks, cinnamon rolls, foccacia, pizza crust) and frozen dough (breadsticks, pizza, rolls) made from manioc (also known as tapioca, yucca or cassava)

CheeCha, CadCan Marketing & Sales, Inc.
7503 35th St. SE, Bay 5
Calgary, AB, Canada T2C 1V3
877-243-3242
www.cheecha.ca
info@cheecha.ca

- Puffed potato snacks
- Many flavors are gluten free

Cherrybrook Kitchen, Healthy Brands Collective
65 East Ave., 3rd Floor
Norwalk, CT, U.S. 06851
888-417-9343 (ext. 1)
www.cherrybrookkitchen.com
info@cherrybrookkitchen.com

- Baking mixes (brownie, cake, cookie, pancake, pancake & waffle) and frostings
- Many products are gluten free

◆ chic-a-peas, LLC.
4545 Center Blvd., Suite 518
Long Island City, NY, U.S. 11109
646-875-8718
www.chicapeas.com

- Gluten-free baked chickpea snacks

◆ Cloud 9 Specialty Bakery
7541 Conway Ave., Unit 6
Burnaby, BC, Canada V5E 2P7
604-249-5010
www.cloud9specialtybakery.com
info@cloud9specialtybakery.com

- Gluten-free baking mixes (all-purpose baking, bread, brownie, cake and cupcake, cookie, granola bar, pancake & waffle) and flours

Club House, McCormick Canada

P.O. Box 5788
London, ON, Canada N6A 4Z2
800-265-2600
www.clubhouse.ca

- Herbs, seasoning blends and spices as well as coatings, mixes (gravy, seasoning), rice flour, sauces and other items
- Many products are gluten free

Conte's Pasta Co., Inc.

310 Wheat Rd.
Vineland, NJ, U.S. 08360
800-211-6607 / 856-697-3400
www.contespasta.com
customerservice@contespasta.com

- Gnocchi, pasta, pasta meals, pierogies, pizza, pizza shells, sauces and other items
- Some products are gluten free

◆ Cooksimple, The Healthy Pantry, Inc.

P.O. Box 1102
Red Lodge, MT, U.S. 59068
877-972-6879
www.cooksimplemeals.com
info@cooksimplemeals.com

- Gluten-free dry pasta, shelf-stable entrées and side dishes with ingredients such as brown rice, buckwheat, pulses, quinoa and/or sorghum

◆ Corn Thins

(see **Real Foods**, p. 282)

◆ Cream Hill Estates (Lara's)

9633 Rue Clément
Lasalle, QC, Canada H8R 4B4
866-727-3628 / 514-363-2066
www.creamhillestates.com
info@creamhillestates.com

- Gluten-free oat products (flour, groats, rolled)
- Regular gluten testing of finished oat products. All products packaged in a dedicated facility free of gluten and the major food allergens

◆ Crunchmaster, TH Foods, Inc.

2134 Harlem Rd.
Loves Park, IL, U.S. 61111
800-896-2396 / 815-636-9500
www.crunchmaster.com

- Baked rice crackers, brown rice crackers with seeds (amaranth, flax, quinoa, sesame) and popped edamame chips

◆ Cuisine Santé, Haco, Ltd.

Worbstrasse 262, Postfach 96
3073 Gümligen, Switzerland
41 (0) 31 950 11 11
www.haco.ch
contact@haco.ch

USA Distributor: Swiss Chalet Fine Foods
9455 NW 40th Street Rd.
Miami, FL, U.S. 33178
305-592-0008
www.scff.com
orders@scff.com

- Cuisine Santé products (dehydrated bases, gravies, sauces, soups, stocks) are gluten free

◆ Cuisine Soleil

8340 Rand du Parc
Rouyn-Noranda, QC, Canada J9Y 0C8
855-637-2444
www.cuisinesoleil.com

- Gluten-free baking mixes (all-purpose, bread, pancake), flours, buckwheat flakes and other items

◆ Cup4Cup, LLC.

1190 Airport Rd., Suite 110
Napa, CA, U.S. 94558
707-754-4263
www.cup4cup.com
info@cup4cup.com

- Gluten-free baking mixes (brownie, cake, multi-purpose flour, pizza crust, pancake & waffle, wholesome flour)

◆ Cybele's, Free To Eat, Inc.

8525 Appian Way
Los Angeles, CA, U.S. 90046
877-895-3729
www.cybelesfreetoeat.com
info@cybelesfreetoeat.com

- Gluten-free cookies

D

◆ Daiya Foods, Inc.
2768 Rupert St.
Vancouver, BC, Canada V5M 3T7
877-324-9211 / 604-569-0530
www.daiyafoods.com
cr@daiyafoods.com

- Gluten-, dairy- and soy-free cheeses (cream cheese-style spreads, shredded, slices, wedges), cheesecakes, mac & cheese entrées, pizzas, salad dressings and yogurts

DeBoles, The Hain Celestial Group, Inc.
4600 Sleepytime Dr.
Boulder, CO, U.S. 80301
800-434-4246
www.deboles.com
customer.care@hain.com

- Pasta products
- Some pastas (made from rice or corn or a combination of rice and quinoa or rice, amaranth and quinoa) are gluten free

Dempster's Bakery, Canada Bread Company, Limited
P.O. Box 61027
Winnipeg, MB, Canada R3M 3X8
800-465-5515
glutenzero.dempsters.ca

- Bagels, breads, buns, English muffins and tortillas
- Gluten-free breads sold under the name "Gluten Zero"

◆ Doctor in the Kitchen, LLC.
P.O. Box 24868
Minneapolis, MN, U.S. 55424
612-728-8905
www.drinthekitchen.com
info@drinthekitchen.com

- Gluten-free flaxseed crackers

◆ Domata
P.O. Box 24074
Minneapolis, MN, U.S. 55424
855-366-2821 / 952-303-5484
www.domataglutenfree.com
domata@domataflour.com

- Gluten-free mixes (pizza crust, recipe-ready flour, seasoned flour)

◆ Dowd & Rogers
1403 N El Camino Real
San Clemente, CA, U.S. 92672
800-232-8619
www.dowdandrogers.com
info@dowdandrogers.com

- Gluten-free baking mixes (brownie, cake, pancake & baking), flours (almond, chia omega, coconut, Italian chestnut, mesquite, quinoa) and peanut powders

Dr. Praeger's Sensible Foods, Inc.
9 Boumar Pl.
Elmwood Park, NJ, U.S. 07407
877-772-3437 / 201-703-1300
www.drpraegers.com
info@drpraegers.com

- Appetizers, entrées and snack products including fish sticks, hash browns, pancakes, potato littles, vegetable cakes, veggie burgers and veggie puffs
- Many items are gluten free

◆ Duinkerken Foods, Inc.
P.O. Box 222
Slemon Park, P.E.I., Canada C0B 2A0
902-888-3604
www.duinkerkenfoods.com
info@duinkerkenfoods.com

- Gluten-free baking mixes (biscuit, bread, brownie, cake, cookie, muffin, pizza crust, waffle/pancake), flours and starches

E

Eden Foods
701 Tecumseh Rd.
Clinton, MI, U.S. 49236
888-424-3336 / 517-456-7424
www.edenfoods.com
info@edenfoods.com

- Extensive line of products such as beans, condiments, flours, fruits and juices, grains, oils, pasta, sauces, snack foods and soy beverages
- Many items are gluten free

Edward & Sons

P.O. Box 1326
Carpinteria, CA, U.S. 93014
805-684-8500
www.edwardandsons.com

- Vegetarian products (bouillon cubes, gravy mixes, ice cream cones, instant soups, instant mashed potatoes, pasta meals, rice crackers, rice toast, sauces)
- Many products are gluten free

◆ Element Snacks, Inc.

133 W 22nd St.
New York, NY, U.S. 10011
855-966-7686
www.elementsnacks.com

- Gluten-free frosted rice and corn snack cakes

◆ El Peto Products

65 Saltsman Dr.
Cambridge, ON, Canada N3H 4R7
800-387-4064 / 519-650-4614
www.elpeto.com
info@elpeto.com

- Gluten-free baked products (breads, brownies, buns, cookies, English muffins, muffins, pies, pie dough, pizza crusts, rolls, tarts, tart shells, waffles), baking mixes (all purpose flour, bread, cake, cookie, muffin, pancake), bread crumbs, cereals, flours, starches and other ingredients

◆ Ener-G Foods, Inc.

5960 1st Ave. S
Seattle, WA, U.S. 98108
800-331-5222 / 206-767-3928
www.ener-g.com
customerservice@ener-g.com

- Gluten-free baked products (biscotti, breads, brownies, buns, cakes, cookies, communion wafers, croûtons, doughnuts, English muffins, focaccia, pizza crust, rolls), baking mixes, flours, starches and other baking ingredients, crackers, pretzels and snack bars

◆ Enjoy Life Foods

3810 N River Rd.
Schiller Park, IL, U.S. 60176
888-503-6569 / 847-260-0300
www.enjoylifefoods.com

- Gluten-free baking mixes (all purpose flour, brownie, muffin, pancake & waffle, pizza crust), baking chocolate, chocolate bars, cookies, lentil chips, snack bars, snack bites and trail mixes

◆ EnviroKidz, Nature's Path Foods

9100 Van Horne Way
Richmond, BC, Canada V6X 1W3
866-880-7284 / 604-248-8777
www.envirokidz.com

- Gluten-free cold cereals, oatmeal and snack bars

◆ Erewhon, Attune Foods, LLC.

2545 Prairie Rd.
Eugene, OR, U.S. 97402
888-720-4367
www.erewhonorganic.com

- Gluten-free cereals

◆ Evol Foods, Boulder Brands USA, Inc.

1600 Pearl St.
Boulder, CO, U.S. 80302
201-421-3970
www.evolfoods.com

- Frozen entrées (breakfast items, burritos, quesadillas, street tacos, meal cups, single-serve meals)
- Many products are gluten free

◆ Explore Cuisine, Inc.

157 Broad St., Suite 308
Red Bank, NJ, U.S. 07701
888-208-9471 / 732-747-8800
www.explorecuisine.com
info@explorecuisine.com

- Gluten-free noodles (rice), pastas (adzuki bean, black bean, chickpea, lentil, rice, soybean) and soups

F

◆ Feel Good Foods

254 36th St.
Brooklyn, NY, U.S. 11232
800-638-8949
www.feel-good-foods.com
info@feelgf.com

- Gluten-free frozen Asian products (dumplings, egg rolls, fried rice)

Flax4Life
468 W Horton Rd.
Bellingham, WA, U.S. 98226
877-352-9487 / 360-715-1944
www.flax4life.net
customerservice@flax4life.net

- Flax-based, gluten-free brownies, buns, cakes, granola and muffins

Food For Life
2991 E Doherty St.
Corona, CA, U.S. 92879
800-797-5090 / 951-279-5090
www.foodforlife.com

- Breads, buns, cereals, English muffins, pasta, pocket breads, tortillas and waffles
- Some breads, English muffins and tortillas are gluten free

Foods By George
3 King St.
Mahwah, NJ, U.S. 07430
201-612-9700
www.foodsbygeorge.com
info@foodsbygeorge.com

- Gluten-free brownies, cakes, English muffins, muffins, pizza, pizza crusts, tarts and tart shells

Freedom Foods North America, Inc.
1921 W Park Ave.
Redlands, CA, U.S. 92373
855-909-1717 / 909-335-1717
www.freedomfoodsus.com
www.freedomfoods.com.au
customerservice@freedomfoodsus.com

- Gluten-free cold cereals, oatmeal, pancake mixes, snack bars and other snacks

Free for All Kitchen, Partners Company
20232–72nd Ave. S
Kent, WA, U.S. 98032
800-632-7477 / 253-867-1580
www.partnerscrackers.com

- Gluten-free brownie thins and crackers

G

Gabriella's Kitchen Inc.
3249 Lenworth Drive
Mississauga, ON L4X 2G6
844-754-6690 / 647-345-5772
www.gkskinnypasta.com
info@gkskinnypasta.com

- Frozen pasta meals and fresh pastas (sold in refrigerated or frozen food section) called "skinnypasta"
- Fresh pastas (made with teff) and frozen pasta meals are gluten free

Garden Lites, Classic Cooking, LLC.
165–35 145th Dr.
Jamaica, NY, U.S. 11434
718-439-0200
www.gardenlites.com
customerservice@garden-lites.com

- Frozen vegetarian items including soufflés, mac & cheese, muffins, veggie bites and veggie cakes
- Most products are gluten free

The GFB: Gluten Free Bar
1314 Leonard St. NW
Grand Rapids, MI, U.S. 49504
616-755-8432
www.theglutenfreebar.com
info@theglutenfreebar.com

- Gluten-free snack bars.

GF Harvest, LLC., GFO, Inc.
578 Lane 9
Powell, WY, U.S. 82435
888-941-9922 / 307-754-7041
www.gfharvest.com
www.canyonoats.com
sales@gfharvest.com

- Gluten-free oats (flour, groats, rolled, quick, steel-cut) and granola sold under the GF Harvest brand as well as oatmeal and granola cups under the Canyon Oats brand
- Oats produced using the gluten-free purity protocol (see p. 28)

gfJules
6400 Baltimore National Pike, #330
Catonsville, MD, U.S. 21228
855-435-8537
www.gfjules.com

- Gluten-free baking mixes (all-purpose flour, bread, brownie, cookie, cornbread, graham cracker / gingerbread, muffin, pancake & waffle, pizza crust)

◆ Glutenberg
2350 Dickson, Local 950
Montreal, QC, Canada H1N 3T1
514-933-2333
www.glutenberg.ca

- Gluten-free beers made from various grains such as amaranth, buckwheat, corn, millet, quinoa and rice

◆ Glutenfree Bakehouse, Whole Foods Market
2800 Perimeter Park Dr., Suite C
Morrisville, NC, U.S. 27560
512-477-4455
www.wholefoodsmarket.com
glutenfree.bakehouse@wholefoods.com

- Gluten-free biscuits, breads, buns, cakes, cookies, cupcakes, muffins, pies, pie crusts, scones and stuffing

◆ The Gluten Free Bistro, LLC.
P.O. Box 17154
Boulder, CO, U.S. 80308
303-257-4000
www.theglutenfreebistro.com

- Gluten-free frozen mini pizzas, pizza crusts and pizza dough

◆ Gluten Free Café, The Hain Celestial Group, Inc.
4600 Sleepytime Dr.
Boulder, CO, U.S. 80301
800-434-4246
www.myglutenfreecafe.com
customer.care@hain.com

- Gluten-free canned soups, frozen entrées and snack bars

◆ Glutenfreeda Foods
P.O. Box 487
Burlington, WA, U.S. 98233
360-755-1300
www.glutenfreeda.com

- Gluten-free burritos, flatbread/pizza crust, pizza wraps, pocket sandwiches as well as cheesecakes and gluten-free oats (granola, instant oatmeal, quick and traditional rolled, steel-cut)

◆ Gluten-Free Naturals, LLC.
P.O. Box 1626
Cranford, NJ, U.S. 07016
866-761-6147 / 917-885-3087
www.gfnfoods.com
info@gfnfoods.com

- Gluten-free baking mixes (all-purpose flour, bread, brownie, cake, cookie, cornbread & corn muffin, pancake, pizza crust)

◆ Gluten-Free Prairie
P.O. Box 325, 116 E Main St.
Manhattan, MT, U.S. 59741
855-684-3711 / 406-282-4280
www.glutenfreeprairie.com
contact@glutenfreeprairie.com

- Gluten-free oats (flour, groats, oatmeal), cookies, granola and baking mixes (all purpose flour, brownie)
- Oats produced using the gluten-free purity protocol (see p. 28)

◆ Glutino, Boulder Brands USA, Inc.
1600 Pearl St., Suite 300
Boulder, CO, U.S. 80302
201-421-3970
www.glutino.com

- Gluten-free baked products (breads, cookies, English muffins, stuffing, toaster pastries), baking mixes (all purpose flour, bread, brownie, cake, cookie, muffin, pancake, pie crust, pizza crust), bread crumbs, chips, crackers, pizzas, pretzels and snack bars

◆ GoGo Quinoa
632 Stinson
St. Laurent, QC, Canada H4N 2E9
888-336-8602 / 438-380-3330
www.gogoquinoa.com
info@gogoquinoa.com

- Quinoa-based products (puffed cereal, flakes, flour, whole grain) as well as cookies, pastas and soups
- Amaranth-based products (puffed cereal, pastas, whole grain)
- Baking mixes (cake, pancake), side dishes and vegetarian burgers made with amaranth, quinoa and/or other grains and legumes

◆ Goldbaum's Natural Foods
54 Freeman St.
Newark, NJ, U.S. 07105
973-854-0688
www.goldbaums.com
info@goldbaums.com

- Gluten-free crackers, couscous, croûtons, ice cream cones, noodles (chow mein), pasta and snacks

◆ Golden Platter Foods, Inc.
37 Tompkins Point Rd.
Newark, NJ, U.S. 07114
973-344-8770
www.goldenplatter.com
contact@goldenplatter.com

- Gluten-free breaded chicken products

◆ GoMacro
415 S Wagoner Ave.
Viola, WI, U.S. 54664
800-788-9540 / 608-627-2310
www.gomacro.com
customercare@gomacro.com

- Gluten-free snack bars

◆ The Good Bean
2980 San Pablo Ave.
Berkeley, CA, U.S. 94702
510-842-7144
www.thegoodbean.com
sayhello@thegoodbean.com

- Gluten-free roasted chickpea snacks, bean chips and snack bars

◆ Goodnessknows, Mars, Inc.,
800 High St.
Hackettstown, NJ, U.S. 07840
800-222-0293
www.goodnessknows.com

- Gluten-free snack squares

GoPicnic
10517 United Parkway
Schiller Park, IL, U.S. 60176
773-328-2490
www.gopicnic.com
cs@gopicnic.com

- Single-serve snack boxes containing individually wrapped products that do not require refrigeration or heating or other preparation
- Many snack boxes are gluten free

◆ Gorilly Goods
N173 W21170 Northwest Passage
Jackson, WI, U.S. 53037
262-423-8000
www.gorillygoods.com

- Gluten-free nut clusters and trail mixes

◆ Grain-Free JK Gourmet, Inc.
635 Petrolia Rd.
North York, ON, Canada M3J 2X8
800-608-0465 / 416-782-0045
www.jkgourmet.com
info@jkgourmet.com

- Gluten-free almond-based items (baking mixes, flour, GG Bites, granola, granola bars)

◆ Grainful
950 Danby Rd., Suite 180
Ithaca, NY, U.S. 14850
607-319-5585
www.grainful.com
info@grainful.com

- Frozen entrées and shelf-stable side dishes made with gluten-free steel-cut oats

H

Habitant, Campbell Company of Canada
60 Birmingham St.
Toronto, ON, Canada M8V 2B8
800-410-7687
www.campbellsoup.ca

- Canned ready-to-serve soups; one product is gluten free

◆ Hail Merry, LLC.
9755 Clifford Dr.
Dallas, TX, U.S. 75220
877-455-4046 / 214-905-5005
www.hailmerry.com
customerservice@hailmerry.com

- Gluten-free coconut macaroons and tarts

◆ Hilary's Eat Well
2205 Haskell Ave.
Lawrence, KS, U.S. 66046
785-856-3399
www.hilaryseatwell.com

- Gluten-free salad dressings, stuffings, veggie bites and vegan burgers

Hodgson Mill, Inc.
1100 Stevens Ave.
Effingham, IL, U.S. 62401
800-525-0177
www.hodgsonmill.com
customerservice@hodgsonmill.com

- Baking mixes, flours and other baking ingredients, grains, seeds and pastas
- Over 60 gluten-free products including baking ingredients and mixes (all purpose, bread, brownie, cake, cookie, cornbread, muffin, multi-purpose, pancake & waffle, pizza crust), coatings, flours, grains, pasta and seeds

Hol•Grain
P.O. Box 10640
New Iberia, LA, U.S. 70562
800-551-3245 / 337-364-7242
www.conradricemill.com
info@conradricemill.com

- Baking mixes (brownie, cookie, pancake & waffle), batters, bread crumbs, crackers, rice, sauces, seasonings, snacks, spices and soups
- Many products are gluten free

◆ Homefree, LLC.
P.O. Box 491
Windham, NH, U.S. 03087
800-552-7172 / 603-898-0172
www.homefreetreats.com
info@homefreetreats.com

- Gluten-free cookies

I

Ian's, Elevation Brands, LLC.
190 Fountain St.
Framingham, MA, U.S. 01702
800-543-6637
www.iansnaturalfoods.com
customerservice@iansnaturalfoods.com

- Bread crumbs and frozen items (chicken [nuggets, patties, tenders], battered vegetables, corn dogs, croûtons, fries, French toast sticks, pancrepes, pasta, pizza, stuffing)
- Most products are gluten free

Imagine Foods, The Hain Celestial Group, Inc.
4600 Sleepytime Dr.
Boulder, CO, U.S. 80301
800-434-4246
www.imaginefoods.com
customer.care@hain.com

- Broths, gravies, sauces, soups and stocks
- Many products are gluten free

J

◆ Joe's Gluten-Free Foods
775 Ross Ave. E
Regina, SK, Canada S4N 4W5
306-347-8221
www.joesglutenfree.com

- Gluten-free baked products (bagels, breads, cakes, cookies, cupcakes, muffins, pies, slices, tarts), mixes and perogies

Jovial Foods, Inc.
P.O. Box 98
North Franklin, CT, U.S. 06254
877-642-0644 / 860-642-6996
www.jovialfoods.com
info@jovialfoods.com

- Ancient grain flours and flour mixes, crackers, cookies, grains, olive oil, pasta and tomato products
- Gluten-free items include ancient grain flour mixes (bread, pastry), cookies (chickpea and rice flours), olive oil, pastas (brown rice) and tomato products

◆ Juno Bar
(see **BumbleBar, Inc.**, p. 267)

K

Kashi Canada, Kellogg Company
5350 Creekbank Rd.
Mississauga, ON, Canada L4W 5S1
866-958-7884
www.kashi.ca

The Kashi Company, Kellogg Company
P.O. Box 8557
La Jolla, CA, U.S. 92308
877-747-2467
www.kashi.com

- Cereals, cookies, crackers, entrées, pilafs, protein powders, snack bars and waffles
- Some products are gluten free

♦ Kay's Naturals
P.O. Box 669, 100 First Ave. SE
Clara City, MN, U.S. 56222
866-873-5499 / 320-847-3220
www.kaysnaturals.com

- Gluten-free high-protein cereals and snacks (made with soy protein)

Kellogg Canada, Inc., Kellogg Company
5350 Creekbank Rd.
Mississauga, ON, Canada L4W 5S1
888-876-3750
www.kelloggs.ca

Kellogg Company
P.O. Box CAMB
Battle Creek, MI, U.S. 49016
800-962-1413
www.kelloggs.com

- Beverages, breakfast sandwiches, cereals, crackers, snack bars, snacks, toaster pastries and waffles
- Some products are gluten free

Kikkoman
P.O. Box 420784
San Francisco, CA, U.S. 94142
415-956-7750
www.kikkomanusa.com
consumer@kikkoman.com

- Breadings, coatings, rice vinegars, sauces (Asian, curry, Hoisin, marinades, oyster, soy, teriyaki), seasoning mixes, soup mixes and soy beverages
- Some products are gluten free

♦ KIND, LLC.
P.O. Box 705
Midtown Station, New York, NY, U.S. 10018
855-884-5463
www.kindsnacks.com
customerservice@kindsnacks.com

- Gluten-free granola grain clusters, popped grain snacks and snack bars

King Arthur Flour
135 US Route 5 S
Norwich, Vermont, U.S. 05055
800-827-6836 / 802-299-2240
www.kingarthurflour.com
customercare@kingarthurflour.com

- Baking mixes, flours and other baking ingredients
- Many gluten-free products including baking mixes (all-purpose, bread, bread & pizza crust, brownie, cake, cookie, doughnut, gingerbread, muffin, pancake, pie crust, scone), flour blends, flours, starches and other baking ingredients

♦ Kinnikinnick
10940 120 St.
Edmonton, AB, Canada T5H 3P7
877-503-4466 / 780-424-2900
www.kinnikinnick.com
info@kinnikinnick.com

- Gluten-free baked products (bagels, breads, buns, cookies, donuts, English muffins, fruit cake, muffins, pie crust, pizza crust, rolls and waffles), stuffings, baking mixes (all purpose flour, cake, cookie, cornbread, bread & bun, pancake & waffle), crumbs (bread, cookie) and graham-style crackers and crumbs

♦ Kitchen Basics, McCormick & Company, Inc.
18 Loveton Circle
Sparks, MD, U.S. 21152
800-967-8424 (U.S.) / 800-209-8707 (CAN)
www.mccormick.com/gourmet

- Gluten-free broths, stock cubes and stocks

♦ Kitchen Table Bakers
41 Princeton Dr.
Syosset, NY, U.S. 11791
800-486-4582 / 516-931-5113
www.kitchentablebakers.com
info@kitchentablebakers.com

- Gluten-free Parmesan cheese crisps

L

Lakefront Brewery, Inc.
1872 N Commerce St.
Milwaukee, WI, U.S. 53212
414-372-8800
www.lakefrontbrewery.com

- Ales, beers and lagers
- "New Grist" beer (made from sorghum and rice) is gluten free

La Messagère, Les bières de la Nouvelle-France
90 Rivière aux Écorces
Saint-Alexis-des Monts, QC, Canada J0K 1V0
819-265-4000
www.lesbieresnouvellefrance.com
info@lesbieresnouvellefrance.com

- Variety of beers
- Gluten-free beers are made from buckwheat and rice or millet

◆ Larabar, Small Planet Foods Canada
5825 Explorer Dr.
Mississauga, ON, Canada L4W 5P6
800-543-2147 / 800-624-4123
www.larabar.ca

◆ Larabar, Small Planet Foods, Inc.
P.O. Box 18932
Denver, CO, U.S. 80218
800-543-2147
www.larabar.com

- Gluten-free snack bars

◆ Lara's
(see **Cream Hill Estates**, p. 269)

Larrowe's
(see **The Birkett Mills**, p. 266)

La Tortilla Factory
3300 Westwind Blvd.
Santa Rosa, CA, U.S. 95403
800-446-1516
www.latortillafactory.com
info@latortillafactory.com

- Tortillas and wraps
- Corn tortillas and some wraps are gluten free

◆ Le Asolane, Molino di Ferro
Via Molino di Ferro 6
31050 Fanzolo di Vedelago TV, Italy
39 0423 487035
www.molinodiferro.com/en
info@molinodiferro.com

- Gluten-free corn-based pastas
- Distributed by Quattrobimbi.com and other online retailers

◆ Leo's Gluten Free
10130 Pacific Ave.
Franklin Park, IL, U.S. 60131
847-233-9211
www.leosglutenfree.com
info@leosglutenfree.com

- Gluten-free fresh pasta and gnocchi

Let's Do... and Let's Do...Organic, Edward & Sons
P.O. Box 1326
Carpinteria, CA, U.S. 93014
805-684-8500
www.edwardandsons.com

- Flours, ice cream cones, sprinkles, starches and other items
- Many products are gluten free.

◆ Le Veneziane, Molino di Ferro
Via Molino di Ferro 6
31050 Fanzolo di Vedelago TV, Italy
39 0423 487035
www.molinodiferro.com/en
info@molinodiferro.com

- Gluten-free breadsticks, cookies, corn-based pastas, gnocchi and sauces
- Distributed by Quattrobimbi.com and other online retailers

◆ Libre Naturals, Inc.
6200 Scott Rd.
Duncan, BC, Canada V9L 6Y8
866-714-5411 / 250-715-1481
www.librenaturals.com
www.librenaturals.ca

- Gluten-free oat products (granola bars, instant oatmeal, granola, quick and rolled oats), seeds and other items

◆ Little Northern Bakehouse

P.O. Box 655, Station A
Abbotsford, BC, Canada V2T 6Z8
888-863-4481
www.littlenorthernbakehouse.com
info@littlenorthernbakehouse.ca

* Gluten-free breads and buns

◆ Lotus Foods, Inc.

5210 Wall Ave.
Richmond, CA, U.S. 94804
510-525-3137
www.lotusfoods.com
info@lotusfoods.com

* Gluten-free ramen noodles (with and without broth), rice, rice-based crackers and heat & eat microwave rice bowls

◆ Lucy's

930 Denison Ave., Suite 101–A
Norfolk, VA, U.S. 23513
757-233-9495
www.drlucys.com
info@drlucys.com

* Gluten-free brownie crisps and cookies

Lundberg Family Farms

P.O. Box 369, 5311 Midway
Richvale, CA, U.S. 95974
888-215-2958 / 530-538-3500
www.lundberg.com

* Brown rice-based items (crackers, pasta, pasta & sauce, rice cakes, side dishes, snacks, syrup) and rice
* Many products are gluten free

M

◆ Manini's

22408 72nd Ave. S
Kent, WA, U.S. 98032
206-686-4600
www.maninis.com
info@maninis.com

* Gluten-free products (buns, fresh pasta, mixes, rolls) made with amaranth, millet, quinoa, sorghum and teff

◆ Mary's Gone Crackers

P.O. Box 965
Gridley, CA, U.S. 95948
888-258-1250
www.marysgonecrackers.com
info@marysgonecrackers.com

* Gluten-free crackers, cookies and pretzels

◆ Mikey's, LLC.

16427 N Scottsdale Rd.
Scottsdale, AZ, U.S. 85254
480-696-2483
www.mikeysmuffins.com
info@mikeysmuffins.com

* Gluten-free products (muffins and pizza crust) made with almond and coconut flours

Milton's Craft Bakers

5875 Avenida Encinas
Carlsbad, CA, U.S. 92008
858-350-9696
www.miltonsbaking.com

* Breads, buns, cookies, crackers, English muffins and rolls
* Some chips, crackers and cookies are gluten free

◆ Modern Table, Inc.

2185 N California Blvd., Suite 215
Walnut Creek, CA, U.S. 94596
866-799-7289
www.moderntable.com

* Gluten-free, legume-based pasta and pasta & veggie kits

◆ Mrs. Leeper's, World Finer Foods

1455 Broad St., 4th Floor
Bloomfield, NJ, U.S. 07003
973-338-0300
www.mrsleepers.com

* Gluten-free pastas, pasta meals and soup mixes

N

◆ Namaste Foods
P.O. Box 3133
Coeur d'Alene, ID, U.S. 83816
866-258-9493/208-266-4136
www.namastefoods.com
admin@namastefoods.com

- Gluten-free flours, baking mixes (blondie, bread & roll, brownie, cake, cookie, flour blend, muffin, muffin & scone, pizza crust, pumpkin baking, waffle & pancake) and other baking ingredients as well as coating mixes, pasta dinners and soup cups

Nature's Path Foods
9100 Van Horne Way
Richmond, BC, Canada V6X 1W3
866-880-7284 / 604-248-8777
www.naturespath.com

- Cereals, cookies, granola and granola bars, oatmeal, oats, snack bars and waffles
- Some products are gluten free

◆ Neat Foods, LLC.
244 N Queen St.
Lancaster, PA, U.S. 17603
888-491-0524
www.eatneat.com
sales@eatneat.com

- Shelf-stable gluten-free meat replacement products (made from nuts, beans and gluten-free oats) and an egg replacer (made from chia seeds and garbanzo beans)

◆ NoGii, SBI Brands
11401 Granite St.
Charlotte, NC, U.S. 28273
800-447-4795
www.nogii.com
info@sbibrands.com

- Gluten-free protein powders and snack bars

◆ NorQuin, Northern Quinoa Corporation
3002 Millar Ave.
Saskatoon, SK, Canada S7K 5X9
866-368-9304 / 306-933-9525
www.quinoa.com

- Gluten-free quinoa-based products (flakes, flour, powder, whole grain)

◆ Nourish Snacks
168A Irving Ave., Suite 401
Port Chester, NY, U.S. 10573
844-466-8747
www.nourishsnacks.com
help@nourishsnacks.com

- Single-serve gluten-free items such as granola bites, fruit and nut snacks, half-popped popcorn and roasted snacks (chickpeas and nuts; corn)
- Products created by dietitian Joy Bauer, RD

◆ Nu Life Market, LLC.
P.O. Box 105, 1202 E 5th St.
Scott City, KS, U.S. 67871
866-962-5236 / 620-872-5236
www.nulifemarket.com

- Gluten-free sorghum-based products including bran, flours, grains and mixes (all-purpose flour, pizza crust) as well as teff flour and grain

O

◆ O'Doughs
320 Oakdale Rd.
Toronto, ON, Canada M3N 1W5
416-342-5700
www.odoughs.com
eatwell@odoughs.com

- Gluten-free bagels, breads, buns, cakes, flatbreads, muffins and pizza crusts with sauce

Olivia's Croutons
1423 North St.
New Haven, VT, U.S. 05472
888-425-3080 / 802-453-2222
www.oliviascroutons.com
info@oliviascroutons.com

- Croûtons and stuffings
- Some products are gluten free

◆ 1-2-3 Gluten-Free
125 Orange Tree Dr.
Chagrin Falls, OH, U.S. 44022
216-378-9233
www.123glutenfree.com
info@123glutenfree.com

- Gluten-free baking mixes (biscuit, brownie, cake, cookie, corn bread, multi-purpose flour, muffin, pan bar, pancake, roll) and brownie chips

◆ Only Oats
(see **Avena Foods, Ltd.**, p. 265)

◆ Orgran
47 53 Aster Ave.
Carrum Downs, Vic 3201, Australia
61 3 9776 9044 (Australia)
877-380-3422 / 845-278-8164 (U.S.)
www.orgran.com
info@orgran.com

- Gluten-free products include baking mixes (bread, brownie, cake, falafel, flour blends, muffin, pancake, pastry, pizza & pastry), biscuits, bread crumbs, cereals, cookies, crackers, crispbreads, croûtons, fruit bars, gravy mix, licorice, pasta, pasta meal and soup mix

P

Pacific Foods
19480 SW 97th Ave.
Tualatin, OR, U.S. 97062
503-692-9666 / 503-924-4570
www.pacificfoods.com

- Broths, soups and stocks as well as gravy, meals and side dishes, non-dairy beverages, purées, sauces and tofu
- Many products are gluten free

◆ Pamela's Products, Inc.
1 Carousel Lane, Suite D
Ukiah, CA, U.S. 95482
707-462-6605
www.pamelasproducts.com
info@pamelasproducts.com

- Gluten-free baking mixes (all-purpose flour, baking & pancake, biscuit & scone, bread, brownie, cake, cookie, cornbread & muffin, flour blend, frosting, pancake, pancake & waffle, pizza crust) as well as biscotti, cookies, fig bars, graham crackers and snack bars

◆ Pasta Legume, LLC.
Box 551
Brewster, NY, U.S. 10509
845-278-8164
www.pastalegume.com

- Gluten-free whole green lentil pasta

◆ Pastariso, Maplegrove Gluten Free Foods, Inc.
5010 Eucalyptus Ave.
Chino, CA, U.S. 91710
909-823-8230
www.pastarisofoods.com

- Gluten-free rice pasta, rice pasta & cheese dinners and mac & cheese cups

◆ Pastato, Maplegrove Gluten Free Foods, Inc.
5010 Eucalyptus Ave.
Chino, CA, U.S. 91710
909-823-8230
www.pastarisofoods.com/pastato

- Gluten-free potato-based pasta and pasta & cheese dinners

◆ PatsyPie
2496 rue Remembrance
Lachine, QC, Canada H8S 1X7
514-695-0707
www.patsypie.com
info@patsypie.com

- Gluten-free baked products (biscotti, brownies, cookies, pie crust) and scone mixes

◆ Perfect Bar
5360 Eastgate Mall, Suite A
San Diego, CA, U.S. 92121
866-628-8548 / 858-795-2650
www.perfectbar.com
service@perfectbar.com

- Gluten-free nut-based refrigerated snack bars

◆ The Piping Gourmets, Batter Up, LLC.
990 Biscayne Blvd., Suite 502
Miami, FL, U.S. 33132
786-233-8660
www.thepipinggourmets.com
info@thepipinggourmets.com

- Gluten-free whoopie pies

◆ **Plum-M-Good, Van Rice Products**
#8–1350 Valmont Way
Richmond, BC, Canada V6V 1Y4
604-273-8038
www.vanrice.com

- Gluten-free rice cakes and brown rice breading crumbs

Pocono
(see **The Birkett Mills**, p. 266)

◆ **Premier Japan, Edward & Sons**
P.O. Box 1326
Carpinteria, CA, U.S. 93014
805-684-8500
www.edwardandsons.com

- Gluten-free sauces (hoisin, teriyaki)

◆ **Premium Gold Flax, Inc.**
1321 12ᵗʰ Ave. NE
Denhoff, ND, U.S. 58430
866-570-1234 / 701-884-2553
www.premiumgoldflax.com
info@premiumgoldflax.com

- Gluten-free flax products (hull lignans, ground, whole), flax-based mixes (all-purpose, brownie, cookie, muffin, pancake & waffle, pizza crust) and a seeds-and-grains mix (made with chia, flax, pumpkin and sunflower seeds; amaranth, buckwheat, mesquite, quinoa)

President's Choice, Loblaw Companies, Ltd.
1 President's Choice Circle
Brampton, ON, Canada L6Y 5S5
888-495-5111
www.presidentschoice.ca

- Thousands of grocery items in numerous product categories
- Extensive variety of gluten-free products

◆ **Promax Nutrition Company**
520 Second St.
Oakmont, PA, U.S. 15139
888-421-2032
www.promaxnutrition.com

- Gluten-free snack bars

◆ **Promise Gluten Free, Cuisine Royale Manufacturing, Ltd.**
Kilmucklin, Tullamore, Co. Offaly, Ireland
www.promiseglutenfree.com
info@promiseglutenfree.com

- Gluten-free breads, buns, bagels, cakes, English muffins, muffins, pancakes, rolls and snack bars

◆ **PureFit**
216 Technology Suite E
Irvine, CA, U.S. 92618
866-787-3348 / 949-679-7997
www.purefit.com
info@purefit.com

- Gluten-free snack bars

◆ **Pure Genius Provisions**
291 Union Street, #PHB
Brooklyn, NY, U.S. 11231
646-820-8074
www.puregeniusprovisions.com
sales@puregeniusprovisions.com

- Gluten-free blondies and brownies made with chickpeas, flax and gluten-free oats

◆ **Purely Elizabeth**
3200 Carbon Pl., Suite 100
Boulder, CO, U.S. 80301
720-242-7525
www.purelyelizabeth.com
info@purelyelizabeth.com

- Gluten-free oat products (cold cereal, granola, muesli, oatmeal)

◆ **Pure Organic, The Pure Bar Company**
P.O. Box 649
Solana Beach, CA, U.S. 92075
888-568-7873 / 949-502-4840
www.thepurebar.com
customerservice@thepurebar.com

- Gluten-free fruit & veggie strips and snack bars

Q

◆ Qrunch Foods
P.O. Box 200128
Denver, CO, U.S. 80220
303-570-4113
www.qrunchfoods.com

- Gluten-free vegan burgers and breakfast "toastables" (made from millet, quinoa, amaranth)

Quaker, PepsiCo Canada
14 Hunter St. E
Peterborough, ON, Canada K9J 7B2
800-267-6287
www.quakeroats.ca

Quaker, PepsiCo, Inc.
P.O. Box 049003
Chicago, IL, U.S. 60604
800-367-6287
www.quakeroats.com

- Bars, cereals, mixes, oatmeal, rice cakes and other snacks
- Some products are gluten free

◆ Quinn Foods, LLC.
2100 Central Ave., Suite 108
Boulder, CO, U.S. 80301
303-927-6655
www.quinnsnacks.com

- Gluten-free popcorn and pretzels

R

◆ Real Foods
47 Campbell Rd.
St. Peters, NSW 2044, Australia
61 2 8595 6600
www.cornthins.com
email@realfoods.com.au

- Gluten-free crispbreads (corn, rice)

◆ The Really Great Food Company
646 Middle Country Rd. #2
St. James, NY, U.S. 11780
800-593-5377
www.reallygreatfood.com
info@reallygreatfood.com

- Gluten-free baking mixes (bread, brownie, cake, muffin, pancake, pizza crust)

◆ Redbridge, Anheuser-Busch
One Busch Place
St. Louis, MO, U.S. 63118
800-342-5283
www.redbridgebeer.com

- Gluten-free beer made from sorghum

◆ Rise Bar
16752 Millikan Ave.
Irvine, CA, U.S. 92606
800-440-6476
www.risebar.com
cs@risebar.com

- Gluten-free snack bars

◆ Rizopia
55 Leek Cres.
Richmond Hill, ON, Canada L4B 3Y2
866-749-6742 / 905-709-8838
www.rizopia.com
info@rizopia.com

- Gluten-free pastas made with rice (brown, white or wild) or quinoa and brown rice

Road's End Organics, Edward & Sons
P.O. Box 1326
Carpinteria, CA, U.S. 93014
805-684-8500
www.edwardandsons.com

- Gravy mixes, sauces and macaroni & cheese dinners
- Some products are gluten free

Ronzoni
85 Shannon Rd.
Harrisburg, PA, U.S. 17112
800-730-5957
www.ronzoni.com

- Variety of pastas
- Some pasta products (made with corn, quinoa and brown and white rice) are gluten free

RP's Pasta Company
1133 E Wilson St.
Madison, WI, U.S. 53703
608-257-7216
www.rpspasta.com
freshpasta@rpspasta.com

- Pastas (fresh and frozen) and pasta sauces
- Some pasta products are gluten free

Rudi's Gluten-Free Bakery, The Hain Celestial Group, Inc.
4600 Sleepytime Dr.
Boulder, CO, U.S. 80301
877-293-0876 / 303-447-0495
www.rudisbakery.com/gluten-free/

* Gluten-free breads, buns, rolls, snack bars and tortillas

Rustic Crust
5 Main St.
Pittsfield, NH, U.S. 03263
888-519-5119 / 603-435-5119
www.rusticcrust.com
info@rusticcrust.com

* Shelf-stable pizza crusts
* One crust is gluten free

S

Saffron Road, American Halal Co., Inc.
1111 Summer St.
Stamford, CT, U.S. 06905
877-425-2587 / 203-961-1954
www.saffronroadfood.com
info@saffronroadfood.com

* Breaded chicken nuggets, broths, chickpea snacks, crackers, desserts, frozen entrées, hors d'oeuvres, lentil chips and simmer sauces
* Many products are gluten free

San-J International
2880 Sprouse Dr.
Henrico, VA, U.S. 23231
800-446-5500 / 804-226-8333
www.san-j.com
info@san-j.com

* Brown rice crackers, Asian cooking sauces, tamari soy sauces, salad dressings and soups
* Most products are gluten free

Savory Choice, Savory Creations International
1900 O'Farrell St., Suite 180
San Mateo, CA, U.S. 94403
866-472-8679 / 650-638-1024
www.savorychoice.com
www.savory-creations.com
info@savorychoice.com

* Gluten-free broth, soup and stock concentrates as well as demi-glaces

Schär
Winkelau 9
I–39014 Postal (BZ), Italy
39 0473 293300
www.schar.com
info@schar.com

Schär USA
125 Chubb Ave.
Lyndhurst, NJ, U.S. 07071
201-355-8470
www.schar.com
info@schar.com

* Gluten-free baked products (baguettes, biscuits, breads, buns, cookies, croissants, pizza crusts, rolls and wafers), baking mixes (bread, pancake & waffle), bread crumbs, breadsticks, crackers, croûtons, pastas, pasta meals and pizza

Sea Fare Pacific, Oregon Seafoods
90428 Metcalf Dr.
Charleston, OR, U.S. 97420
541-266-8862
www.seafarepacific.com
sales@oregonseafoods.com

* Gluten-free fish and seafood products (chowders, entrées, soups) in shelf-stable pouches as well as canned Albacore tuna

Silver Hills Bakery
P.O. Box 2250
Abbotsford, BC, Canada V2T 4X2
888-853-6466 / 604-850-5600
www.silverhillsbakery.ca
info@silverhillsbakery.ca

* Bagels, breads and buns
* Some breads are gluten free

Simple Mills
444 N Wells St., Suite 204
Chicago, IL, U.S. 60654
312-600-6196
www.simplemills.com
info@simplemills.com

* Gluten-free almond-based baking mixes (bread, cake, cookie, muffin & bread, muffin & cake, pancake & waffle, pizza dough) and crackers

Simply Asia, Simply Asia Foods, Inc.
P.O. Box 13242
Berkley, CA, U.S. 94712-4242
800-967-8424 (U.S.) / 800-209-8707 (CAN)
www.simplyasia.com

- Asian products (coconut milk, noodle bowls, noodles & sauces, noodle soup bowls, sauces, seasoning blends)
- Some products are gluten free

♦ SimplyProtein, Wellness Foods
301–721 Bloor St. W
Toronto, ON, Canada M6G 1L5
800-547-5790
www.simplyprotein.ca
customerservice@thesimplybar.com

- Gluten-free snacks and snack bars

♦ Simply Shari's
P.O. Box 8186
Scottsdale, AZ, U.S. 85252
805-320-3880
www.simplysharis.com
info@simplysharis.com

- Gluten-free cookies

♦ Smart Flour Foods
4020 S Industrial Dr., Suite 110
Austin, TX, U.S. 78744
888-660-6564 / 512-706-1775
www.smartflourfoods.com
info@smartflourfoods.com

- Gluten-free buns, pizza and pizza crusts as well as pancake & waffle mix (made with amaranth, sorghum, tapioca, teff)

Sol Cuisine
1201 Fewster Dr.
Mississauga, ON, Canada L4W 1A2
905-502-8500
www.solcuisine.com
info@solcuisine.com

- Vegan and vegetarian products including burgers, falafel, meatless beef and chicken, tofu, tofu ribs, veggie breakfast sausages)
- Most products are gluten free

♦ SOYJOY
P.O. Box 9606
Mission Hills, CA, U.S. 91346
888-676-9569
us.soyjoy.com

- Gluten-free snack bars

♦ Sunshine Burger and Specialty Food Company, Inc.
701 Jones Ave.
Fort Atkinson, WI, U.S. 53538
920-568-1100
www.sunshineburger.com
info@sunshineburger.com

- Gluten-free vegan burgers

Swanson, Campbell Soup Company
1 Campbell Pl.
Camden, NJ, U.S. 08103-1701
800-257-8443
www.campbellsoup.com

- Broths and stocks
- Many are gluten free

T

Taste Adventure, Will-Pak Foods, Inc.
9431 Haven Ave., Suite 105
Rancho Cucamonga, CA, U.S. 91730
909-912-1888
www.tasteadventure.com
taste_adv@earthlink.net

- Shelf-stable products (chilies, side dishes, soups)
- Most products are gluten free

♦ Taste of Nature
230 Ferrier St.
Markham, ON, Canada L3R 2Z5
905-415-8218
www.tasteofnature.ca
info@tasteofnature.ca

- Gluten-free snack bars

♦ The Teff Company
P.O. Box A
Caldwell, ID, U.S. 83606
888-822-2221 / 208-461-5634
www.teffco.com
questions@teffco.com

- Teff flour and grain

Thai Kitchen, Simply Asia Foods, Inc.
P.O. Box 13242
Berkeley, CA, U.S. 94712-4242
800-967-8424 (U.S.) / 800-209-8707(CAN)
www.thaikitchen.com
www.thaikitchencanada.ca
- Asian products (coconut milk, rice meal kits, rice noodles, rice side dishes, sauces, soups, Thai herbs and spices)
- Many products are gluten free

◆ Three Bakers, Gluten Free Food Group, LLC.
360 J & J Rd.
Moscow, PA, U.S. 18444
570-689-9694
www.threebakers.com
contact@threebakers.net
- Gluten-free breads, buns, pizzas, pizza crust, rolls, snack crackers and stuffing mix

◆ Tinkyada
120 Melford Dr., Unit 8
Scarborough, ON, Canada M1B 2X5
416-609-0016
www.tinkyada.com
- Gluten-free pastas made from brown or white rice

The Tofurky Company
P.O. Box 176
Hood River, OR, U.S. 97031
800-508-8100
www.tofurky.com
info@tofurky.com
- Vegan products such as meat substitutes (burgers, chick'n, deli slices, hot dogs, sausages), pizzas, pocket sandwiches and tempeh
- Some products are gluten free

◆ Tolerant Foods, MXO Global, Inc.
220 Appin Ave.
Mount Royal, QC, Canada H3P 1V8
888-653-7268
www.tolerantfoods.com
cs@tolerantfoods.com
- Gluten-free pastas made from legumes (beans, lentils, peas)

◆ Tonya's Gluten Free Kitchen
167 Sinclair Rd.
Newmanstown, PA, U.S. 17073
717-949-4175
www.tonyasglutenfree.com
tonya@tonyasglutenfree.com
- Gluten-free soft pretzels and pretzel bites

Toufayan Bakeries, Inc.
175 Railroad Ave.
Ridgefield, NJ, U.S. 07657
800-328-7482 / 201-941-2000
www.toufayan.com
info@toufayan.com
- Bagels, breadsticks, croissants, flatbreads, pita breads, pita chips, tortillas and wraps
- Some wraps and pita chips are gluten free

◆ TruRoots, The JM Smuckers Company
1 Strawberry Lane
Orrville, OH, U.S. 44667
800-288-3637
www.truroots.com
- Gluten-free products including pasta (made with quinoa, amaranth, brown rice), pilafs, quinoa, quinoa blends, rice, seeds and legumes

U

◆ Udi's Gluten Free, Boulder Brands USA, Inc.
1600 Pearl St., Suite 300
Boulder, CO, U.S. 80302
201-421-3970
www.udisglutenfree.com
- Gluten-free baked products (bagels, baguettes, breads, brownies, buns, cinnamon rolls, cookies, muffins, pizza crusts, rolls, tortillas), entrées, granola, granola bars, steel-cut oats, pizzas and snacks

V

Van's, Van's International Foods, Inc.
P.O. Box 3901
Peoria, IL, U.S. 61612
855-258-5685
www.vansfoods.com
info@vansfoods.com
- Cereals, chips, crackers, French toast sticks, pancakes, pasta entrées, snack bars and waffles
- Many products are gluten free

◆ Viki's Foods
999 S Oyster Bay Rd., Suite 403
Bethpage, NY, U.S. 11714
516-767-8700
www.vikisfoods.com
info@vikisgourmet.com

- Gluten-free granola

W

◆ Watusee Foods
1201 New York Ave. NW, Suite 400
Washington, DC, U.S. 20005
202-281-8245
www.watuseefoods.com

- Gluten-free products (bread crumbs and roasted snacks) made with chickpeas

◆ Whole Note Food Company
2900 Katy Hockley Cut Off Rd., Unit A111
Katy, TX, U.S. 77493
713-806-5294
www.wholenotegf.com
customerservice@wholenotegf.com

- Gluten-free baking mixes (crêpe, muffin, multi-purpose flour, pancake, pizza crust, pumpkin bread and muffin, waffle) made from whole-grain flours (brown rice, buckwheat, millet, oat, sorghum, teff), flaxseed meal, garbanzo bean flour and fava bean flour

The Wizard's, Edward & Sons
P.O. Box 1326
Carpinteria, CA, U.S. 93014
805-684-8500
www.edwardandsons.com

- Worcestershire and hot sauces
- Gluten-free version of each sauce

Wolff's
(see **The Birkett Mills**, p. 266)

◆ Wondergrain, Nature2Kitchen
7209 NW 41st St.
Miami, FL, U.S. 33166
877-307-0253
www.wondergrain.com
wondergrain@nature2kitchen.com

- Gluten-free products including pearled and whole-grain sorghum, sorghum flour and baking mixes (all-purpose flour, cookie)

◆ Woodstock Mini Me's, Blue Marble Brands
313 Iron Horse Way
Providence, RI, U.S. 02908
888-534-0246
www.minimes.com

- Gluten-free frosted mini rice cakes

◆ WOW Baking Company
7032 S 188th St.
Kent, WA, U.S. 98032
425-251-0541
www.wowbaking.com

- Gluten-free brownies, cake mixes, cookies and cookie dough

X

◆ XO Baking Co.
21781 Ventura Blvd., Suite 323
Woodland Hills, CA, U.S. 91364
818-883-1702
www.xobakingco.com
info@xobakingco.com

- Gluten-free mixes (all-purpose flour, biscuit and scone, blondie, bread, brownie, cake, cookie, frosting, muffin, pancake and waffle, pie crust)

Z

◆ Zing, Northwest Nutritional Foods, LLC.
10228 Fischer Pl. NE
Seattle, WA, U.S. 98125
877-600-9402 / 206-362-3989
www.zingbars.com
info@zingbars.com

- Gluten-free snack bars

Gluten-Free Specialty Retailers

17

The following is a select list of businesses in the U.S. and Canada that sell *only* gluten-free products in their retail stores. Most offer an extensive range of shelf-stable, fresh, refrigerated and frozen items as well as related products such as baking equipment, books and supplements. Some of these stores have an on-site dedicated gluten-free bakery. If shopping in person is not a possibility, contact the company to see if there are other ways to purchase their products.

Gluten-free products also can be purchased from online retailers who do not have a storefront. There are many online retailers and two of these who offer gluten-free products exclusively are included after the list of gluten-free stores.

Gluten-Free Stores

Against The Grain, LLC.
2292 West 5400 South
Taylorsville, UT, U.S. 84129
801-955-4418
www.againstthegrainslc.com
imglutenfree@againstthegrainslc.com

G-Free NYC
77A W 85th St.
New York, NY, U.S. 10024
646-781-9770
www.g-freenyc.com
info@g-freenyc.com

Goodbye Gluten
2066 Avenue Rd.
Toronto, ON, Canada M5M 4A6
416-781-9191
www.goodbyegluten.com
info@goodbyegluten.com

Herbalicious
612 West Main St.
Mount Pleasant, PA, U.S. 15666
724-542-9745
www.everythingnutritious.com
herbalicious@verizon.net

Jake's Gluten-Free Market & Bakery
12570 W Fairview Ave., Suite 102
Boise, ID, U.S. 83713
208-322-5935
http://jakesglutenfreestore.com
jakesglutenfreemarket@gmail.com

Janell's Gluten-Free Market
13342 NE 175th St.
Woodinville, WA, U.S. 98072
425-892-8677
www.janellsglutenfreemarket.com

Lorenzo's Specialty Foods, Ltd.
1060 St. Mary's Road
Winnipeg, MB, Canada R2M 3S9
866-639-1711 / 204-253-1300
www.lorenzosfoods.ca
hello@lorenzosfoods.ca

Louise Sans Gluten Free
475 Dumont, #109
Dorval, QC Canada H9S 5W2
514-631-3434
www.louisesansgluten.com
info@louisesansgluten.com

Specialty Food Shop
555 University Ave.
Toronto, ON, Canada M5G 1X8
800-737-7976 / 416-813-5294
www.specialtyfoodshop.com
sfs.admin@sickkids.ca

Strictly Gluten Free
396A Larkfield Road
East Northport, NY, U.S. 11731
855-435-4846 / 631-486-6835
www.strictlyglutenfree.com
info@strictlyglutenfree.com

Gluten-Free Online Retailers

Gluten-Free Mall, Inc.
191 Commerce Dr.
New Holland, PA, U.S. 17557
866-575-3720 / 707-509-4528
www.glutenfreemall.com
info@glutenfreemall.com

Gluten Free Palace, LLC.
1616 52nd St.
Brooklyn, NY, U.S. 11219
888-945-8836 / 718-483-8663
www.glutenfreepalace.com
customercare@glutenfreepalace.com

Quattrobimbi Imports, Inc.
48 Lawridge Dr.
Rye Brook, NY, U.S. 10573
866-618-7759 / 914-819-0494
www.quattrobimbi.com
info@quattrobimbi.com

Resources

American Celiac Organizations

Celiac Disease Foundation (CDF)
20350 Ventura Blvd., Suite 240
Woodland Hills, CA, U.S. 91364
818-716-1513
www.celiac.org
cdf@celiac.org

Celiac Support Association, Inc. (CSA)
413 Ash St.
Seward, NE, U.S. 68434
877-272-4272 / 402-643-4101
www.csaceliacs.org
celiacs@csaceliacs.org

Gluten Intolerance Group of North America (GIG)
31214 – 124th Ave. SE
Auburn, WA, U.S. 98092
253-833-6655
www.gluten.org
customerservice@gluten.org

Beyond Celiac (formerly the National Foundation for Celiac Awareness)
P.O. Box 544
224 South Maple St.
Ambler, PA, U.S. 19002
844-856-6692 / 215-325-1306
www.beyondceliac.org/
info@beyondceliac.org

North American Society for the Study of Celiac Disease (NASSCD)
3300 Woodcreek Dr.
Downers Grove, IL, U.S. 60515
630-522-7886
www.nasscd.org/
info@nasscd.org

Canadian Celiac Organizations

Canadian Celiac Association (CCA)
5025 Orbitor Dr., Bldg. 1, Suite 400
Mississauga, ON, Canada L4W 4Y5
800-363-7296 / 905-507-6208
www.celiac.ca
info@celiac.ca

Fondation Québécoise de la Maladie Coeliaque (Quebec Celiac Disease Foundation)
4837 rue Boyer, Bureau 230
Montreal, QC, Canada H2J 3E6
514-529-8806
www.fqmc.org
info@fqmc.org

International Celiac Organizations

Country	Website (www.)
Argentina	celiaco.org.ar
Australia	coeliacsociety.com.au
Austria	zoeliakie.or.at
Belgium	coeliakie.be | sbc-asbl.be
Brazil	acelbra.org.br
Chile	coacel.cl
Croatia	celijakija.hr
Czech Republic	coeliac.cz/en | celiac.cz
Denmark	coeliaki.dk
Estonia	tsoliaakia.ee
Finland	keliakialiitto.fi
France	afdiag.org
Germany	dzg-online.de
Greece	koiliokaki.com | coeliac.gr
Hungary	coeliac.hu
India	celiacsocietyrajasthan.com
Iran	celiac.ir/en
Ireland	coeliac.ie
Italy	celiachia.it
Luxembourg	alig.lu
Mexico	acelmex.org.mx
Netherlands	glutenvrij.nl
New Zealand	coeliac.org.nz
Norway	ncf.no
Pakistan	celiac.com.pk
Paraguay	fupacel.org.py
Poland	celiakia.org.pl
Portugal	celiacos.org.pt
Romania	celiachie.ro
Russia	celiac.spb.ru
Saudi Arabia	saudiceliac.com/ar/
Slovakia	celiakia.sk
Slovenia	drustvo-celiakija.si
Spain	celiacos.org
Spain (Catalunya)	celiacscatalunya.org
Sweden	celiaki.se
Switzerland	zoeliakie.ch | coeliakie.ch | celiachia.ch
Tunisia	atmc.org.tn
Turkey	colyak.org.tr
United Arab Emirates	glutenfreeuae.com
United Kingdom	coeliac.co.uk
Uruguay	acelu.org

American Celiac Disease Centers and Programs

Eastern U.S.

Celiac Center, Beth Israel Deaconess Medical Center
Boston, MA
617-667-1272
www.celiacnow.org

Celiac Center, Paoli Hospital
Paoli, PA
866-225-5654 / 484-580-1000
www.mainlinehealth.org/paoliceliac

Celiac Disease Center, Columbia University
New York, NY
212-342-4529
www.celiacdiseasecenter.columbia.edu

Celiac Disease Program, Children's National Health System
Washington, DC
202-476-3032
www.childrensnational.org/departments/celiac-disease-program

Celiac Disease Program, Gastroenterology and Nutrition Division, Boston Children's Hospital
Boston, MA
617-355-6058
www.childrenshospital.org/celiac

Center for Celiac Disease, Children's Hospital of Philadelphia
Philadelphia, PA
215-590-3076
www.chop.edu/centers-programs/center-celiac-disease/

Center for Celiac Research and Treatment, Massachusetts General Hospital
Boston, MA
617-724-8476
www.celiaccenter.org

Jefferson Celiac Center, Thomas Jefferson University Hospital
Philadelphia, PA
800-533-3669 / 215-923-5422
www.hospitals.jefferson.edu/departments-and-services/celiac-center/

Kogan Celiac Center, Barnabas Health Ambulatory Care Center
Livingston, NJ
888-724-7123 / 973-322-7272
www.barnabashealth.org/Ambulatory-Care/Our-Services/Celiac-Disease-Center.aspx

Midwestern and Southern U.S.

Bonnie Lynn Mechanic Celiac Disease Clinic, Children's Hospital of Wisconsin
Milwaukee, WI
414-607-5280
www.chw.org/medical-care/gastroenterology-and-hepatology-program/specialty-programs/bonnie-lynn-mechanic-celiac-disease-clinic/

Celiac Center, University of Tennessee Medical Center
Knoxville, TN
865-305-6970
www.utmedicalcenter.org/departments/gastroenterology/medical-services/celiac-center/

Celiac Disease Center, Nationwide Children's Hospital
Columbus, OH
614-722-3450
www.nationwidechildrens.org/celiac-disease

Celiac Disease Clinic, Center for Digestive Diseases, University of Iowa Hospitals and Clinics
Iowa City, IA
319-356-4060
www.uihealthcare.org/celiacdisease/

Celiac Disease Clinic, Mayo Clinic
Rochester, MN
507-284-5255
www.mayoclinic.org/departments-centers/
gastroenterology-hepatology

Digestive Health Center, University of Virginia Health System
Charlottesville, VA
434-924-2959 / 434-243-3090
www.uvahealth.com/services/digestive-health

University of Chicago Celiac Disease Center
Chicago, IL
888-824-0200 / 773-702-7593
www.uchospitals.edu/specialties/celiac
www.cureceliacdisease.org

Western U.S.

Celiac Disease Program, Digestive Health Center at Blake Wilbur Building, Stanford Health Care
Palo Alto, CA
650-736-5555
www.stanfordhealthcare.org/medical-clinics/
celiac-disease-program.html

Celiac Disease Clinic at Rady Children's Hospital
San Diego, CA
858-966-4003
www.rchsd.org/programs-services/
gastroenterology-hepatology-nutrition/services/
celiac-disease-clinic/

Celiac Disease Clinic, University of California San Diego
San Diego, CA
619-543-2347
https://health.ucsd.edu/specialties/gastro/areas-
expertise/Pages/celiac-disease-clinic.aspx

Celiac Disease Program, Division of Digestive Diseases, University of California Los Angeles
Los Angeles, CA
310-206-6279
www.gastro.ucla.edu/site.cfm?id=20

Celiac Disease Program, Lucile Packard Children's Hospital, Stanford Children's Health
Palo Alto, CA
650-723-5070
www.stanfordchildrens.org/en/service/celiac-
disease

Colorado Center for Celiac Disease, Children's Hospital Colorado
Aurora, CO
720-777-3825 / 720-777-6669
www.childrenscolorado.org/doctors-and-
departments/departments/digestive/programs/
colorado-center-for-celiac-disease/

Certification of Gluten-Free Products

Gluten-Free Certification Organization (GFCO)
Gluten Intolerance Group
253-218-2956
www.gfco.org

Gluten-Free Certification Program (GFCP)
Canadian Celiac Association
866-817-0952
www.glutenfreecert.com

Gluten-Free Certification Program (GFCP)
Beyond Celiac Disease (formerly the National Foundation for Celiac Awareness
844-856-6692 / 215-325-1306
www.beyondceliac.org/gluten-free-certification/

CSA Recognition Seal Program
Celiac Support Association
877-272-4272
www.csaceliacs.info/csa_recognition_seal.jsp

Websites: Celiac Disease and the Gluten-Free Diet

Academy of Nutrition and Dietetics Celiac Disease Evidence Analysis Project
www.andeal.org/topic.cfm?menu=5279

Beyond Celiac Webinars
www.beyondceliac.org/webinars/archive/

Celiac Center at Beth Israel Deaconess Medical Center, Harvard Medical School
www.celiacnow.org

Celiac Disease Center at Columbia University
www.celiacdiseasecenter.columbia.edu/

Dietitians in Gluten Intolerance Diseases (DIGID), Medical Nutrition Practice Group DPG of the Academy of Nutrition and Dietetics
www.mnpgdpg.org/page/dietitians-in-gluten-intolerance-diseases

Dietitians of Canada Practice-Based Evidence in Nutrition (PEN): "Celiac Disease" section
www.pennutrition.com/toc_public.aspx

GI Kids
www.gikids.org/content/3/en/celiac-disease

Gluten Free Drugs
www.glutenfreedrugs.com

Gluten Free Watchdog
www.glutenfreewatchdog.org

Health Canada Celiac Disease Links
www.hc-sc.gc.ca/fn-an/securit/allerg/cel-coe/index-eng.php
www.hc-sc.gc.ca/fn-an/pubs/securit/gluten_conn-lien_gluten-eng.php
www.hc-sc.gc.ca/fn-an/consult/2014-cel-oats-contam-avoine-coel/document-consultation-eng.php

NASPGHAN Children's Digestive Health
www.naspghan.org/content/51/en/Celiac-Disease

National Institutes of Health Celiac Disease Research Studies
www.clinicaltrials.gov/ct2/results?cond="Celiac+Disease"

Shelley Case, RD (dietitian) Websites
www.shelleycase.com
www.glutenfreediet.ca

Tricia Thompson, RD (dietitian) Websites
www.glutenfreedietitian.com
www.glutenfreewatchdog.org

University of Chicago Celiac Disease Center
www.cureceliacdisease.org/

University of Chicago Celiac Disease Center Resources
www.cureceliacdisease.org/fact-sheets/
www.cureceliacdisease.org/preceptorship-program/

Books

Gluten Freedom: The Leading Expert Offers the Essential Guide to a Healthy, Gluten-Free Lifestyle
- Dr. Alessio Fasano, MD (Director of the Center for Celiac Research and Treatment, Boston, MA) and Susie Flaherty (Director of Communications, Center for Celiac Research, Boston, MA)
- Provides the latest scientific research about gluten-related disorders including symptoms, diagnosis, gluten-free diet, some recipes, prevention strategies and alternative treatments; also includes resources, references and dietary management for children, pregnancy, college students and seniors
- ISBN 978-1-118-42310-3 | Turner Publishing Company | www.turnerpublishing.com |

Mayo Clinic Going Gluten Free: Essential Guide to Managing Celiac Disease and Related Conditions
- Dr. Joseph A. Murray, MD (gastroenterologist at Mayo Clinic in Rochester, MN) with contributions from other health professionals
- In a consumer-friendly style, features detailed information about celiac disease, non-celiac gluten sensitivity and wheat allergy including symptoms, diagnosis, the gluten-free diet and emotional aspects
- ISBN 978-0-8487-4388-8 | Oxmoor House, Time Home Entertainment, Inc. | www.timeinc.com |

Celiac Disease: A Hidden Epidemic (Newly Revised and Updated Edition)
- Dr. Peter H. R. Green, MD (Director, Celiac Disease Center at Columbia University, New York, NY) and Rory Jones, MS (Science Writer and Adjunct Professor, Barnard College)
- Features information about celiac disease including symptoms, diagnostic tests, related conditions and complications, treatment, lifestyle issues and resources
- ISBN 978-0-06-07669-4-8 | William Morrow (an imprint of HarperCollins Publishers) | www.harpercollins.com |

Gluten Exposed: The Science Behind the Hype and How to Navigate to a Healthy, Symptom-Free Life
- Dr. Peter H. R. Green, MD (Director, Celiac Disease Center at Columbia University, New York, NY) and Rory Jones, MS (Science Writer and Adjunct Professor Barnard College)
- Includes an examination of the effect of gluten on the body and brain; the different food-gut-brain conditions; how to isolate, test for and treat symptoms; who should follow a gluten-free diet; and the long-term effects of a gluten-free diet
- ISBN 978-0-06-23942-8-6 | William Morrow (an imprint of HarperCollins Publishers) | www.harpercollins.com |

Celiac Disease for Dummies
- Dr. Ian Blumer, MD (internal medicine) and Dr. Sheila Crowe, MD (gastroenterologist)
- Offers very comprehensive and practical information about celiac disease including symptoms, diagnostic tests, associated conditions, complications, treatment, nutritional considerations, alternate and complementary therapies, follow-up, frequently asked questions and resources
- ISBN 978-0-470-16036-7 | Dummies | www.dummies.com |

Real Life with Celiac Disease: Troubleshooting and Thriving Gluten-Free

- Melinda Dennis, RD (dietitian and Nutrition Director, Celiac Center at Beth Israel Deaconess Medical Centre, Boston, MA), Dr. Daniel Leffler, MD (Director of Clinical Research, Celiac Center at Beth Israel Deaconess Medical Center in Boston) and more than 50 international celiac experts
- Includes 53 chapters addressing a wide variety of topics on celiac disease and gluten-related disorders, each chapter featuring a patient case study with a specific problem and/or questions followed by a discussion about treatment recommendations, lifestyle changes and outcomes
- ISBN 978-1-60356-008-5 | American Gastroenterology Association Press | www.reallifewithceliacdisease.com |

Academy of Nutrition and Dietetics *Celiac Disease Nutrition Guide – Third Edition*

- Tricia Thompson, RD (dietitian)
- Provides a short overview of celiac disease and non-celiac gluten sensitivity; also includes information about the gluten-free diet (foods and ingredients, label reading, eating out, nutrition tips, resources, two recipes, supplements and medications)
- ISBN 978-0-88091-483-3 | Academy of Nutrition and Dietetics | www.eatright.org |

Complete Gluten-Free Diet and Nutrition Guide: With a 30-Day Meal Plan and Over 100 Recipes

- Alexandra Anca, RD (dietitian) and Theresa Santandrea-Cull (culinary expert)
- Includes information about celiac disease including symptoms, diagnosis and management, as well as foods allowed and to avoid, shopping tips, substitutions, nutritional considerations, healthy meal plans and recipes
- ISBN 978-0-7788-0252-5 | Robert Rose | www.robertrose.ca |

The Complete Guide to Living Well Gluten-Free: Everything You Need to Know to Go from Surviving to Thriving

- Beth Hillson (founder of the Gluten-Free Pantry and food editor of *Gluten-Free and More* magazine)
- Features detailed information about celiac disease, non-celiac gluten sensitivity and the gluten-free diet, along with personal stories and a dose of humor
- ISBN 978-0-7382-1708-6 | Da Capo Press | www.dacapopress.com |

Celiac Disease: A Guide to Living with Gluten Intolerance (Second Edition)

- Sylvia Llewelyn Bower, RN (nurse), Mary Kay Sharrett, RD (dietitian) and Dr. Steve Plogsted, PharmD (pharmacist)
- Includes information on symptoms, diagnosis, dermatitis herpetiformis, complications, healthy gluten-free diet guidelines, GF baking, recipes, medications, resources and the emotional aspects of celiac disease
- ISBN 978-1-936303-63-2 | Demos Health | www.demosmedpub.com |

Canadian Celiac Association's *Acceptability of Foods and Food Ingredients for the Gluten-Free Diet* pocket dictionary

- Written by dietitians with expertise in celiac disease who did extensive research into ingredient manufacturing practices and food-labeling regulations in the U.S., Canada and Europe
- Features pocket-size dictionary of more than 300 foods and food ingredients and over 300 food additives listed in alphabetical order for easy reference, easy-to-understand description of each item and food ingredients classified by category (Allowed, Not Allowed or To Check)
- Print version ISBN 0-921026-21-8
- Canadian Celiac Association, 5025 Orbitor Drive, Bldg. 1, Suite 400, Mississauga, ON, Canada L4W 4Y5 | 800-363-7296 / 905-507-6208 | www.celiac.ca |

Growing Up Gluten Free: A Lifestyle Guide for Raising Your Gluten-Free Child
- Amy Macklin, RD (dietitian)
- Written from the perspective of a dietitian whose son was diagnosed with celiac disease
- Includes information about the emotional aspects of celiac disease and its impact on the family, as well as practical information about the gluten-free diet, labeling, eating out, birthday parties, sleepovers, traveling, school issues and helpful resources
- ISBN 978-1-51713-880-6 | CreateSpace | www.glutenfreeroots.com |

Academy of Nutrition and Dietetics *Pocket Guide to Gluten-Free Strategies for Clients with Multiple Diet Restrictions – Second Edition*
- Tricia Thompson, RD (dietitian)
- Offers evidence-based information for dietitians who counsel clients on a gluten-free diet with other pre-existing conditions (food allergies, diabetes, lipid disorders, lactose intolerance, weight issues and vegetarianism); includes potential nutrient deficiencies and provides food lists, menus, resources and references
- ISBN 978-0-88091-020-0 (print)   ISBN 978-0-88091-021-7 (e-book) | Academy of Nutrition and Dietetics | www.eatrightstore.org/products/books-publications |

Academy of Nutrition and Dietetics *Celiac Disease Toolkit*
- Celiac expert dietitians Melinda Dennis, RD; Cynthia Kupper, RD; Anne Roland Lee, RD; Mary K. Sharrett, RD and Tricia Thompson, RD
- Designed for dietitians for application of the Academy's Celiac Disease Evidence-Based Nutrition Practice Guidelines
- Includes pediatric and adult case studies, sample documentation and outcome monitoring forms and a variety of client education materials (e.g., dining out, adding oats, cross-contamination and more)
- Download and print the materials at www.eatrightstore.org/products/practitioner-tools/toolkits

Magazines

Allergic Living
- Quarterly publication for those with food allergies, celiac disease, gluten sensitivity and environmental allergies; includes insightful articles on the social and psychological impacts of diet restrictions as well as latest research and advocacy news, recipes, advice from specialists and product reviews
- Website includes a wide variety of information and a special section on celiac disease, the gluten-free diet and gluten-free recipes
- Subscriptions: U.S. $19.99 (U.S. funds, 1 year, 4 issues); $29.99 (2 years, 8 issues)
  Canada $17.69 plus tax (CA funds, 1 year, 4 issues); $26.54 plus tax (2 years, 8 issues)
- Allergic Living U.S., P.O. Box 1042, Niagara Falls, NY, U.S. 14304
- Allergic Living Canada, 2100 Bloor St. W, Suite 6-168, Toronto, ON, Canada M6S 5A5
- (Access for both) 888-771-7747 / 416-604-0110 | www.allergicliving.com |

Gluten-Free Living
- Bimonthly national publication devoted to the gluten-free lifestyle; includes articles on celiac disease, gluten intolerance, gluten-free diet and ingredient concerns, lifestyle and savings tips, recipes, other allergies combined with a gluten-free diet, chef's menus, interviews, profiles, new products and medical and research information; reviewed by a medical and dietetic advisory board
- Subscriptions: U.S. $34 (1 year, 6 issues); $61 (2 years, 12 issues)
  Canada $40 (U.S. funds, 1 year, 6 issues); $66 (2 years, 12 issues)
  International $45 (U.S. funds, 1 year, 6 issues); $76 (2 years, 12 issues)
- Gluten-Free Living, Madavor Media, LLC., 25 Braintree Hill Office Park, Suite 404, Braintree, MA, U.S. 02184
- 855-367-4813 / 903-636-4308 ⏐ www.glutenfreeliving.com ⏐

Delight Gluten-Free
- Bimonthly international food and lifestyle publication for people living with gluten sensitivities and food allergies; contains in-depth articles, glossy photographs and gourmet recipes; reviewed by a medical advisory board
- Subscriptions: U.S. $24 (1 year, 6 issues); $40 (2 years, 12 issues)
  Canada $35 (U.S. funds, 1 year, 6 issues); $51 (U.S. funds, 2 years, 12 issues)
  International $53 (U.S. funds, 1 year, 6 issues)
- Delight Gluten-Free, 3140 Neil Armstrong Blvd., Suite 307, Eagen, MN, U.S. 55121
- 800-305-6964 ⏐ www.delightglutenfree.com ⏐

Gluten Free & More
- Bimonthly national magazine featuring inspirational and educational articles about food allergies and intolerances, as well as celiac disease; all recipes gluten-free; ingredient substitutions provided for common food allergies; published by Belvoir Media Group and reviewed by an advisory board (MDs, dietitians and directors of American Celiac organizations)
- Subscriptions: U.S. $23 (1 year, 6 issues); $42 (2 years, 12 issues); $19 (digital, 1 year, 6 issues)
  Canada $33 (CA funds, 1 year, 6 issues); $19 (CA funds, digital, 1 year, 6 issues)
- Gluten Free & More, Belvoir Media Group, P.O. Box 8535, Big Sandy, TX, U.S. 75755
- 800-474-8614 ⏐ www.glutenfreeandmore.com ⏐

Cookbooks

Carol Fenster

100 Best Gluten-Free Recipes
ISBN 978-0-470-47583-6 ⏐ Houghton Mifflin Harcourt ⏐

1,000 Gluten-Free Recipes
ISBN 978-0-470-06780-2 ⏐ Houghton Mifflin Harcourt ⏐

100 Best Quick Gluten-Free Recipes
ISBN 978-0-544-26371-0 ⏐ Houghton Mifflin Harcourt ⏐

125 Gluten-Free Vegetarian Recipes
ISBN 978-1-58333-425-6 ⏐ Avery/Penguin Group ⏐

Gluten-Free Quick & Easy
ISBN 978-1-58333-278-8 ⏐ Avery/Penguin Group ⏐

Gluten-Free 101: The Essential Beginner's Guide to Easy Gluten-Free Cooking
ISBN 978-1-118-53912-5 | Houghton Mifflin Harcourt |

Cooking Free: 220 Flavorful Recipes for People with Food Allergies and Multiple Food Sensitivities
ISBN 978-1-58333-215-3 | Avery/Penguin Group |

Wheat-Free Recipes & Menus: Delicious, Healthful Eating for People with Food Sensitivities
ISBN 978-1-58333-191-3 | Avery/Penguin Group |

Author Contact: Carol Fenster, PhD
President/Founder, Savory Palate, LLC.
5397 E Mineral Circle, Centennial, CO, U.S. 80122
303-741-5408 | www.carolfenstercooks.com |

Heather Butt and Donna Washburn

Easy Everyday Gluten-Free Cooking
ISBN 978-0-7788-0462-8 | Robert Rose |

Great Gluten-Free Whole-Grain Bread Machine Recipes
ISBN 978-0-7788-0463-5 | Robert Rose |

125 Best Gluten-Free Bread Machine Recipes
ISBN 978-0-7788-0238-9 | Robert Rose |

The Gluten-Free Baking Book
ISBN 978-0-77880-274-7 | Robert Rose |

Complete Gluten-Free Cookbook: 150 Gluten-Free, Lactose-Free Recipes, Many with Egg-Free Variations
ISBN 978-0-7788-0158-0 | Robert Rose |

250 Gluten-Free Favorites
ISBN 978-0-7788-0225-9 | Robert Rose |

Authors Contact: Heather Butt, PHEc. and Donna Washburn, PHEc.
Quality Professional Services
1655 County Rd. 2, Mallorytown, ON, Canada K0E 1R0
www.bestbreadrecipes.com | bread@bestbreadrecipes.com |

Bette Hagman

The Gluten-Free Gourmet Bakes Bread: More Than 200 Wheat-Free Recipes
ISBN 978-0805060782 | Henry Holt and Company, Macmillan |

The Gluten-Free Gourmet Cooks Fast and Healthy: Wheat-Free and Gluten-Free with Less Fuss and Less Fat
ISBN 978-0805065251 | Henry Holt and Company, Macmillan |

The Gluten-Free Gourmet Cooks Comfort Foods: Creating Old Favorites with the New Flours
ISBN 978-0805078084 | Henry Holt and Company, Macmillan |

More from the Gluten-Free Gourmet: Delicious Dining without Wheat
ISBN 978-0805065244 | Henry Holt and Company, Macmillan |

The Gluten-Free Gourmet: Living Well without Wheat (Revised Edition)
ISBN 978-0805064841 | Henry Holt and Company, Macmillan |

The Gluten-Free Gourmet Makes Dessert: More Than 200 Wheat-Free Recipes for Cakes, Cookies, Pies and Other Sweets
ISBN 978-0805072761 | Henry Holt and Company, Macmillan |

Beth Hillson
Gluten-Free Makeovers
ISBN 978-0738214610 | Da Capo Press |

Robert Landolphi
Gluten-Free Every Day Cookbook: More Than 100 Recipes from the Gluten-Free Chef
ISBN 978-0-7407-7813-1 | Andrews McMeel Publishing |

Cooking Light Gluten-Free Baking: Delectable From-Scratch Sweet and Savory Treats
ISBN 978-084874-2409 | Oxmoor House |

Judith Finlayson
The Complete Gluten-Free Whole Grains Cookbook: 125 Delicious Recipes from Amaranth to Quinoa to Wild Rice
ISBN 978-07788-04383 | Robert Rose |

Patricia Green and Carolyn Hemming
Grain Power: Over 100 Delicious Gluten-Free Ancient Grains & Superblend Recipes
ISBN 978-0-14-3186908 | Penguin Group |

Marlissa Brown
The Gluten-Free, Hassle-Free Cookbook
ISBN 978-1936303793 | Demos Health |

Nancy Hughes and Lara Rondinelli-Hamilton
Gluten-Free Recipes for People with Diabetes
ISBN 978-158040-4952 | American Diabetes Association |

Sheri Sanderson
Incredible Edible Gluten-Free Foods for Kids
ISBN 978-1-890627-28-7 | Woodbine House |

Online Cooking Resources

Pulse Canada, Shelley Case and Carol Fenster
Pulses and the Gluten-Free Diet
- www.pulsecanada.com/pulses-and-the-gluten-free-diet

Karen Robertson
Cooking Gluten Free! A Food Lover's Collection of Chef and Family Recipes without Gluten or Wheat – 4th Edition
- 174 recipes can be downloaded (desktop, tablet, mobile phone); shared with two other people
- Available from www.cookingglutenfree.com

Prep Dish
- Online gluten-free and paleo menu planning service by chef/dietitian Allison Stevens; includes weekly menu, grocery list and instructions for prepping meals
- Slogan: "Shop once, prep once, enjoy healthy, stress-free meals all week!"
- Cost: $14/month or $99/year or premium plan $149/year
- Site also includes free recipes, videos and blog
- www.prepdish.com | 512-431-8989 |

Gluten-Free Product Information

Gluten Free Watchdog, LLC.
- Company founded and managed by dietitian Tricia Thompson, RD
- Conducts gluten testing of products labeled gluten-free, as well as products not labeled gluten-free but appearing to be free of gluten-containing ingredients
- General product information and test results are reported on the website
- Subscribers have full access to the database of product reports and testing information, including the ppm level of gluten in each product
- Subscription costs: Watchdog Level $4.99/month (includes new reports and three-month history); Premium Level Full Access $29.99 for the first month, then $4.99/month
- www.glutenfreewatchdog.org

Eating Out and Travel Resources

Gluten-Free Passport Resources
- Offers an extensive variety of resources (books, dining translation cards, e-books, Apple apps), services and blog articles by Kim Koeller that focus on gluten- and allergy-free dining and travel
- www.glutenfreepassport.com | www.glutenfreeblog.com
- GlutenFree Passport, 80 Burr Ridge Parkway, Suite 141, Burr Ridge, IL, U.S. 60527
- 708-792-3702

Let's Eat Out Around the World Gluten Free and Allergy Free – Fourth Edition
- Features travel checklists, sample menus, ingredients and menu item descriptions with precise questions to ask about gluten, wheat, dairy, eggs, fish, shellfish, peanuts, tree nuts, soy and corn; includes information about French, Indian, Italian, Mexican, Chinese and Thai cuisines, plus steak and seafood restaurants
- ISBN 978-1-9363036-0-1
- Also available as an e-book: eISBN 978-1-617052-04-0

Multi-Lingual Phrase Passport for Gluten & Allergy Free Travel: part of the ***Let's Eat Out!*** series
- Pocket-size guide provides over 1500 phrase translations from English to French, German, Italian and Spanish; details gluten and other food concerns with all phrases translated by professional language services and quality tested by native speakers
- ISBN 978-0-9764845-4-7
- Also available as an e-book: eISBN 978-0-615-34449-2

Language Phrase Guides for Gluten-Free and Food Allergy Travel: part of the ***Let's Eat Out!*** series
- Downloadable gluten-free and food allergy guide with over 300 phrases in various languages: French/English, German/English, Italian/English and Spanish/English

Gluten-Free Dining Translation Cards
- Downloadable gluten-free restaurant and travel cards in various languages: English, Arabic/English, Czech/English, Dutch/English, French/English, German/English, Greek/English, Hebrew/English, Italian/English, Latvian/English, Norwegian/English, Portuguese/English, Russian/English, Spanish/English, Swedish/English

Country-Specific Travel Paks
- Downloadable PDFs of the Gluten-Free Dining Translation Cards, specific language phrase guide and ethnic restaurant cuisine dishes / cooking preparation advice for Argentina, Australia, Austria, Belgium, Brazil, Canada, Caribbean, Central America, Cuba, Europe (six-country pack), France, Germany, Greece, Ireland, Israel, Italy, Latvia, Mexico, Middle East, Netherlands, New Zealand, Peru, Portugal, Russia, South America, Spain, Switzerland, U.K. and U.S.

Gluten-Free Ethnic Restaurant Paperback Passports: part of the ***Let's Eat Out!*** series
- Restaurant cuisine menu choices from the *Let's Eat Out!* book packaged into three pocket-sized guides for easy reference: American Steak & Mexican; Chinese, Indian and Thai; French and Italian
- ISBN 0-9764845-1-X; 0-9764845-3-6; 0-9764845-2-8

Gluten-Free Dining e-books by Ethnic Restaurant Cuisines: part of the ***Let's Eat Out!*** series
- Sample restaurant menu items, descriptions and questions to ask restaurant staff from the *Let's Eat Out!* series packaged into individual e-books for easy reference: Steak & Seafood, French, Indian, Italian, Mexican and Thai
- eISBN: 978-0-9829599-4-7; 978-0-9829599-5-4; 978-0-9829599-7-8; 978-0-9829599-3-0; 978-0-9830577-0-3; 978-0-9829599-6-1

Gluten- and Wheat-Free Toolbox for Local Dining and Global Travel e-book
- Based on the *Let's Eat Out!* book, this gluten- and wheat-free e-book features a gluten-free travel checklist, cuisine-specific meal choices in ethnic restaurants around the world and discussion about possible hidden presence of gluten and wheat in various dishes
- eISBN 978-0-9830577-3-4

EatOut Gluten & Allergy Free Apple App
- Identifies hundreds of menu items (description, ingredients, preparation, specific considerations) from seven ethnic cuisines; customizes menu options based on any combination of ten common food allergens; includes over 300 pages from the book *Let's Eat Out!*
- Works 100% off-line without any connectivity or roaming charges

iCanEat Fast Food Gluten & Allergy Free Apple App
- Includes menus from 40 U.S. fast food chains
- Allows an individual to enter their allergen and/or gluten-free requirements; suitable menu choices will be displayed
- Works 100% off-line without any roaming charges

Bob & Ruth's Gluten-Free Dining & Travel Club
- Company specializing in gluten-free travel including escorted "Gluten-Free Getaways," destination resorts, cruises and tours of exotic places all over the world
- www.bobandruths.com
- Bob & Ruth's, 205 Donerail Crt., Havre de Grace, MD, U.S. 21078
- 410-939-3218

The Celiac Scene
- Comprehensive listing of celiac-endorsed restaurants in Victoria, Vancouver Island and the Gulf Islands in British Columbia, Canada; interactive free maps can be searched by city and district; recommendations are reviewed and restaurants must meet specific standards in order to be listed
- Owned, operated and maintained by individuals with celiac disease
- Site also features over 260 fast-food chains across North America that make an online commitment to serving the gluten-free consumer, with links to nutrition and allergen statements, gluten-free options and menus
- www.theceliacscene.com

Gluten-Free Food Service Training and Accreditation Programs

Gluten-Free Food Program (GFFP)
- Program designed for food service and hospitality sector including restaurants, caterers, camps, hotels, convention centers and health care and educational institutions
- Developed in partnership with and endorsed by the Canadian Celiac Association and Fondation Québécoise de la Maladie Coeliaque
- The GFFP program includes:
  - *GF-Smart*: Course for food handlers and managers to help understand what is involved in offering gluten-free food, why avoiding gluten contamination is essential and how to plan and operate a gluten-management system once it is in place. Available online or in a classroom setting for larger groups customized by sector and customer.
  - *GF-Verified* program: Membership-based marketing program for food service and hospitality establishments that participate in the inspection program. Facilities must implement the necessary training, standards and menu reviews, in addition to undergoing an annual third-party inspection. Inspection verifies facility's conformance to the requirements of the GF-Verified program.
- GF-Finder tool on GFFP website allows consumers to search for GF-Verified establishments in their area
- For more information see www.gf-verified.com and www.gf-smart.com

Gluten-Free Food Service (GFFS) Training and Accreditation Program

- Program of the Gluten Intolerance Group of North America (GIG) designed for a wide range of food service establishments (e.g., restaurants, health care facilities, schools, colleges, camps, bakeries)
- GFFS experts review the food service establishment's menu, as well as policies, procedures and practices; facility documentation is compared to GFFS Core Standards of Practices for Gluten-Free Food Production and Service
- Facility receives the GFFS Certification Program Manual that includes core standards of safe gluten-free food preparation from procurement of ingredients/foods to storage, production and delivery of gluten-free foods, as well as staff training materials
- Third-party GFFS auditors conduct on-site facility inspection
- Successful audit and completion of the GFFS training and management certification allows the GFFS logo to be displayed in the facility, on menus or other appropriate locations, for a one-year certification indicating the establishment has met the strict gluten-free standards, and facility subsequently is inspected annually
- Certified facilities will be listed on GFFS and GIG websites. Consumers can search restaurants by location in the certified directory on these websites
- On-site customized training also available
- For more information see www.gffoodservice.org

Gluten-Free Resource Education Awareness Training (GREAT) Kitchens

- Gluten-free training courses (online modules, on-site training) from Beyond Celiac (formerly the National Foundation for Celiac Awareness [NFCA]) designed for the food service sector
- Includes various online modules:
  - GREAT Kitchens Standard: for food service staff
  - GREAT Kitchens Management: for owners, general managers, chefs and key staff members; also comprehensive manual with review of content and other resources
  - GREAT Schools Standard: for food service staff
  - GREAT Schools, Colleges and Camps: for food service directors, dining managers, chefs, dietitians and camp directors
  - Individual Kitchen Modules: The Gluten-Free Guest, Gluten-Free Ingredients, Back-of House, Front-of House, Implementation
  - Individual School Modules: The Gluten-Free Student, Gluten-Free Ingredients, Back-of-House, Serving the Gluten-Free Student, Gluten-Free Action Plan
  - Supplemental materials: Spanish manual and exam
- On-site GREAT training customized for the facility by expert Beyond Celiac facilitator
- Successful completion of the GREAT Kitchens/Schools modules, implementation of the course standards and approval of application for GREAT accreditation allows use of the GREAT Kitchens/ Schools logo to be displayed in a facility and on its menus and website for two years; facility will be listed on the Beyond Celiac website and GREAT Kitchens newsletter, as well as on the Find Me Gluten-Free app
- For more information see www.greatgfkitchens.org

Children's Books

Adam's Gluten-Free Surprise: Helping Others Understand Gluten Free
- Debbie Simpson
- 34-page illustrated book for children, parents, grandparents, babysitters, teachers and others. A story about a boy named Adam with newly diagnosed celiac disease, whose teacher and classmates learn about gluten free and surprise him by making the Valentine's Day party completely gluten free.
- ISBN 978-1478396543 | CreateSpace |

Eating Gluten-Free with Emily: A Story for Children with Celiac Disease
- Bonnie Kruszka
- Illustrated book for children ages three to seven. A story about a five-year-old girl who develops celiac disease and how she makes positive lifestyle changes to manage her disease. The author and her daughter have celiac disease.
- ISBN 978-1-4392-1226-4 | CreateSpace |

Hailey's Gluten-Free Surprise: Helping Others Understand Gluten Free
- Debbie Simpson
- 34-page illustrated book for children, families, babysitters, teachers and others. A story about a girl named Hailey with newly diagnosed celiac disease whose teacher and classmates learn about gluten free and surprise her by making the Valentine's Day party completely gluten free.
- ISBN 978-1491044773 | CreateSpace |

Mommy, What Is Celiac Disease?: A Look at the Sunny Side of Being a Gluten-Free Kid
- Katie Chalmers
- 32-page illustrated book for young children, families, teachers and caregivers. The story is a conversation between a mother and daughter about celiac disease and the gluten-free diet, presented in a positive and empowering manner. The author (a graphic designer) and her daughter both have celiac disease, which brings a unique perspective to this story.
- ISBN 978-0982871102 | Awareness Press, LLC. |

Other Children's Resources

Celiac Disease Foundation – Gluten-Free Kids Resources
www.celiac.org/live-gluten-free/resources/for-parents-and-children/

Gluten Intolerance Group – Generation GF
www.gluten.org/community/kids/

Beyond Celiac Disease – Kids Central
www.beyondceliac.org/living-with-celiac-disease/kids/

College/University Resources

Beyond Celiac – Going to College Gluten-Free
www.beyondceliac.org/living-with-celiac-disease/college/toolkit/

Gluten-Free Guide to College: A Student's Guide to Navigating the Gluten-Free Diet in College by Rebecca Panzer, RD
www.tinyurl.com/GFGuide2College

Medication Resource

Gluten Free Drugs
- Online resource containing information about over-the-counter and prescription medications listed by therapeutic category or alphabetical product name
- Site developed and managed by pharmacist Dr. Steve Plogsted, PharmD, Nutrition Support Services, Children's Hospital, Columbus, OH
- www.glutenfreedrugs.com

Appendices

Appendix A

Companies with Gluten-Free Oat Products

A growing number of companies sell gluten-free oats (whole groats, steel-cut, rolled, flour and bran) and/or a wide array of gluten-free products with oat-based ingredients. Many gluten-free cereals, granola, cookies and snack bars contain these specialty oats and they also are found in breads, muffins, baking mixes, entrées, side dishes, veggie burgers, crackers and other foods. Gluten-free products featured in chapter 15 on pages 205–262 will have an asterisk symbol (*) if they contain oats.

The following companies use oats in some or all of their gluten-free products. Please note this is not an all-inclusive list and manufacturers may change product formulations at any time.

Aleias	Garden Lites	Pamela's
Amy's	The GFB: Gluten Free Bar	PureFit
Ancient Harvest	GF Harvest	Pure Genius Provisions
Annie's Homegrown	gfJules	Purely Elizabeth
Avena Foods – Only Oats	Glutenfree Bakehouse	Quaker
	Glutenfreeda Foods	
Bakery on Main	Gluten-Free Prairie	Rudi's Gluten-Free Bakery
Barbara's	GoMacro	
Blue Diamond	GoPicnic	Schär
Bobo's Oat Bars	Grainful	
Bob's Red Mill		Taste of Nature
	Hodgson Mill	
Canyon Oats	Homefree	Udi's Gluten Free
Cloud 9 Specialty Bakery		
Cream Hill Estates – Lara's	Kellogg Company	Van's
Crunchmaster	KIND	Viki's
Cybele's	King Arthur Flour	
		Whole Note Food Company
Dr. Praeger's Sensible Foods	Libre Naturals	WOW Baking Company
	Lucy's	
EnviroKidz		XO Baking Co.
Erewhon	Modern Table	
		Zing
Flax4Life	Nature's Path	
Freedom Foods	Neat Foods	
	Nourish Snacks	

Product and manufacturer information, exhaustively researched between January and July 2016, was from sources believed to be reliable at the time of printing. **The author assumes no liability for any errors, omissions or inaccuracies.**

Appendix B

Canadian Celiac Association Professional Advisory Council Position Statement on Consumption of Oats by Individuals with Celiac Disease

The safety of oats in individuals with celiac disease has been extensively investigated. Health Canada has reviewed the clinical evidence from numerous international studies and has concluded that the consumption of oats, uncontaminated with gluten from wheat, rye or barley, is safe for the vast majority of patients with celiac disease. A 2015 review entitled *Celiac Disease and Gluten-Free Claims on Uncontaminated Oats* is available on Health Canada's web page **Celiac Disease and Gluten-Free Claims on Uncontaminated Oats (www.hc-sc.gc.ca/fn-an/consult/2014-cel-oats-contam-avoine-coel/document-consultation-eng.php)**.

Most commercially available oats in North America are contaminated with gluten-containing grains (wheat, rye, barley). This has been confirmed in various studies including one by **Health Canada scientists (www.ncbi.nlm.nih.gov/pmc/articles/PMC3118497/)**.

We are fortunate in Canada and the USA that specially-produced pure, uncontaminated oats have been available in the marketplace for many years. These oats are grown on dedicated fields and are harvested, stored, transported and processed in dedicated gluten-free facilities. In addition, they are accurately tested for their gluten content to be under 20 ppm. This entire process is often referred to as a purity protocol.

Health Canada's Food and Drug Regulations include oats, along with wheat, rye and barley, in the list of gluten-containing grains, so even pure, uncontaminated oats were prohibited from making a gluten-free claim. However, on May 29, 2015, the Minister of Health issued a Marketing Authorization that permits the use of gluten-free claims for specially produced oats and foods containing these oats as ingredients. The **Marketing Authorization (www.hc-sc.gc.ca/fn-an/securit/allerg/cel-coe/avoine-gluten-oats-eng.php)** provision allows for an exemption from the Food and Drug Regulations provided these oats do not contain more than 20 parts per million (ppm) of gluten from wheat, rye, barley or their hybridized strains.

Health Canada does not specify the methods or controls oat producers should use in order to meet the Marketing Authorization requirements. Many producers of gluten-free oats use the purity protocol which has been proven to be effective. Some producers may use other methods such as mechanical and/or optical sorting to remove gluten-containing grains from oats rather than a purity protocol. The Professional Advisory Council is not aware of any published North American data that demonstrates the levels of gluten in oats that have been cleaned using mechanical and/or optical sorting.

The Marketing Authorization and other important information about oats can be found on Health Canada's web page **Gluten-Free Labelling Claims for Specially Produced Oats (www.hc-sc.gc.ca/fn-an/securit/allerg/cel-coe/avoine-gluten-oats-eng.php)**.

The Canadian Celiac Association supports Health Canada's decision to allow gluten-free claims for specially produced gluten-free oats and products containing such oats. Also, the Professional Advisory Council recommends the following guidelines for individuals with celiac disease and other gluten-related disorders who wish to add pure, uncontaminated oats or oat products in their diet:

1. The individual should be stabilized on the gluten-free diet and their celiac antibody levels should have normalized. This process may take 6–18 months, although there is considerable variation among individuals.

2. The fibre content of an oat-containing diet is often higher than the typical gluten-free diet. When adding oats to the diet, individuals may experience a change in stool pattern or mild gastrointestinal symptoms, including abdominal bloating and gas. These symptoms should resolve within a few days. Therefore, it is advised to start with a small amount of oats per day [adults 25–70 grams ($1/4$–$3/4$ cup dry rolled oats) and children 10–25 grams ($1/8$–$1/4$ cup)] and gradually increase as tolerated.

3. There are case reports of individuals with celiac disease relapsing from the consumption of pure, uncontaminated oats. Individuals should be aware of this possibility. If symptoms occur and/or persist, they should discontinue consuming oats.

4. If a reaction to oats has occurred, it is worthwhile to do a re-challenge if the individual wants to try oats again. Development of symptoms at the time of the second challenge would strongly suggest intolerance to oats. Research suggests that intolerance to oats occurs but is quite rare. The mechanism for this intolerance is unknown at this time.

5. A consultation with a dietitian who can carefully review the diet to ensure that the individual is not consuming foods that contain gluten is highly recommended.

6. If a reaction occurs with a re-challenge of gluten-free oats, notify your physician, as well as the Canadian Food Inspection Agency (CFIA) about the reaction. The CFIA requires contact information of the individual, brand name, package size, UPC code, best-before date, name and address of store where product was purchased, date of purchase and concern. See www.inspection.gc.ca or call 800-442-2342. The Canadian Celiac Association would also appreciate notification about the product details at askthecca@celiac.ca

7. The safety of oats in non-celiac gluten sensitivity has not been studied. The Canadian Celiac Association will continue to monitor the scientific developments in the area of oats in celiac disease and other gluten-related disorders and will keep its members updated.

Professional Advisory Council
Canadian Celiac Association
May 29, 2015

Appendix C

American and Canadian Regulations and Guidance Documents

Code of Federal Regulations (CFR)

www.ecfr.gov/

Code of Federal Regulations (CFR) Title 21 Food and Drugs

www.ecfr.gov/ (scroll down to Title 21)

Food and Drug Administration's Compliance Policy Guides (CPG): Chapter 5 – Food, Colors, and Cosmetics

www.fda.gov/ICECI/ComplianceManuals/CompliancePolicyGuidanceManual/ucm119194.htm

---

Code of Federal Regulations (CFR) Title 9 Animals and Animal Products

www.ecfr.gov/ (scroll down to Title 9)

United States Department of Agriculture (USDA) Food Safety Inspection Service (FSIS)

Labeling guidance documents and other policies can be found at various web links (see following pages and in the labeling reference section [see p. 333]. Also, the FSIS uses specific regulations from CFR Title 21.

Code of Federal Regulations Title 27 Alcohol, Tobacco Products and Firearms

www.ecfr.gov/ (scroll down to Title 27)
www.ttb.gov/other/regulations.shtml

Health Canada's Food and Drug Regulations (FDR)

www.laws-lois.justice.gc.ca/eng/regulations/c.r.c.,_c._870/index.html

Ingredients

The chart below lists the regulatory code number(s), compliance policy guidance documents (CPGs) and/or web links pertaining to specific ingredients from the FDA, USDA and Health Canada.

Ingredient Name	FDA (CFR)	FSIS of the USDA	Health Canada (FDR)
Autolyzed Yeast and Autolyzed Yeast Extract / Yeast Extract	21 CFR 184.1983 (Baker's Yeast Extract) 21 CFR 102.22	www.fsis.usda.gov/wps/portal/fsis/topics/food-safety-education/get-answers/food-safety-fact-sheets/food-labeling/natural-flavorings-on-meat-and-poultry-labels	B.01.009 (2) #10 B.01.010.1 (1 and 2)
Malt	21 CFR Sec. 184.1443a CPG Sec. 515.200	21 CFR Sec. 184.1443a CPG Sec. 515.200	B.01.010.1 (1 and 2)
Malt Syrup / Malt Extract	21 CFR Sec. 184.1445 CPG Sec. 515.200	21 CFR Sec. 184.1445 CPG Sec. 515.200	B.01.010.1 (1 and 2)
Malt Flavoring	CPG Sec. 515.200	CPG Sec. 515.200	B.10.005 [S] B.01.010.1 (1 and 2)
Caramel	21 CFR Sec. 73.85	21 CFR Sec. 73.85	B.16.100 Table III #2 B.01.010.1 (1 and 2)
Hydrolyzed Plant/Vegetable Proteins	21 CFR Sec. 102.22 21 CFR Sec. 101.22 (h)(7)	www.fsis.usda.gov/wps/portal/fsis/topics/food-safety-education/get-answers/food-safety-fact-sheets/food-labeling/natural-flavorings-on-meat-and-poultry-labels	B.01.009 (1) #30 B.01.009 (3)(c) B.01.010 (3)(a) #8 B.01.010.1 (1 and 2)
Natural Flavor	21 CFR Sec. 101.22	www.fsis.usda.gov/wps/portal/fsis/topics/food-safety-education/get-answers/food-safety-fact-sheets/food-labeling/natural-flavorings-on-meat-and-poultry-labels	B.10.005 [S] B.01.009 (2) #2 B.01.010 (3)(b) #4 B.01.010.1 (1 and 2)
Spices, Herbs and Seasonings	21 CFR Sec. 182.10 21 CFR Sec. 101.22 (a)(2) 21 CFR Sec. 170.3 (n)(26) CPG Sec. 525.650 CPG Sec. 525.750	www.fsis.usda.gov/wps/portal/fsis/topics/food-safety-education/get-answers/food-safety-fact-sheets/food-labeling/natural-flavorings-on-meat-and-poultry-labels	B.01.009 (2) #4 B.01.009 (2) #5 B.01.010 (3)(b) #6 B.01.010.1 (1 and 2) B.07.001 [S] – B.07.039 [S]

Ingredients

Ingredient Name	FDA (CFR)	FSIS of the USDA	Health Canada (FDR)
Smoke Flavoring	21 CFR Sec. 101.22 (h)(6) CPG Sec. 525.650	www.fsis.usda.gov/OPPDE/larc/Policies/Labeling_Policy_Book_082005.pdf (page 174–175) 9 CFR Sec. 317.2(j)(3) 9 CFR Sec. 381.119(a)	B.10.005 [S] B.10.006 [S] B.16.100 Table XI Part 1 W.1 B.01.009 (2) #2 B.01.010.1 (1 and 2) www.inspection.gc.ca/food/labelling/food-labelling-for-industry/meat-and-poultry-products/eng/13939 7911498 3/13939791624757chap=3
Starch	CPG Sec. 578.100	www.fsis.usda.gov/OPPDE/larc/Policies/Labeling_Policy_Book_082005.pdf (page 179)	B.01.009 (1) #9 B.01.010 (3)(a) #20 B.13.011 [S] B.01.010.1 (1 and 2)
Modified Food Starch	21 CFR Sec. 172.892 CPG Sec. 578.100	21 CFR Sec. 172.892	B.01.009 (1) #9 B.01.010 (3)(a) #21 B.01.010.1 (1 and 2)
Dextrin	21 CFR Sec.184.1277	21 CFR Sec.184.1277	B.01.010.1 (1 and 2)
Maltodextrin	21 CFR Sec. 184.1444	21 CFR Sec. 184.1444	B.01.010.1 (1 and 2)
Glucose Syrup	21 CFR Sec. 184.1865 21 CFR Sec. 168.120	21 CFR Sec. 184.1865	B.18.016 [S] B.18.017 [S] B.01.010.1 (1 and 2)
Rice Syrup	21 CFR Sec. 168.120	21 CFR Sec. 168.120	B.18.018 [S] B.01.010.1 (1 and 2)
Vinegar	CPG Sec. 525.825	CPG Sec. 525.825 Distilled vinegar can be labeled as "vinegar"	B.01.009 (1) # 21 B.01.010 (3)(b) #23 B.19.001- B.19.009 B.01.010.1 (1 and 2)
Malt Vinegar	CPG Sec. 525.825	CPG Sec. 525.825	B.19.005 [S]

Alcoholic Beverages

Beverage	FDA	TTB	Health Canada
Beer	Regulated By TTB	27 CFR 7.22 27 CFR 7.22a 27 CFR 25.15	B.02.130 – B.02.135 www.hc-sc.gc.ca/fn-an/label-etiquet/allergen/project_1220_qa_qr-eng.php (Question 19)
Gluten-Free Beer	www.fda.gov/Food/GuidanceRegulation/GuidanceDocumentsRegulatoryInformation/LabelingNutrition/ucm166239.htm	Regulated by FDA	www.inspection.gc.ca/food/labelling/food-labelling-for-industry/allergens-and-gluten/eng/1388152325341/1388152326591?chap=2#s4c2
Distilled Alcohols and Liqueurs	Regulated By TTB	27 CFR 5.22 27 CFR 5.32 27 CFR 5.32a	B.01.009 (1) #21 B.02.001 – B.02.108 www.hc-sc.gc.ca/fn-an/label-etiquet/allergen/project_1220_qa_qr-eng.php (Question 20)
Wine	CPG 510.450	27 CFR 4 27 CFR 24	B.01.009 (1) #21 B.02.100 [S] – B.02.108 www.hc-sc.gc.ca/fn-an/label-etiquet/allergen/project_1220_qa_qr-eng.php (Questions 20, 22)

Appendix D

Codex Alimentarius Standard for Foods for Special Dietary Use for Persons Intolerant to Gluten

CODEX STAN 118-1979 Adopted in 1979.
Amendment: 1983 and 2015. Revision: 2008.

1.   SCOPE

1.1   This standard applies to foods for special dietary uses that have been formulated, processed or prepared to meet the special dietary needs of people intolerant to gluten.

1.2   Foods for general consumption which by their nature are suitable for use by people with gluten intolerance may indicate such suitability in accordance with the provisions of Section 4.3.

2.   DESCRIPTION

2.1   Definitions

The products covered by this standard are described as follows:

2.1.1   *Gluten-free foods*

Gluten-free foods are dietary foods

a)   consisting of or made only from one or more ingredients which do not contain wheat (i.e., all Triticum species, such as durum wheat, spelt, and khorasan wheat, which is also marketed under different trademarks such as KAMUT), rye, barley, oats[1] or their crossbred varieties, and the gluten level does not exceed 20 mg/kg in total, based on the food as sold or distributed to the consumer, and/or

b)   consisting of one or more ingredients from wheat (i.e., all Triticum species, such as durum wheat, spelt, and khorasan wheat, which is also marketed under different trademarks such as KAMUT), rye, barley, oats[1] or their crossbred varieties, which have been specially processed to remove gluten, and the gluten level does not exceed 20 mg/kg in total, based on the food as sold or distributed to the consumer.

2.1.2   *Foods specially processed to reduce gluten content to a level above 20 up to 100 mg/kg*

These foods consist of one or more ingredients from wheat (i.e., all Triticum species, such as durum wheat, spelt, and khorasan wheat, which is also marketed under different trademarks such as KAMUT), rye, barley, oats[1] or their crossbred varieties, which have been specially processed to reduce the gluten content to a level above 20 up to 100 mg/kg in total, based on the food as sold or distributed to the consumer.

Decisions on the marketing of products described in this section may be determined at the national level.

2.2   Subsidiary Definitions

2.2.1   *Gluten*

For the purpose of this standard, "gluten" is defined as a protein fraction from wheat, rye, barley, oats[1] or their crossbred varieties and derivatives thereof, to which some persons are intolerant and that is insoluble in water and 0.5M NaCl.

2.2.2   *Prolamins*

Prolamins are defined as the fraction from gluten that can be extracted by 40%–70% of ethanol. The prolamin from wheat is gliadin, from rye is secalin, from barley hordein and from oats[1] avenin.

It is, however, an established custom to speak of gluten sensitivity. The prolamin content of gluten is generally taken as 50%.

---

1   Oats can be tolerated by most but not all people who are intolerant to gluten. Therefore, the allowance of oats that are not contaminated with wheat, rye or barley in foods covered by this standard may be determined at the national level.

3. ESSENTIAL COMPOSITION AND QUALITY FACTORS

3.1 For products referred to in 2.1.1 a) and b), the gluten content shall not exceed 20 mg/kg in the food as sold or distributed to the consumer.

3.2 For products referred to in 2.1.2, the gluten content shall not exceed 100 mg/kg in the food as sold or distributed to the consumer.

3.3 Products covered by this standard substituting important basic foods, should supply approximately the same amount of vitamins and minerals as the original foods they replace.

3.4 The products covered by this standard shall be prepared with special care under Good Manufacturing Practice (GMP) to avoid contamination with gluten.

4. LABELLING

In addition to the general labelling provisions contained in the *General Standard for the Labelling of Prepackaged Foods* (CODEX STAN 1-1985) and the *General Standard for the Labelling of and Claims for Prepackaged Foods for Special Dietary Uses* (CODEX STAN 146-1985), and any specific labelling provisions set out in a Codex standard applying to the particular food concerned, the following provisions for the labelling of "gluten-free foods" shall apply:

4.1 The term "gluten-free" shall be printed in the immediate proximity of the name of the product in the case of products described in section 2.1.1.

4.2 The labelling of products described in section 2.1.2 should be determined at the national level. However, these products must not be called gluten free. The labelling terms for such products should indicate the true nature of the food, and shall be printed in the immediate proximity of the name of the product.

4.3 A food which, by its nature, is suitable for use as part of a gluten-free diet, shall not be designated "special dietary," "special dietetic" or any other equivalent term. However, such a food may bear a statement on the label that "this food is by its nature gluten-free" provided that it complies with the essential composition provisions for gluten-free as set out in section 3.1 and provided that such a statement does not mislead the consumer. More detailed rules in order to ensure that the consumer is not misled may be determined at the national level.

5. METHODS OF ANALYSIS AND SAMPLING
5.1 General outline of the methods

- The quantitative determination of gluten in foods and ingredients shall be based on an immunologic method or other method providing at least equal sensitivity and specificity.
- The antibody used should react with the cereal protein fractions that are toxic for persons intolerant to gluten and should not cross-react with other cereal proteins or other constituents of the foods or ingredients.
- Methods used for determination should be validated and calibrated against a certified reference material, if available.
- The detection limit has to be appropriate according to the state of the art and the technical standard. It should be 10 mg gluten/kg or below.
- The qualitative analysis that indicates the presence of gluten shall be based on relevant methods (e.g., ELISA-based methods, DNA methods).

5.2 Method for determination of gluten

Enzyme-linked Immunoassay (ELISA) R5 Mendez Method.

Appendix E

History of Gluten-Free Labeling Regulations:
United States, Canada and the Codex Alimentarius Commission

United States

A directive in the *Food Allergen and Consumer Protection Act of 2004 (FALCPA)* required the Secretary of Health and Human Services to issue a final rule to define the food-labeling term "gluten free" by 2008. The Secretary designated the Food and Drug Administration (FDA) to undertake this rule-making as the FDA is responsible for ensuring the safety of and establishing food labeling requirements for the vast majority of foods sold in the U.S. The following is a summary of the development of the final rule on "Gluten-free labeling of foods" that was issued on August 5, 2013, with a compliance date of August 5, 2014, by which FDA-regulated foods labeled "gluten free" were required to meet the agency's definition of gluten-free foods. FDA's definition of gluten-free foods is published in Title 21 of the *Code of Federal Regulations* (CFR), Part 101, Section 101.91 (21 CFR 101.91).

The FDA's Center for Food Safety and Applied Nutrition (CFSAN) consulted with appropriate experts and stakeholders to help develop its regulation to define and permit the voluntary use of the term "gluten free" on food labels. Two key meetings were held to examine this issue.

FDA's CFSAN Food Advisory Committee Meeting on Thresholds for Major Food Allergens and for Gluten in Food

The FDA/CFSAN Food Advisory Committee (FAC) met July 13–15, 2005, to discuss the agency's June 2005 draft report entitled "Approaches to Establish Thresholds for Major Food Allergens and for Gluten in Food." The July 14 session brought together scientific experts and stakeholders representing federal government agencies, trade associations and the food industry, as well as celiac consumers and their families. A panel of experts listened to presentations addressing the characteristics and treatment of celiac disease, quality of life issues faced by patients and their families, the relationship between gluten proteins in various grains and celiac disease, analytical methods for measuring gluten levels in food, the value and use of prospective and retrospective gluten tolerance studies, and examples of existing national and international definitions of "gluten-free" standards for food labeling.

Two presentations examined the broad question of safe gluten threshold levels: the first by Dr. Alessio Fasano, MD, Professor of Pediatrics, Medicine and Physiology and Director of the Mucosal Biology Research Center affiliated with the Center for Celiac Research at the University of Maryland; the second by Dr. Pekka Collin, MD, PhD, Assistant Professor of Medicine, Tampere University Hospital, Tampere, Finland.

Dr. Fasano highlighted preliminary results of the Italian gluten micro-challenge study (conducted by Dr. Carlo Catassi, MD, and colleagues) that examined the consequences of prolonged ingestion of minimal gluten intakes of either 10 or 50 mg/day for three months by adults with celiac disease (see p. 330 for the reference of the completed study published in 2007). The study revealed a trend toward an increase in inflammatory cells in the villi (intraepithelial lymphocytes) at 50 mg/day; thus researchers concluded that "ingestion of contaminating gluten should be kept lower than 50 mg/d in the treatment of CD." Based upon the results of this study and also taking into account that in Italy foods marketed as gluten free allow a gluten contamination level of up to 20 ppm (i.e., less than 20 ppm gluten), Dr. Fasano suggested that a threshold level of 20 ppm gluten for "special celiac foods" is safe for most people with celiac disease provided that they do not exceed a maximum gluten intake of 50 mg per day. In comparison, Dr. Collin presented retrospective data conducted by him and his colleagues, that a safe threshold level of 100 ppm gluten for wheat starch-based gluten-free food products is safe for most people with celiac disease, if the daily intake of such foods is less than 300 grams/day (equivalent to a maximum intake of 30 mg gluten/day – see the calculations in table E.1).

Using the values in the table published in the study by Collin et al., 2004, one can estimate that a 300 gram/day intake of wheat starch-based gluten-free foods that contained 20 ppm gluten (the gluten threshold level recommended by Catassi et al., 2007) would provide a total of daily intake of 6 mg gluten, which is well below the maximum of 50 mg/day gluten intake suggested by Catassi et al., 2007.

Based on these two presentations, it appears that there is a range of gluten tolerance levels in people with celiac disease. Further research is necessary to determine safe gluten threshold levels for gluten-free specialty products and the amounts of these foods that can safely be consumed by the celiac population at large (see pp. 43–48).

The entire agenda, speaker presentations, slides and meeting summary for the July 2005 FAC meeting can be accessed at a link on FDA's website (see p. 333).

Table E.1   Daily gluten intake based on varying concentrations of gluten (in ppm) in different quantities (in grams) of gluten-free products*

Gluten content in products (in ppm)	Amount of gluten-free foods (in grams) per day			
	50 grams	100 grams	200 grams	300 grams
20 ppm	1 mg	2 mg	4 mg	6 mg
50 ppm	2.5 mg	5 mg	10 mg	15 mg
100 ppm	5 mg	10 mg	20 mg	30 mg
200 ppm	10 mg	20 mg	40 mg	60 mg

* Adapted from: Collin P, Thorell L, Kaukinen K, et al. The safe threshold for gluten contamination in gluten-free products: Can trace amounts be accepted in the treatment of coeliac disease? *Aliment Pharmacol Ther* 2004; 19:1277–83.

Calculation Facts for Table E.1:

20 ppm gluten = 2 mg gluten/100 grams of food

$$\frac{2 \text{ mg gluten}}{100 \text{ grams of food}} = \frac{6 \text{ mg gluten}}{300 \text{ grams of food}}$$

100 ppm = 10 mg gluten/100 grams of food

$$\frac{10 \text{ mg gluten}}{100 \text{ grams of food}} = \frac{30 \text{ mg gluten}}{300 \text{ grams of food}}$$

CFSAN Public Meeting on Gluten-Free Food Labeling

The CFSAN held a meeting on August 19, 2005, that included presentations from representatives of federal government agencies as well as the food industry, scientific community and celiac disease groups. The purpose of the meeting was to help the FDA gain a better understanding of:

1) How manufacturers produce gluten-free foods

2) The analytical methods used to verify that foods are gluten free

3) The costs of producing gluten-free foods

4) The food-purchasing practices of consumers with celiac disease as related to products marketed or labeled "gluten free" compared to those products without a "gluten-free" designation

In addition to the presentations at the meeting, individuals and groups not able to attend had been invited to submit comments to the FDA. Website links from the public meeting can be found on page 333.

FDA Proposed and Final Rule on Gluten-Free Food Labeling

The FDA published a proposed gluten-free food labeling rule in the *Federal Register* on January 23, 2007, with a 90-day comment period. Also, the FDA announced in this proposal that it was going to conduct a safety assessment for gluten exposure in individuals with celiac disease. The draft report, entitled *Health Hazard Assessment for Gluten Exposure in Individuals with Celiac Disease: Determination of Tolerable Daily Intake Levels and Levels of Concern for Gluten* (Gluten Report), addressed FDA's safety assessment that was completed in 2008. This Gluten Report was reviewed by an external group of scientific experts that shared their feedback with the FDA in a peer review report issued in December 2010. The FDA reviewed the expert comments, made further revisions in the Gluten Report and released it in final form in May 2011.

On August 3, 2011, a *Federal Register* notice announced that the FDA was reopening the public comment period on the proposed gluten-free food labeling rule previously issued in January 2007. In this notice, the FDA made available and sought comments on its May 2011 Gluten Report.

In the August 2011 *Federal Register* notice, the FDA also stated that it "continues to believe the proposed definition of 'gluten free' is the correct one." The then-current analytical methods that could reliably and consistently detect gluten at levels of 20 ppm or more in a variety of foods were described.

The 60-day public comment period closed on October 3, 2011. The FDA reviewed the submitted comments and stated it would be issuing a final rule that defined "gluten free" for the labeling of food products and dietary supplements, anticipated to be available by the end of 2012. References for these documents are included on pages 332 and 333.

On August 5, 2013, the FDA published the final rule, titled "Gluten-free labeling of food" found in Title 21 of the *Code of Federal Regulations*, Part 101, Section 101.91 (21 CFR 101.91), see pages 53 and 332. A summary of this gluten-free food labeling rule is included in chapter 7, table 7.1 "Gluten-free labeling regulations in the United States and Canada," on pages 56–58.

Canada

Food and Drug Regulation B.24.018

The federal *Food and Drug Regulations (FDR)*, Division 24 (Foods for Special Dietary Use), regulate foods that have been specially processed or formulated to meet the particular needs of individuals for whom specific physical and/or physiological conditions exist. Canada's first gluten-free regulation came into effect in 1995 and in Section B.24.018 the *FDR* defined the terms for food labeled as "gluten free" as follows: "No person shall label, package, sell or advertise a food in a manner likely to create an impression that it is a gluten-free food unless the food does not contain wheat, including spelt and kamut, or oats, barley, rye or triticale or any part thereof."

Due to subsequent advances in the understanding of celiac disease and the gluten-free diet (including the safety of pure, uncontaminated oats), Health Canada acknowledged that the gluten-free regulation needed revising. On May 13, 2010, *Health Canada's Proposed Policy Intent for Revising Canada's Gluten-Free Labelling Requirements* was released for comments from consumers, industry and other stakeholders. After extensive consultation, a document entitled *Summary of Comments Received on Health Canada's Proposed Policy Intent for Revising Canada's Gluten-Free Labelling Requirements* was published in July 2012. More information about these documents can be found on pages 53, 54 and 334.

The 1995 gluten-free regulation B.24.018 was later further revised (see pp. 54, 334) in order to harmonize with the amendments to the Food and Drug Regulations entitled *Enhanced Labelling for Allergen Sources and Gluten Sources and Added Sulphites* that were passed in 2011.

Codex Alimentarius Commission

In addition to country-specific regulations, there is a "gluten-free" standard from the Codex Alimentarius Commission. In 1963, the World Health Organization (WHO) and the Food and Agriculture Organization (FAO) formed this commission with a mandate to develop internationally agreed-upon food standards to ensure fair trade practices. The organization includes representatives from around the world including the United States, Canada, most European countries and many African, Asian and Latin American countries. However, not all participating countries adopt the standards developed by the commission and many have their own separate, and often different, standards and specific regulations.

The Codex Committee on Nutrition and Foods for Special Dietary Uses (CX/NFSDU) developed a *Codex Standard for Gluten-Free Foods* in 1976 that was adopted in 1981. This standard is referred to as "Codex Stan 118–1981." In 1983, amendments to the section on labeling of this standard were adopted.

The Codex Stan 118–1981 applied to products made from gluten-containing grains that were specially processed to remove most of the toxic protein fraction from the starch component. The nitrogen content for this initial definition had been based upon analysis that used an indirect method to determine the protein content of cereals and wheat starch. Section 2.2.2 of this Codex standard states that the nitrogen content of the grain used in the product must not exceed 0.05 grams per 100 grams of grain on a dry-matter basis. At the time when this definition was established, the newer ELISA-based methods for detecting and estimating the gluten content of foods were not available. Using the earlier indirect method, it was estimated that specially prepared wheat starch used in gluten-free foods that met this Codex standard could contain approximately 40–60 mg of gluten per 100 grams.

A proposal to revise the *Codex Standard for Gluten-Free Foods* was adopted in 1993. The *Draft Revised Standard for Gluten-Free Foods* was first published in 1998, with additional changes incorporated in 2006. In November 2007 the name was changed to *Draft Revised Codex Standard for Foods for Special Dietary Use for Persons Intolerant to Gluten*, and further changes and additions were made including definitions of gluten-free foods and foods specially processed to reduce gluten content, levels of gluten expressed as mg/kg, use of oats, labeling specifications and methods of analysis and sampling.

At the 31st session of the Codex Alimentarius Commission, held in Geneva, Switzerland, during June 30–July 4, 2008, the *Draft Revised Codex Standard for Foods for Special Dietary Use for Persons Intolerant to Gluten* was officially adopted. This new standard was renumbered to "Codex Stan 118–1979." In 2015, further amendments were made to this standard (see appendix D on p. 312). It also can be accessed on the Codex website (see p. 336).

Appendix F

Nutrient Composition of Gluten-Free Grains, Flours, Starches, Gums, Legumes, Nuts and Seeds

Food Item	Weight (in grams for 1 cup)	Thiamin B₁ (mg)	Riboflavin B₂ (mg)	Niacin B₃ (mg)	Pyridoxine B₆ (mg)	Folate (mcg)	Calcium (mg)	Iron (mg)	Magnesium (mg)	Zinc (mg)	Protein (grams)	Carbohydrates (grams)	Dietary Fiber (grams)
Gluten-Free Flours and Starches													
Almond Flour (blanched)	112	0.21	0.80	3.9	0.13	55	264	3.7	300	3.3	24	21	11
Almond Meal (natural with skins)	100	0.21	1.14	3.6	0.14	44	269	3.7	270	3.1	21	22	13
Amaranth Flour	120	0.07	0.19	1.3	0.68	344	203	8.2	280	3.6	17	81	10
Arrowroot Starch/Flour	128	0.00	0.00	0.0	0.01	9	51	0.4	4	0.1	0.4	113	4
Black Bean Flour (whole)	129	0.92	0.32	3.4	0.49	245	181	9.0	281	3.3	32	80	34
Buckwheat Flour (whole groat)	120	0.50	0.23	7.4	0.70	65	49	4.9	301	3.7	15	85	12
Chestnut Flour	102	0.82	0.39	3.6	0.67	111	73	3.5	117	2.6	5	83	17
Chickpea / Garbanzo Bean Flour (whole)	111	0.64	0.14	1.7	0.50	309	85	6.3	157	3.2	26	67	18
Corn Bran (crude)	76	0.01	0.08	2.1	0.12	3	32	2.1	49	1.2	6	65	60
Corn Flour – Yellow (masa, enriched)	114	1.68	0.92	11.3	0.54	382	157	9.7	106	2.1	10	87	7
Corn Flour – Yellow (degermed, unenriched)	126	0.09	0.07	3.3	0.12	60	3	1.2	23	0.5	7	104	2
Corn Flour – Yellow (whole grain)	117	0.29	0.09	2.2	0.43	29	8	2.8	109	2.0	8	90	9
Cornmeal – Yellow (degermed, enriched)	157	0.87	0.60	7.8	0.29	526	5	6.9	50	1.0	11	125	6
Cornmeal – Yellow (degermed, unenriched)	157	0.22	0.08	1.6	0.29	47	5	1.7	50	1.0	11	125	6
Cornmeal – Yellow (whole grain)	122	0.47	0.25	4.4	0.37	30	7	4.2	155	2.2	10	94	9
Cornstarch	128	0.00	0.00	0.0	0.00	0	3	0.6	4	0.1	0.3	117	1
Flaxseed Meal / Ground Flax	112	1.84	0.18	3.5	0.53	97	286	6.4	439	4.9	21	32	31
Garfava™ Flour	157	NA	NA	NA	NA	NA	104	7.9	NA	NA	35	92	12
Hazelnut Flour	112	0.72	0.13	2.0	0.63	127	128	5.3	183	2.7	17	19	11
Lentil Flour (whole)	180	0.40	0.56	4.9	0.94	215	99	17.0	187	6.9	47	110	31
Mesquite Flour	146	0.28	0.09	4.5	0.34	26	196	5.1	125	3.1	12	122	46
Millet Flour	119	0.49	0.09	7.2	0.44	50	17	4.7	142	3.1	13	89	4
Navy Bean Flour (whole)	149	0.49	0.21	0.6	2.00	161	238	8.9	250	4.5	38	91	35
Oat Bran (gluten free, raw)	94	1.10	0.21	0.9	0.16	49	55	5.1	221	2.9	16	62	15
Oat Flour (gluten free)	120	0.80	0.13	1.6	0.12	65	66	7.7	83	2.6	18	79	11
Pea Flour – Yellow (whole)	166	1.08	0.22	4.5	0.18	23	134	8.0	214	5.4	41	105	21
Peanut Flour (defatted)	60	0.42	0.29	16.2	0.30	149	84	1.3	222	3.1	31	21	10

Food Item (cont'd)	Weight (in grams for 1 cup)	Thiamin B₁ (mg)	Riboflavin B₂ (mg)	Niacin B₃ (mg)	Pyridoxine B₆ (mg)	Folate (mcg)	Calcium (mg)	Iron (mg)	Magnesium (mg)	Zinc (mg)	Protein (grams)	Carbohydrates (grams)	Dietary Fiber (grams)
Peanut Flour (low-fat)	60	0.27	0.10	6.9	0.18	80	78	2.8	29	3.6	20	19	10
Pinto Bean Flour (whole)	130	0.43	0.18	2.0	0.56	242	96	7.8	218	3.9	31	80	21
Potato Flour	160	0.37	0.08	5.6	1.23	40	104	2.2	104	0.9	11	133	9
Potato Starch	192	0.00	0.00	0.0	NA	NA	19	2.9	NA	NA	0.2	158	0
Quinoa Flour	112	0.63	0.34	1.5	0.43	308	52	4.5	213	3.8	14	76	8
Rice Bran (crude)	118	3.20	0.34	40.1	4.80	74	67	21.9	922	7.1	16	59	25
Rice Flour – Brown	158	0.70	0.13	10.0	1.20	25	17	3.1	177	3.9	11	121	7
Rice Flour – Sweet	160	NA	NA	NA	NA	NA	6	0.0	NA	NA	10	132	2
Rice Flour – White	158	0.22	0.03	4.1	0.69	6	16	0.6	55	1.3	9	127	4
Sorghum Flour – White (whole grain)	121	0.40	0.07	5.4	0.39	30	15	3.8	149	2.0	10	93	8
Sorghum Flour – White (refined, unenriched)	161	0.15	0.01	2.1	0.11	N/A	10	1.6	50	0.8	15	124	3
Soy Flour (defatted)	105	0.73	0.27	2.7	0.60	320	253	9.7	304	2.6	54	36	18
Soy Flour (low-fat)	88	0.96	0.25	2.6	0.92	254	251	7.2	251	3.6	44	27	14
Soy Flour (full-fat)	84	0.49	0.97	3.6	0.39	290	173	5.4	360	3.3	32	27	8
Tapioca Starch/Flour	120	NA	NA	NA	NA	NA	28	0.0	NA	NA	0	106	0
Teff Flour	160	1.07	0.38	4.4	0.53	139	254	9.7	275	7.1	17	116	12
Gluten-Containing Flours													
Wheat Bran (crude)	58	0.30	0.34	7.9	0.76	46	42	6.1	354	4.2	9	37	25
Whole Wheat Flour (whole grain)	120	0.60	0.20	6.0	0.49	53	41	4.3	164	3.1	16	86	13
All-Purpose White Flour (enriched)	125	0.98	0.62	7.4	0.06	364	19	5.8	28	0.9	13	95	3
Gluten-Free Gums													
Guar Gum (1 Tbsp.)	10	0.00	0.00	0.0	0.00	0	29	0.0	0	0.0	0.5	8	8
Xanthan Gum (1 Tbsp.)	9	NA	NA	NA	NA	NA	5.4	0.1	NA	NA	0.5	7	7
Gluten-Free Grains													
Amaranth (raw)	193	0.22	0.39	1.8	1.14	158	307	14.7	479	5.5	26	126	13
Amaranth (cooked)	246	0.04	0.05	0.6	0.28	54	116	5.2	160	2.1	9	46	5
Buckwheat Groats (roasted, raw)	164	0.37	0.44	8.4	0.58	69	28	4.1	362	4.0	19	123	17
Buckwheat Groats (roasted, cooked)	168	0.07	0.07	1.6	0.13	24	12	1.3	86	1.0	6	34	5

Food Item (cont'd)	Weight (in grams for 1 cup)	Thiamin B₁ (mg)	Riboflavin B₂ (mg)	Niacin B₃ (mg)	Pyridoxine B₆ (mg)	Folate (mcg)	Calcium (mg)	Iron (mg)	Magnesium (mg)	Zinc (mg)	Protein (grams)	Carbohydrates (grams)	Dietary Fiber (grams)
Millet (raw)	200	0.84	0.58	9.4	0.77	170	16	6.0	228	3.4	22	146	17
Millet (cooked)	174	0.18	0.14	2.3	0.19	33	5	1.1	77	1.6	6	41	2
Oats – Steel-Cut (gluten free, raw)	180	1.37	0.25	1.7	0.21	101	97	8.5	319	7.2	30	119	19
Oats – Steel-Cut (gluten free, cooked)	245	0.46	0.08	0.6	0.07	34	32	2.8	106	2.4	10	40	6
Oatmeal – Regular, Quick, Rolled Oats (gluten free, unenriched, raw)	81	0.37	0.13	0.9	0.08	26	42	3.4	112	3.0	11	55	8
Oatmeal – Regular, Quick, Rolled Oats (gluten free, unenriched, cooked)	234	0.18	0.04	0.5	0.01	14	21	2.1	63	2.3	6	28	4
Quinoa (raw)	170	0.61	0.54	2.6	0.83	313	80	7.8	335	5.3	24	109	12
Quinoa (cooked)	185	0.20	0.20	0.8	0.23	78	31	2.8	118	2.0	8	39	5
Rice – Brown (long grain, raw)	185	1.00	0.18	12.0	0.89	43	17	2.4	215	3.9	14	141	7
Rice – Brown (long grain, cooked)	202	0.36	0.14	5.2	0.25	18	6	1.1	79	1.2	6	52	3
Rice – White (long grain, enriched, raw)	185	1.07	0.10	7.8	0.30	716	52	8.0	46	2.0	13	148	2
Rice – White (long grain, enriched, cooked)	158	0.26	0.02	2.3	0.15	153	16	1.9	19	0.8	4	45	<1
Rice – White (long grain, unenriched, raw)	185	0.13	0.09	3.0	0.25	15	52	1.5	46	2.0	13	148	2
Rice – White (long grain, unenriched, cooked)	158	0.03	0.02	0.6	0.15	5	16	0.3	19	0.8	4	45	<1
Rice – White (long grain, parboiled, enriched, raw)	185	1.10	0.09	9.3	0.84	797	131	6.2	50	1.9	14	150	3
Rice – White (long grain, parboiled, enriched, cooked)	158	0.34	0.03	3.7	0.25	215	30	2.9	14	0.6	5	41	<1
Rice – White (long grain, parboiled, unenriched, raw)	185	0.41	0.09	9.3	0.84	15	131	1.4	50	1.9	14	150	3
Rice – White (long grain, parboiled, unenriched, cooked)	158	0.12	0.03	3.7	0.25	5	30	0.4	14	0.6	5	41	<1
Rice – Wild (raw)	160	0.18	0.42	10.8	0.63	152	34	3.1	283	9.5	24	120	10
Rice – Wild (cooked)	164	0.09	0.14	2.1	0.22	43	5	1.0	52	2.2	7	35	3
Sorghum – White (refined/pearled, raw)	192	0.17	0.01	2.6	0.13	N/A	12	1.9	60	0.9	18	148	4
Sorghum – White (refined/pearled, cooked)	187	0.05	0.00	0.7	0.04	N/A	3	0.5	17	0.3	5	42	1
Sorghum – White (whole grain, raw)	192	0.64	0.18	7.1	0.85	38	25	6.5	317	3.2	20	138	13
Sorghum – White (whole grain, cooked)	170	0.21	0.06	2.4	0.28	13	8	2.2	106	1.1	7	46	4
Teff (raw)	193	0.75	0.52	6.5	0.93	145	347	14.7	355	7.0	26	141	15
Teff (cooked)	252	0.46	0.08	2.3	0.24	45	123	5.2	126	2.8	10	50	7

Food Item (cont'd)	Weight (in grams for 1 cup)	Thiamin B₁ (mg)	Riboflavin B₂ (mg)	Niacin B₃ (mg)	Pyridoxine B₆ (mg)	Folate (mcg)	Calcium (mg)	Iron (mg)	Magnesium (mg)	Zinc (mg)	Protein (grams)	Carbo-hydrates (grams)	Dietary Fiber (grams)
Gluten-Free Beans, Peas and Lentils (cooked)													
Black Beans	172	0.42	0.10	0.9	0.12	256	46	3.6	120	1.9	15	41	15
Chickpeas / Garbanzo Beans	164	0.19	0.10	0.9	0.23	282	80	4.7	79	2.5	15	45	13
Cranberry/Romano Beans	177	0.37	0.12	0.9	0.14	366	88	3.7	88	2.0	17	43	15
Fava/Broad Beans	170	0.17	0.15	1.2	0.12	177	61	2.6	73	1.7	13	33	9
Kidney Beans – Red	177	0.28	0.10	1.0	0.21	230	50	5.2	80	1.9	15	40	13
Lentils	198	0.34	0.15	2.1	0.35	358	38	6.6	71	2.5	18	40	16
Navy Beans	182	0.43	0.12	1.2	0.25	255	126	4.3	96	1.9	15	47	19
Pinto Beans	171	0.33	0.11	0.5	0.39	294	79	3.6	86	1.7	15	45	15
Soybeans – Edamame	155	0.31	0.24	1.4	0.16	482	98	3.5	99	2.1	19	14	8
Soybeans – Mature	172	0.27	0.49	0.7	0.40	93	175	8.8	148	2.0	31	14	10
Split Peas	196	0.37	0.11	1.7	0.10	127	27	2.5	71	2.0	16	41	16
White Beans	179	0.21	0.08	0.3	0.17	145	161	6.6	113	2.5	17	45	11
Nuts													
Almonds (whole, natural with skins)	143	0.29	1.63	5.2	0.20	63	385	5.3	386	4.5	30	31	18
Almonds (whole, blanched)	145	0.28	1.03	5.1	0.17	71	342	4.8	389	4.3	31	27	14
Brazil Nuts (unblanched)	133	0.82	0.05	0.4	0.13	29	213	3.2	500	5.4	19	16	10
Hazelnuts/Filberts	135	0.87	0.15	2.4	0.76	153	154	6.3	220	3.3	20	23	13
Peanuts (dry-roasted)	146	0.22	0.29	21.0	0.68	142	85	2.3	260	4.0	36	31	12
Pecans (halves)	99	0.65	0.13	1.2	0.21	22	69	2.5	120	4.5	9	14	10
Walnuts – English (shelled, halves)	100	0.34	0.15	1.1	0.54	98	98	2.9	158	3.1	15	14	7
Seeds													
Chia Seeds	227	1.41	0.39	20.0	NA	NA	1432	17.5	760	10.4	38	96	78
Flaxseed	168	2.76	0.27	5.2	0.80	146	428	9.6	659	7.3	31	49	46
Flaxseed Meal / Ground Flax	112	1.84	0.18	3.5	0.53	97	286	6.4	439	4.9	21	32	31
Hemp Seeds (hulled)	160	2.04	0.46	14.7	0.96	176	112	12.7	1120	15.8	51	14	6
Pumpkin Seeds (kernels, dried)	129	0.35	0.20	6.4	0.18	75	59	11.4	764	10.1	39	14	8
Pumpkin Seeds (whole, roasted)	64	0.02	0.03	0.2	0.02	6	35	2.1	168	6.6	12	34	12
Sesame Seeds (kernels, dried, decorticated)	150	1.05	0.14	8.7	0.60	172	90	9.5	518	10.1	31	18	17
Sesame Seeds (whole, dried)	144	1.14	0.36	6.5	1.14	140	1404	21.0	505	11.2	26	34	17
Sunflower Seeds (hulled kernels, dry-roasted)	128	0.14	0.32	9.0	1.00	303	90	4.9	165	6.8	25	31	14

Appendix G

Carbohydrate Content of Flours, Starches, Grains, Legumes and Seeds: Highest to Lowest

Carbohydrate Content of Flours and Starches (highest to lowest)

Flour or Starch	Weight in Grams (1 cup)	Carbohydrates (grams)	Fiber (grams)
Potato Starch	192	158	0
Potato Flour	160	133	9
Rice Flour – Sweet	160	132	2
Rice Flour – White	158	127	4
Cornmeal – Yellow (degermed, enriched)	157	125	6
Cornmeal – Yellow (degermed, unenriched)	157	125	6
Sorghum Flour – White (refined, unenriched)	161	124	3
Mesquite Flour	146	122	46
Rice Flour – Brown	158	121	7
Cornstarch	128	117	1
Teff Flour	160	116	12
Arrowroot Starch/Flour	128	113	4
Lentil Flour (whole)	180	110	31
Tapioca Starch/Flour	120	106	0
Pea Flour – Yellow (whole)	166	105	21
Corn Flour – Yellow (degermed, unenriched)	126	104	2
Cornmeal – Yellow (whole grain)	122	94	9
Sorghum Flour – White (whole grain)	121	93	8
Garfava™ Flour	157	92	12
Navy Bean Flour (whole)	149	91	35
Corn Flour – Yellow (whole grain)	117	90	9
Millet Flour	119	89	4
Corn Flour – Yellow (masa, enriched)	114	87	7
Buckwheat Flour (whole groat)	120	85	12
Chestnut Flour	102	83	17
Amaranth Flour	120	81	10
Black Bean Flour (whole)	129	80	34
Pinto Bean Flour (whole)	130	80	21
Oat Flour (gluten free)	120	79	11
Quinoa Flour	112	76	8
Chickpea / Garbanzo Bean Flour (whole)	111	67	18
Corn Bran (crude)	76	65	60
Oat Bran (gluten free, raw)	94	62	15
Rice Bran (crude)	118	59	25
Soy Flour (defatted)	105	36	18
Flaxseed Meal / Ground Flax	112	32	31
Soy Flour (low-fat)	88	27	14
Soy Flour (full-fat)	84	27	8
Almond Meal (natural with skins)	100	22	13
Almond Flour (blanched)	112	21	11
Peanut Flour (defatted)	60	21	10
Hazelnut Flour	112	19	11
Peanut Flour (low-fat)	60	19	10

Carbohydrate Content of Grains (highest to lowest)

Grain	Weight in Grams (1 cup cooked)	Carbohydrates (grams)	Fiber (grams)
Rice – Brown (long grain)	202	52	3
Teff	252	50	7
Amaranth	246	46	5
Sorghum – White (whole grain)	170	46	4
Rice – White (long grain, enriched)	158	45	<1
Rice – White (long grain, unenriched)	158	45	<1
Sorghum – White (refined/pearled)	187	42	1
Millet	174	41	2
Rice – White (long grain, parboiled, enriched)	158	41	<1
Rice – White (long grain, parboiled, unenriched)	158	41	<1
Oats – Steel-Cut (gluten free)	245	40	6
Quinoa	185	39	5
Rice – Wild	164	35	3
Buckwheat Groats (roasted)	168	34	5
Oatmeal – Regular, Quick, Rolled Oats (gluten free, unenriched)	234	28	4

Carbohydrate Content of Legumes (highest to lowest)

Bean, Lentil or Pea	Weight in Grams (1 cup cooked)	Carbohydrates (grams)	Fiber (grams)
Navy Beans	182	47	19
Chickpeas / Garbanzo Beans	164	45	13
Pinto Beans	171	45	15
White Beans	179	45	11
Cranberry/Romano Beans	177	43	15
Black Beans	172	41	15
Split Peas	196	41	16
Kidney Beans – Red	177	40	13
Lentils	198	40	16
Fava/Broad Beans	170	33	9
Soybeans – Edamame	155	14	8
Soybeans – Mature	172	14	10

Carbohydrate Content of Seeds (highest to lowest)

Seed	Weight in Grams (1 cup)	Carbohydrates (grams)	Fiber (grams)
Chia Seeds	227	96	78
Flaxseed	168	49	46
Pumpkin Seeds (whole, roasted)	64	34	12
Sesame Seeds (whole, dried)	144	34	17
Flaxseed Meal / Ground Flax	112	32	31
Sunflower Seeds (hulled kernels, dry-roasted)	128	31	14
Sesame Seeds (kernels, dried, decorticated)	150	18	17
Hemp Seeds (hulled)	160	14	6
Pumpkin Seeds (kernels, dried)	129	14	8

References

This section includes a selection of references from various scientific journals and books as well as government, celiac and other organizations' websites and other pertinent sources.

Celiac Disease

Abu Daya H, Lebwohl B, Lewis S, et al. Celiac disease patients presenting with anemia have more severe disease than those presenting with diarrhea. *Clin Gastroenterol Hepatol* 2013; 11:1472–7.

Bai J, Fried M, Corazza G, et al. World Gastroenterology Organisation global guidelines on celiac disease. *J Clin Gastroenterol* 2013; 47:121–6.

Bao F, Bhagat G. Histopathology of celiac disease. *Gastrointest Endosc Clin N Am* 2012; 22:679–94.

Case S. The gluten-free diet: How to provide effective education and resources. *Gastroenterol* 2005; 128 (4 Suppl 1):S128–34.

Catassi C, Anderson R, Hill I, et al. World perspective on celiac disease. *J Pediatr Gastroenterol Nutr* 2012; 55:494–9.

Catassi C, Kryszak D, Bhatti B, et al. Natural history of celiac disease autoimmunity in a USA cohort followed since 1974. *Ann Med* 2010; 42:530–8.

Cranney A, Zarkadas M, Graham I, et al. The Canadian celiac health survey. *Dig Dis Sci* 2007; 52:1087–95.

Fasano A, Berti I, Gerdarduzzi T, et al. Prevalence of celiac disease in at-risk and not-at-risk groups in the United States: A large multicenter study. *Arch Intern Med* 2003; 163:286–92.

Guandalini S, Assiri A. Celiac disease: A review. *JAMA Pediatr* 2014; 168:272–8.

Hollon J, Cureton P, Martin M, et al. Trace gluten contamination may play a role in mucosal and clinical recovery in a subgroup of diet-adherent non-responsive celiac disease patients. *BMC Gastroenterol* 2013; 13:40.

Kang J, Kang A, Green A, et al. Systematic review: Worldwide variation in the frequency of coeliac disease and changes over time. *Aliment Pharmacol Ther* 2013; 38:226–45.

Kasarda D. Can an increase in celiac disease be attributed to an increase in the gluten content of wheat as a consequence of wheat breeding? *J Agric Food Chem* 2013; 61:1155–9.

Lebwohl B, Granath F, Ekbom A, et al. Mucosal healing and mortality in coeliac disease. *Aliment Pharmacol Ther* 2013; 37:332–9.

Lebwohl B, Kapel R, Neugut A, et al. Adherence to biopsy guidelines increases celiac disease diagnosis. *Gastrointest Endosc* 2011; 74:103–9.

Lebwohl B, Murray J, Rubio-Tapia A, et al. Predictors of persistent villous atrophy in coeliac disease: A population-based study. *Aliment Pharmacol Ther* 2014; 39:488–95.

Lee A, Ng D, Diamond B, et al. Living with coeliac disease: Survey results from the U.S.A. *J Hum Nutr Diet* 2012; 25:233–8.

Leffler D, Schuppan D, Pallav K, et al. Kinetics of the histological, serological and symptomatic responses to a gluten challenge in adults with coeliac disease. *Gut* 2013; 62:996–1004.

Ludvigsson J, Bai J, Biagi F, et al. Diagnosis and management of adult coeliac disease: Guidelines from the British Society of Gastroenterology. *Gut* 2014; 63:1210–28.

Ludvigsson J, Leffler D, Bai J, et al. The Oslo definitions for coeliac disease and related terms. *Gut* 2013; 62:43–52.

Pulido O, Zarkadas M, Dubois S, et al. Clinical features and symptom recovery on a gluten-free diet in Canadian adults with celiac disease. *Can J Gastroenterol* 2013; 27:449–53.

Rashid M, Cranney A, Zarkadas M, et al. Celiac disease: Evaluation of the diagnosis and dietary compliance in Canadian children. *Pediatrics* 2005; 116:e754–9.

Rashid M, Lee J. Serologic testing in celiac disease: Practical guide for clinicians. *Can Fam Physician* 2016; 62:38–43.

Rashid M, Zarkadas M, Anca A, et al. Oral manifestations of celiac disease: A clinical guide for dentists. *J Can Dent Assoc* 2011; 77:b39.

Rubio-Tapia A, Hill I, Kelly C, et al. ACG clinical guidelines: Diagnosis and management of celiac disease. *Am J Gastroenterol* 2013; 108:656–76.

Rubio-Tapia A, Ludvigsson J, Brantner T, et al. The prevalence of celiac disease in the United States. *Am J Gastroenterol* 2012; 107:1538–44.

Rubio-Tapia A, Rahim M, See J, et al. Mucosal recovery and mortality in adults with celiac disease after treatment with a gluten-free diet. *Am J Gastroenterol* 2010; 105:1412–20.

Sapone A, Bai J, Ciacci C, et al. Spectrum of gluten-related disorders: Consensus on new nomenclature and classification. *BMC Med* 2012; 10:13.

Singh P, Arora S, Lal S, et al. Risk of celiac disease in the first- and second-degree relatives of patients with celiac disease: A systematic review and meta-analysis. *Am J Gastroenterol* 2015; 110:1539–48.

Tapsas D, Hollén E, Stenhammar L, et al. The clinical presentation of coeliac disease in 1030 Swedish children: Changing features over the past four decades. *Dig Liver Dis* 2016; 48:16–22.

Zarkadas M, Cranney A, Case S, et al. The impact of a gluten-free diet on adults with coeliac disease: Results of a national survey. *J Hum Nutr Diet* 2006; 19:41–9.

Zarkadas M, Dubois S, MacIsaac K, et al. Living with coeliac disease and a gluten-free diet: A Canadian perspective. *J Hum Nutr Diet* 2013; 26:10–23.

Infant Feeding and Celiac Disease

Henriksson C, Boström A, Wiklund I. What effect does breastfeeding have on coeliac disease? A systematic review update. *Evid Based Med* 2013; 18:98–103.

Lebwohl B, Murray J, Verdu E, et al. Gluten introduction, breastfeeding, and celiac disease: Back to the drawing board. *Am J Gastroenterol* 2016; 111:12–4.

Lionetti E, Castellaneta S, Francavilla R, et al. Introduction of gluten, HLA status, and the risk of celiac disease in children. *N Engl J Med* 2014; 371:1295–303.

Pinto-Sánchez M, Verdu E, Liu E, et al. Gluten introduction to infant feeding and risk of celiac disease: Systematic review and meta-analysis. *J Pediatr* 2016; 168:132–43.e3.

Vriezinga S, Auricchio R, Bravi E, et al. Randomized feeding intervention in infants at high risk for celiac disease. *N Engl J Med* 2014; 371:1304–15.

Dermatitis Herpetiformis

Antiga E, Caproni M. The diagnosis and treatment of dermatitis herpetiformis. *Clin Cosmet Investig Dermatol* 2015; 23:257–65.

Collin P, Reunala T. Recognition and management of the cutaneous manifestations of celiac disease: A guide for dermatologists. *Am J Clin Dermatol* 2003; 4:13–20.

Non-Celiac Gluten Sensitivity

Aziz I, Hadjivassiliou M, Sanders D. Does gluten sensitivity in the absence of coeliac disease exist? *BMJ* 2012; 345:e7907.

Aziz I, Lewis N, Hadjivassiliou M, et al. A UK study assessing the population prevalence of self-reported gluten sensitivity and referral characteristics to secondary care. *Eur J Gastroenterol Hepatol* 2014; 26:33–9.

Aziz I, Sanders D. The irritable bowel syndrome-celiac disease connection. *Gastrointest Endosc Clin N Am* 2012; 22:623–37.

Biesiekierski J, Newnham E, Irving P, et al. Gluten causes gastrointestinal symptoms in subjects without celiac disease: A double-blind randomized placebo-controlled trial. *Am J Gastroenterol* 2011; 106:508–14.

Biesiekierski J, Newnham E, Shepherd S, et al. Characterization of adults with a self-diagnosis of nonceliac gluten sensitivity. *Nutr Clin Pract* 2014; 29:504–9.

Biesiekierski J, Peters S, Newnham E, et al. No effects of gluten in patients with self-reported non-celiac gluten sensitivity after dietary reduction of fermentable, poorly absorbed short-chain carbohydrates. *Gastroenterology* 2013; 145:320–8.e1–3.

Caio G, Volta U, Tovoli F, et al. Effect of gluten free diet on immune response to gliadin in patients with non-celiac gluten sensitivity. *BMC Gastroenterol* 2014; 14:26.

Carroccio A, Mansueto P, Iacono G, et al. Non-celiac wheat sensitivity diagnosed by double-blind placebo-controlled challenge: Exploring a new clinical entity. *Am J Gastroenterol* 2012; 107:1898–1906.

Catassi C, Bai K, Bonaz B, et al. Non-celiac gluten sensitivity: The new frontier of gluten related disorders. *Nutrients* 2013; 5:3839–53.

Catassi C, Elli L, Bonaz B, et al. Diagnosis of non-celiac gluten sensitivity (NCGS): The Salerno experts' criteria. *Nutrients* 2015; 7:4966–77.

Cooper B, Holmes G, Ferguson R, et al. Gluten-sensitive diarrhea without evidence of celiac disease. *Gastroenterology* 1980; 79:801–6.

Di Sabatino A, Volta U, Salvatore C, et al. Small amounts of gluten in subjects with suspected nonceliac gluten sensitivity: A randomized, double-blind, placebo-controlled, cross-over trial. *Clin Gastroenterol Hepatol* 2015; 13:1604–12.e3.

Elli L, Tomba C, Branchi F, et al. Evidence for the presence of non-celiac gluten sensitivity in patients with functional gastrointestinal symptoms: Results from a multicenter randomized double-blind placebo-controlled gluten challenge. *Nutrients* 2016; 8:84.

Fasano A. Leaky gut and autoimmune diseases. *Clin Rev Allergy Immunol* 2012; 42:71–8.

Fasano A, Sapone A, Zevallos V, et al. Nonceliac gluten sensitivity. *Gastroenterology* 2015; 148:1195–1204.

Halmos E, Power V, Shepherd S, et al. A diet low in FODMAPs reduces symptoms of irritable bowel syndrome. *Gastroenterology* 2014; 146:67–75.e5.

Kabbani T, Vanga R, Leffler D, et al. Celiac disease or non-celiac gluten sensitivity? An approach to clinical differential diagnosis. *Am J Gastroenterol* 2014; 109:741–6.

Lebwohl B, Ludvigsson J, Green P. Celiac disease and non-celiac gluten sensitivity. *BMJ* 2015; 351:h4347.

Lundin K, Alaedini A. Non-celiac gluten sensitivity. *Gastrointest Endosc Clin N Am* 2012; 22:723–34.

Mansueto P, Seidita A, D'Alcamo A, et al. Non-celiac gluten sensitivity: Literature review. *J Am Coll Nutr* 2014; 33:39–54.

Molina-Infante J, Santolaria S, Sanders D, et al. Systematic review: Noncoeliac gluten sensitivity. *Aliment Pharmacol Ther* 2015; 41:807–20.

Newnham E. Does gluten cause gastrointestinal symptoms in subjects without coeliac disease? *J Gastroenterol Hepatol* 2011; 26 Suppl 3:132–4.

Sanders D, Aziz I. Non-celiac wheat sensitivity: Separating the wheat from the chat! *Am J Gastroenterol* 2012; 107:1908–12.

Sapone A, Lammers K, Casolaro V, et al. Divergence of gut permeability and mucosal immune gene expression in two gluten-associated conditions: Celiac disease and gluten sensitivity. *BMC Med* 2011; 9:23.

Sapone A, Lammers K , Mazzarella G, et al. Differential mucosal IL-17 expression in two gliadin-induced disorders: Gluten sensitivity and the autoimmune enteropathy celiac disease. *Int Arch Allergy Immunol* 2010; 152:75–80.

Tavakkoli A, Lewis S, Tennyson C, et al. Characteristics of patients who avoid wheat and/or gluten in the absence of celiac disease. *Dig Dis Sci* 2014; 59:1255–61.

Uhde M, Ajamian M, Caio G, et al. Intestinal cell damage and systemic immune activation in individuals reporting sensitivity to wheat in the absence of coeliac disease. *Gut Online First*: July 25, 2016 doi:10.1136/gutjnl-2016-311964.

Volta U, Bardella M, Calabro A, et al. An Italian prospective multicenter survey on patients suspected of having non-celiac gluten sensitivity. *BMC Med* 2014; 12:85.

Zanini B, Baschè R, Ferraresi C, et al. Randomised clinical study: Gluten challenge induces symptom recurrence in only a minority of patients who meet clinical criteria for non-celiac gluten sensitivity. *Aliment Pharmacol Ther* 2015; 42:968–76.

Oats

Health Canada has conducted two major reviews on the safety of oats for individuals with celiac disease. The following two publications include an extensive list of references on oats. In addition, other key references are listed below.

Celiac Disease and Gluten-Free Claims on Uncontaminated Oats – 2015.
www.hc-sc.gc.ca/fn-an/consult/2014-cel-oats-contam-avoine-coel/document-consultation-eng.php

Celiac Disease and the Safety of Oats: Health Canada's Position on the Introduction of Oats to the Diet of Individuals Diagnosed with Celiac Disease (CD) – 2007.
www.hc-sc.gc.ca/fn-an/securit/allerg/cel-coe/oats_cd-avoine-eng.php

Comino I, Bernado D, Bancel E, et al. Identification and molecular characterization of oat peptides implicated on coeliac immune response. *Food & Nutrition Research* 2016; 60:10.3402/fnr.v60.30324.

Comino I, Moreno M de L, Sousa C. Role of oats in celiac disease. *World J Gastroenterol* 2015; 21:11825–31.

Dicke W, Weigers H, Kamer J. Coeliac disease II: The presence in wheat of a factor having a deleterious effect in cases of coeliac disease. *Acta Paediatrica* 1953; 42:34–42.

Gélinas P, McKinnon C, Méndez E. Gluten contamination of cereal foods in Canada. *Int J Food Sci Technol* 2007; 43:1245–52.

Guttormsen V, Løvik A, Bye A, et al. No induction of anti-avenin IgA by oats in adult, diet-treated coeliac disease. *Scand J Gastroenterol* 2008; 43:161–5.

Hernando A, Mujico J, Mena M, et al. Measurement of wheat gluten and barley hordeins in contaminated oats from Europe, the United States and Canada by sandwich R5 ELISA. *Eur J Gastroenterol Hepatol* 2008; 20:545–54.

Janatuinen E, Kemppainen T, Julkunen R, et al. No harm from five year ingestion of oats in coeliac disease. *Gut* 2002; 50:332–5.

Janatuinen E, Kemppainen T, Pikkarainen P, et al. Lack of cellular and humoral immunological responses to oats in adults with coeliac disease. *Gut* 2000; 46:327–31.

Kamer J, Weijers H, Dicke W. Coeliac disease: An investigation into the injurious constituents of wheat in connection with their action on patients with coeliac disease. *Acta Paediatr* 1953; 42:223–31.

Koerner T, Cléroux C, Poirier C, et al. Gluten contamination in the Canadian commercial oat supply. *Food Addit Contam Part A Chem Anal Control Expo Risk Assess* 2011; 28:705–10.

La Vielle S, Pulido O, Abbott M, et al. Celiac disease and gluten-free oats: A Canadian position based on a literature review. *Can J Gastroenterol Hepatol* 2016 [advance online publication].

Thompson T. Do oats belong in a gluten-free diet? *J Am Diet Assoc* 1997; 97:1413–6.

Thompson T. Oats and the gluten-free diet. *J Am Diet Assoc* 2003; 103:376–9.

Thompson T. Gluten contamination of commercial oat products in the United States. *N Engl J Med* 2004; 351:2021–2.

Thompson T. Contaminated oats and other gluten-free foods in the United States. *J Am Diet Assoc* 2005; 105:348.

Foods, Beverages and Ingredients

General

Canadian Celiac Association's *Acceptability of Foods and Food Ingredients for the Gluten-Free Diet* pocket dictionary. Mississauga, ON: 2014.

Cifuentes, A (Ed). *Foodomics: Advanced Mass Spectrometry in Modern Food Science and Nutrition* Vol. 52. New York: John Wiley & Sons, 2013.

Top 10 ingredients you really don't need to worry about. *Gluten-Free Living* magazine 2016. www.glutenfreeliving.com/gluten-free-foods/ingredients/top-10-ingredients-you-really-dont-need-to-worry-about/

Thompson T. *Pocket Guide to Gluten-Free Strategies for Clients with Multiple Diet Restrictions,* 2nd ed. Academy of Nutrition and Dietetics, 2016.

Thompson T, Rubin E. Dispelling Gluten-Free Labeling and Ingredient Myths Webinar. *National Foundation for Celiac Awareness*. 2014.

Distilled Alcohol

Buglass A (Ed). *Handbook of Alcoholic Beverages: Technical, Analytical and Nutritional Aspects.* West Sussex, UK: John Wiley & Sons, 2011.

U.S. International Trade Commission. *Industry & trade summary: Distilled spirits.* USITC Publication 3373, November 2000.

Wine

Harbertson J. A Guide to the Fining of Wine. *Washington State University Extension Manual EM016*, 2009. http://cru.cahe.wsu.edu/CEPublications/em016/EM016.pdf

Health Canada. Vintage Wines and Application of Enhanced Allergen Regulations. 2012. www.hc-sc.gc.ca/fn-an/label-etiquet/allergen/vintage-wine-vin-millesimes-eng.php

Marchal R, Marchal-Delahaut L, Lallement A, et al. Wheat gluten used as a clarifying agent of red wines. *J Agr Food Chem* 2002; 50:177–84.

Mobley E. Should I be worried about wine if I have a gluten allergy? Wine Spectator 2013. www.winespectator.com/webfeature/show/id/48789

Simonato B, Mainente F, Tolin S, et al. Immunochemical and mass spectrometry detection of residual proteins in gluten fined red wine. *J Agr Food Chem* 2011; 59:3101–10.

Szymanski E. The problem of gluten in wine. Wineoscope 2011.
www.wineoscope.com/2011/11/16/189/

Thompson T. Gluten content of wine aged in oak barrels sealed with wheat paste. Gluten Free Dietitian 2012.
www.glutenfreedietitian.com/gluten-content-of-wine-aged-in-oak-barrels-sealed-with-wheat-paste/

Thompson T. It's not just food anymore: An update on gluten-free alcoholic beverage labeling webinar. *National Foundation for Celiac Awareness*. 2013.

Beer

Canadian Food Inspection Agency. Gluten-Free Claims: Gluten-Free Beer. 2016.
www.inspection.gc.ca/food/labelling/food-labelling-for-industry/allergens-and gluten/eng/1388152325341/1388152326591?chap=2#s4c2

Colgrave M, Goswami H, Blundell M, et al. Using mass spectrometry to detect hydrolysed gluten in beer that is responsible for false negatives by ELISA. *J Chromatogr A* 2014; 1370:105–14.

Department of Treasury and Tobacco Tax and Trade Bureau. Revised Interim Policy on Gluten Content Statements in the Labeling and Advertising of Wine, Distilled Spirits, and Malt Beverages. 2014.
http://www.ttb.gov/rulings/2014-2.pdf

Ratner A. GF Barley Beer: It's here, but is it safe? *Gluten-Free Living* magazine 2012; 2:37–39.

Thompson T. Beer: Why is it so hard to assess fermented and hydrolyzed products for gluten?
Gluten Free Dietitian 2012.
www.glutenfreedietitian.com/beer-why-it-is-so-hard-to-assess-fermented-and-hydrolyzed-products-for-gluten/

Thompson T. Gluten-free labeling of beer. Gluten Free Watchdog and Gluten Free Dietitian [a compilation of articles].
www.glutenfreewatchdog.org/news/?s=beer
www.glutenfreedietitian.com/category/gluten-free-labeling-of-beer/

Thompson T. Is barley-based "gluten-removed" beer safe for people with celiac disease?
Gluten Free Watchdog 2014.
www.glutenfreewatchdog.org/reports/Gluten_Removed_Barley_Based_Beers_Jan_14.pdf
www.glutenfreewatchdog.org/news/category/gluten-free-beer

Vinegars

Marcason W. Can a patient with celiac disease have distilled vinegar? *J Am Diet Assoc* 2004; 104:1183.

The Vinegar Institute. Frequently Asked Questions. 2015.
www.versatilevinegar.org/faqs/

Thompson T. Vinegar! Gluten Free Dietitian 2009.
www.glutenfreedietitian.com/vinegar/

Barley Grass and Wheat Grass

Thompson T. Can products containing wheat and barley grass be labeled gluten free? Gluten Free Dietitian 2010.
www.glutenfreedietitian.com/can-products-containing-wheat-and-barley-grass-be-labeled-gluten-free/

Blue Cheese

Anca A. Blue cheese in the gluten-free diet: A research update. *Celiac News* 2009; 23:1–5.

Thompson T. Blue cheese. Gluten Free Dietitian 2008.
www.glutenfreedietitian.com/blue-cheese/

Flavorings and Smoke Flavoring

Thompson T. Flavorings & extracts: Are they gluten free? Gluten Free Dietitian 2009.
www.glutenfreedietitian.com/flavorings-extracts-are-they-gluten-free/

Autolyzed Yeast and Autolyzed Yeast Extract / Yeast Extract

Ratner A. Can celiacs say "yes" to yeast? *Gluten-Free Living* magazine 2003; 9:3,8.

Thompson T. Update on gluten-free status of yeast extract. Gluten Free Dietitian 2013.
www.glutenfreedietitian.com/update-on-gluten-free-status-of-yeast-extract/

Waffle V. Yeast extract questioned: New GF labeling laws in Canada prompt a closer look at this food flavoring. *Gluten-Free Living* magazine November/December 2013; 39–41.

Barley Malt, Barley Malt Extract/Syrup, Barley Malt Flavoring

Thompson T. Attention gluten-free manufacturers: Important information about malt. Gluten Free Watchdog 2016.
www.glutenfreewatchdog.org/news/attention-gluten-free-manufacturers-important-information-about-malt/

Caramel

Kamuf W, Nixon A, Parker L, et al. Overview of caramel colors. *Cereal Foods World* 2003; 48:64–9.

Thompson T. Caramel color. Gluten Free Dietitian 2009.
www.glutenfreedietitian.com/caramel-color/

Spices, Herbs and Seasonings

Canadian Food Inspection Agency. Food Safety Action Plan Report: 2010-2011 Targeted Surveys: Allergens. 2011.
www.allergicliving.com/wp-content/uploads/2013/08/Gluten_Report-FSAP-FY301-FINAL-FORMATTED-EN.pdf

Case S. Are spices safe? *Allergic Living* magazine Fall 2013; 41.

Tainter D, Grenis A. *Spices and Seasonings in Food Technology Handbook*. New York: John Wiley & Sons, 2001: 198–232.

Thompson T. Special report: Gluten contamination of spices. Gluten Free Watchdog 2013.
www.glutenfreewatchdog.org/reportUploads/Gluten_Free_Watchdog_Special_Report_on_Spices_Public.pdf

Wheat Starch

Association des Amidonneeries de Céréales de l'Union Européene. Communication on EU Allergen Labelling of Wheat Starch and Wheat Starch Derivatives and Their Use in Gluten-Free Foods. 2010.
www.starch.eu/wp-content/uploads/2012/09/2009-02-13-Communication-on-EU-allergen-labelling.pdf

Chartrand L, Russo P, Duhaime A, et al. Wheat starch intolerance in patients with celiac disease. *J Am Diet Assoc* 1997; 97:612–8.

Faulkner-Hogg K, Selby W, Loblay R. Dietary analysis in symptomatic patients with coeliac disease on a gluten-free diet: The role of trace amounts of gluten and non-gluten food intolerances. *Scand J Gastroenterol* 1999; 34:784–9.

Kaukinen K, Collin P, Holm K, et al. Wheat starch-containing gluten-free flour products in the treatment of coeliac disease and dermatitis herpetiformis: A long-term follow-up study. *Scand J Gastroenterol* 1999; 34:163–9.

Kaukinen K, Salmi T, Collin P, et al. Clinical trial: Gluten microchallenge with wheat-based starch hydrolysates in coeliac disease patients - a randomized double-blind, placebo-controlled study to evaluate safety. *Aliment Pharmacol Ther* 2008; 28:1240–8.

Lohiniemi S, Mäki M, Kaukinen K, et al. Gastrointestinal symptoms rating scale in coeliac disease patients on wheat starch-based gluten-free diets. *Scand J Gastroenterol* 2000; 35:947–9.

Peraaho M, Kaukinen K, Paasikivi K, et al. Wheat-starch-based gluten-free products in the treatment of newly detected coeliac disease: Prospective and randomized study. *Aliment Pharmacol Ther* 2003; 17:587–94.

Thomspon T. Using wheat starch in gluten-free foods. Gluten Free Watchdog 2015.
www.glutenfreewatchdog.org/news/using-wheat-starch-in-gluten-free-foods/

Thompson T. Wheat starch, gliadin, and the gluten-free diet. *J Am Diet Assoc* 2001; 101:1456–9.

Waffle V. The new word on wheat starch. *Gluten-Free Living* magazine 2015.
www.glutenfreeliving.com/gluten-free-foods/ingredients/new-word-on-wheat-starch/

Dextrin

Thompson T. Dextrin from wheat. Gluten Free Dietitian 2012.
www.glutenfreedietitian.com/dextrin-from-wheat/

Thompson T. Wheat-based dextrin: How much gluten does it contain? Gluten Free Dietitian 2011.
www.glutenfreedietitian.com/wheat-based-dextrin-how-much-gluten-does-it-contain/

Maltodextrin

EFSA Panel on Dietetic Products, Nutrition and Allergies. Opinion of the Scientific Panel on Dietetic Products, Nutrition and Allergies, Wheat-Based Maltodextrin and Glucose Syrups, European Food Safety Authority. EFSA-Q-2004-091 and 092. *The EFSA Journal* 2004; 126:1–6.

EFSA Panel on Dietetic Products, Nutrition and Allergies. Opinion of the Scientific Panel on Dietetic Products, Nutrition and Allergies [NDA] Related to a Notification from AAC on Wheat-Based Maltodextrins Pursuant to Article 6, paragraph 11 of Directive 2000/13/EC. *The EFSA Journal* 2007; 487:1–7.

Permanent Exemption Obtained for "Allergen Labelling" of Wheat-Based Maltodextrins, Glucose Syrups, Dextrose. Starch Europe 2007.
www.starch.eu/wp-content/uploads/2012/09/Statement-on-permanent-exemption-obtained-for-allergen-labelling11-2007.pdf

Thompson T. Maltodextrin. Gluten Free Dietitian 2007.
www.glutenfreedietitian.com/maltodextrin/

Glucose Syrup

EFSA Panel on Dietetic Products, Nutrition and Allergies. Opinion of the Scientific Panel on Dietetic Products, Nutrition and Allergies [NDA] Related to a Notification from Finnsugar Ltd. on Glucose Syrups Produced from Barley Starch Pursuant to Article 6, paragraph 11 of Directive 2000/13/EC. *The EFSA Journal* 2007; 456:1–6.

Opinion of the Scientific Panel on Dietetic Products, Nutrition and Allergies [NDA] Related to a Notification from AAC on Wheat-Based Glucose Syrups including Dextrose Pursuant to Article 6, paragraph 11 of Directive 2000/13/EC. *The EFSA Journal* 2007; 488:1-8.

Gluten Threshold Levels, PPM and Testing

Gluten Threshold Levels

Akobeng A, Thomas A. Systematic review: Tolerable amount of gluten for people with coeliac disease. *Aliment Pharmacol Ther* 2008; 27:1044–52.

Catassi C, Fabiani E, Iacono G, et al. A prospective, double-blind, placebo-controlled trial to establish a safe gluten threshold for patients with celiac disease. *Am J Clin Nutr* 2007; 85:160–6.

Catassi C, Rossini M, Rätsch I, et al. Dose dependent effects of protracted ingestion of small amounts of gliadin in coeliac disease children: A clinical and jejunal morphometric study. *Gut* 1993; 34:1515–9.

Ciclitira P, Evans D, Fagg N, et al. Clinical testing of gliadin fractions in coeliac patients. *Clin Sci* 1984; 66:357–64.

Collin P, Thorell L, Kaukinen K, et al. The safe threshold for gluten contamination in gluten-free products: Can trace amounts be accepted in the treatment of coeliac disease? *Aliment Pharmacol Ther* 2004; 19:1277–83.

Fassano A, Flaharty S. *Gluten Freedom: The Nation's Leading Expert Offers the Essential Guide to a Healthy Gluten-Free Lifestyle.* Nashville, TN: Wiley, 2014.

Gibert A, Espadaler M, Canela M, et al. Consumption of gluten-free products: Should the threshold value for trace amounts of gluten be at 20, 100 or 200 ppm? *Eur J Gastroenterol Hepatol* 2006; 18:1187–95.

Gibert A, Kruizinga A, Neuhold S, et al. Might gluten traces in wheat substitutes pose a risk in patients with celiac disease? A population-based probabilistic approach to risk estimation. *Am J Clin Nutr* 2013; 97:109–16.

Hischenhuber C, Crevel R, Jarry B, et al. Review article: Safe amounts of gluten for patients with wheat allergy or coeliac disease. *Aliment Pharmacol Ther* 2006; 23:559–75.

La Vieille S, Dubois S, Hayward S, et al. Estimated levels of gluten incidentally present in a Canadian gluten-free diet. *Nutrients* 2014; 6:881–96.

Gluten Content of Naturally Gluten-Free Foods and Gluten-Free Specialty Products

Gélinas P, McKinnon C, Mena M, et al. Gluten contamination of cereal foods in Canada. *Int J Food Sci Tech* 2008; 43:1245–52.

Gendel S, Zhu J. Analysis of U.S. Food and Drug Administration food allergen recalls after implementation of the food allergen labeling and consumer protection act. *J Food Prot* 2013; 76:1933–8.

Koerner T, Cleroux C, Poirier C, et al. Gluten contamination in the Canadian commercial oat supply. *Food Addit Contam Part A Chem Anal Control Expo Risk Assess* 2011; 28:705–10.

Koerner T, Cleroux C, Poirier C, et al. Gluten contamination of naturally gluten-free flours and starches used by Canadians with celiac disease. *Food Addit Contam Part A Chem Anal Control Expo Risk Assess* 2013; 30:2017–21.

Koerner T, Poirier C, Cleroux C, et al. Cross contamination of grains: Canadian exposure assessment for naturally gluten-free grains. Food Research Division, Food Directorate, Health Canada. From British Columbia Food Protection Association. 2014.
www.goo.gl/FXLePm

Ratner A. Gluten in GF grains: The risk and steps taken to prevent it. *Gluten-Free Living* magazine 2010; 3:21–4,47.

Sharma G, Pereira M, Williams K. Gluten detection in foods available in the United States – A market survey. *Food Chem* 2015; 169:120–6.

Thompson T. Five percent of tested foods making gluten-free claims are not gluten-free study finds. Gluten Free Watchdog 2014.
www.glutenfreewatchdog.org/news/five-percent-of-tested-foods-making-gluten-free-claims-are-not-gluten-free-study-finds/

Thompson T. Gluten contamination of commercial oat products in the United States. *New Engl J Med* 2004; 351:2021–2.

Thompson T, Grace T. Gluten content of selected labeled gluten-free foods sold in the US. *Pract Gastroenterol* 2013; 37:10–6.
https://med.virginia.edu/ginutrition/wp-content/uploads/sites/199/2014/06/Parrish_Oct_13-2.pdf

Thompson T, Lee A, Grace T. Gluten contamination of grains, seeds, and flours in the United States: A pilot study. *J Am Diet Assoc* 2010; 110:937–40.

Thompson T, Rubin E. Dispelling gluten-free labeling and ingredient myths webinar. *National Foundation for Celiac Awareness*. 2014.

Thompson T, Simpson S. A comparison of gluten levels in labeled gluten-free and certified gluten-free foods sold in the United States. *Eur J Clin Nutr* 2015; 69:143–6.

Gluten Testing Methods

Colgrave M, Goswami H, Blundell M, et al. Using mass spectrometry to detect hydrolysed gluten in beer that is responsible for false negatives by ELISA. *J Chromatogr A* 2014; 1370:105–14.

Garcia E, Llorente M, Hernando A, et al. Development of a general procedure for complete extraction of gliadins for heat processed and unheated foods. *Eur J Gastroenterol Hepatol* 2005; 17:529–39.

Gessendorfer B, Koehler P, Wieser H. Preparation and characterization of enzymatically hydrolyzed prolamins from wheat, rye, and barley as references for the immunochemical quantitation of partially hydrolyzed gluten. *Anal Bioanal Chem* 2009; 395:1721–8.

Méndez E, Vela C, Immer U, et al. Report of a collaborative trial to investigate the performance of the R5 enzyme linked immunoassay to determine gliadin in gluten-free food. *Eur J Gastroenterol Hepatol* 2005; 17:1053–63.

Scherf K, Poms R. Recent developments in analytical methods for tracing gluten. *J Cereal Sci* 2016; 67:112–22.

Tanner G, Colgrave M, Blundell M. Measuring hordein (gluten) in beer – A comparison of ELISA and mass spectrometry. *PLoS One* 2013; 8:e56452.

Thompson T. Testing food for gluten. Gluten Free Dietitian [a compilation of articles].
www.glutenfreedietitian.com/category/testing-food-for-gluten/

Thompson T, Méndez E. Commercial assays to assess gluten content of gluten-free foods: Why they are not created equal. *J Am Diet Assoc* 2008; 108:1682–7.

Valdés L, García E, Llorente M, et al. Innovative approach to low-level gluten determination in foods using a novel sandwich enzyme-linked immunosorbent assay protocol. *Eur J Gastroenterol Hepatol* 2003; 15:465–74.

Working Group on Prolamin Analysis and Toxicity (PWG). Proceedings of the 28th Meeting. Ed. Koehler, P. September 2014.
www.wgpat.com/proceeding_28th.pdf

Gluten-Free Labeling Regulations

United States

Food and Drug Administration (FDA)

FDA: About and What the Agency Regulates
www.fda.gov/AboutFDA/WhatWeDo/

Food, Drug and Cosmetic Act (FD&C Act)
www.fda.gov/regulatoryinformation/legislation/federalfooddrugandcosmeticactfdcact/

FDA Title 21 Code of Federal Regulations (CFR)
www.accessdata.fda.gov/scripts/cdrh/cfdocs/cfcfr/cfrsearch.cfm
www.ecfr.gov

A Food Labeling Guide: Guidance for Industry
www.fda.gov/downloads/food/guidanceregulation/ucm265446.pdf

U.S. Food and Drug Administration Manual of Compliance Policy Guides
www.fda.gov/ICECI/ComplianceManuals/CompliancePolicyGuidanceManual/default.htm

U.S. Food and Drug Administration Manual of Compliance Policy Guides: Chapter 5 – Food, Colors, and Cosmetics
www.fda.gov/ICECI/ComplianceManuals/CompliancePolicyGuidanceManual/ucm119194.htm

FDA Food Allergen Labeling and Consumer Protection Act (FALCPA)

Food Allergen Labeling and Consumer Protection Act of 2004 (Public Law 108-282, Title II)
www.fda.gov/Food/GuidanceRegulation/GuidanceDocumentsRegulatoryInformation/Allergens/ucm106187.htm

Food Allergen Labeling and Consumer Protection Act of 2004 Questions and Answers
www.fda.gov/Food/GuidanceRegulation/GuidanceDocumentsRegulatoryInformation/Allergens/ucm106890.htm

Guidance for Industry: Questions and Answers Regarding Food Allergens, including the FALCPA 2004 (Edition 4); Final Guidance
www.fda.gov/food/guidanceregulation/guidancedocumentsregulatoryinformation/allergens/ucm059116.htm

Establishment of Dockets: Risk Assessment for Establishing Food Allergen Thresholds; Requests for Comments December 2012
www.regulations.gov/document?D=FDA-2012-N-0711-0001

FDA Gluten-Free Labeling of Foods Final Rule

Federal Register August 5, 2013 Food Labeling: Gluten-Free Labeling of Foods (Final Rule)
www.federalregister.gov/articles/2013/08/05/2013-18813/food-labeling-gluten-free-labeling-of-foods

Code of Federal Regulations Title 21 Gluten-Free Labeling of Food (CFR 101.91)
www.accessdata.fda.gov/scripts/cdrh/cfdocs/cfcfr/CFRSearch.cfm?fr=101.91

Questions and Answers: Gluten-Free Labeling Final Rule
www.fda.gov/Food/GuidanceRegulation/GuidanceDocumentsRegulatoryInformation/Allergens/ucm362880.htm

Guidance for Industry: Gluten-Free Labeling of Foods; Small Entity Compliance Guide
www.fda.gov/Food/GuidanceRegulation/GuidanceDocumentsRegulatoryInformation/ucm402549.htm

Gluten-Free Labeling of Foods: Overview
www.fda.gov/Food/GuidanceRegulation/GuidanceDocumentsRegulatoryInformation/Allergens/ucm362510.htm

Gluten and Food Labeling: FDA's Regulation of Gluten-Free Claims
www.fda.gov/Food/ResourcesForYou/Consumers/ucm367654.htm

History of the Development of the Final Gluten-Free Rule

FDA's Response to Comments on the Report Titled "Health Hazard Assessment for Gluten Exposure in Individuals with Celiac Disease." December 2012.
www.fda.gov/downloads/Food/FoodScienceResearch/RiskSafetyAssessment/UCM362401.pdf

Federal Register Food Labeling; Gluten-Free Labeling of Foods; Reopening of the Comment Period. August 3, 2011.
www.gpo.gov/fdsys/pkg/FR-2011-08-03/pdf/2011-19620.pdf

Health Hazard Assessment for Gluten Exposure in Individuals with Celiac Disease: Determination of Tolerable Daily Intake Levels and Levels of Concern for Gluten. May 2011.
www.fda.gov/downloads/Food/ScienceResearch/ResearchAreas/RiskAssessmentSafetyAssessment/UCM264152.pdf

External Peer Review of the FDA/CFSAN Draft Health Hazard Assessment for Gluten in Individuals with Celiac Disease: Determination of Tolerable Daily Intake Levels and Levels of Concern for Gluten. December 2010.
www.fda.gov/downloads/Food/FoodScienceResearch/UCM264150.pdf

Proposed Rule: Food Labeling; Gluten-Free Labeling of Foods. January 23, 2007.
www.gpo.gov/fdsys/pkg/FR-2007-01-23/html/E7-843.htm

Approaches to Establish Thresholds for Major Food Allergens and for Gluten in Food. March 2006.
www.fda.gov/Food/GuidanceRegulation/GuidanceDocumentsRegulatoryInformation/Allergens/ucm106108.htm

FDA's Responses to Public Comments on the Draft Report "Approaches to Establish Thresholds for Major Food Allergens and for Gluten in Food." March 2006.
www.fda.gov/Food/GuidanceRegulation/GuidanceDocumentsRegulatoryInformation/Allergens/ucm106042.htm

Transcript of Public Meeting: Gluten-Free Food Labeling. August 19, 2005.
www.fda.gov/Food/GuidanceRegulation/GuidanceDocumentsRegulatoryInformation/Allergens/ucm107204.htm

Food Labeling; Gluten-Free Labeling of Foods; Public Meeting; Request for Comments. July 19, 2005.
www.gpo.gov/fdsys/pkg/FR-2005-07-19/pdf/05-14196.pdf

Draft Report to Establish Thresholds for Major Food Allergens and for Gluten in Food. June 2005.
www.fda.gov/downloads/Food/GuidanceRegulation/UCM316632.pdf

U.S. Department of Agriculture (USDA)

Federal Inspection Acts (Meat, Poultry and Egg Products)
www.fsis.usda.gov/wps/portal/fsis/topics/rulemaking

A Guide To Federal Food Labeling Requirements for Meat, Poultry and Egg Products
www.fsis.usda.gov/shared/PDF/Labeling_Requirements_Guide.pdf?redirecthttp=true

USDA Food Standards and Labeling Policy Book
www.fsis.usda.gov/OPPDE/larc/Policies/Labeling_Policy_Book_082005.pdf

USDA Labeling/Label Approval
www.fsis.usda.gov/wps/portal/fsis/topics/regulatory-compliance/labeling

Allergens – Voluntary Labeling Statements
www.fsis.usda.gov/wps/portal/fsis/topics/regulatory-compliance/labeling/ingredients-guidance/allergens-voluntary-labeling-statements/allergens-voluntary-labeling-statements

Allergies and Food Safety
www.fsis.usda.gov/wps/portal/fsis/topics/food-safety-education/get-answers/food-safety-fact-sheets/food-labeling/allergies-and-food-safety/allergies-and-food-safety

USDA Ingredients Guidance
www.fsis.usda.gov/wps/portal/fsis/topics/regulatory-compliance/labeling/Ingredients-Guidance

Natural Flavorings on Meat and Poultry Labels
www.fsis.usda.gov/wps/portal/fsis/topics/food-safety-education/get-answers/food-safety-fact-sheets/food-labeling/natural-flavorings-on-meat-and-poultry-labels

Alcohol

Alcohol and Tobacco Tax and Trade Bureau (TTB) Alcohol Beverage Labeling and Advertising
www.ttb.gov/consumer/labeling_advertising.shtml

TTB Regulations
www.ttb.gov/other/regulations.shtml

TTB Allergen Labeling FAQ's
www.ttb.gov/faqs/allergen.shtml

Revised Interim Policy on Gluten Content Statements in the Labeling and Advertising of Wine, Distilled Spirits, and Malt Beverages
www.ttb.gov/rulings/2014-2.pdf

Guidance for Industry: Labeling of Certain Beers Subject to the Labeling Jurisdiction of the Food and Drug Administration
www.fda.gov/Food/GuidanceRegulation/GuidanceDocumentsRegulatoryInformation/LabelingNutrition/ucm166239.htm

FDA Labeling CPG Sec. 510.450 Labeling – Diluted Wines and Cider with Less Than 7% Alcohol
www.fda.gov/ICECI/ComplianceManuals/CompliancePolicyGuidanceManual/ucm074431.htm

Information for Consumers

Ingredient List and Contains Statement on the Food Label: U.S. Food and Drug Administration Guidance for Industry
www.fda.gov/downloads/Food/GuidanceRegulation/UCM265446.pdf (page 23)

To report adverse reactions or other problems with FDA-regulated products
www.fda.gov/Safety/ReportaProblem/ucm059044.htm#food

Consumer Complaint Coordinators, contact the following:
www.fda.gov/Safety/ReportaProblem/ConsumerComplaintCoordinators/default.htm

Canada

Health Canada

Canadian Food and Drug Act
www.laws-lois.justice.gc.ca/eng/acts/f-27/

Food and Drug Regulations (FDR)
www.laws-lois.justice.gc.ca/eng/regulations/c.r.c.,_c._870/index.html

Canadian Food Inspection Agency (CFIA)

Acts and Regulations
www.inspection.gc.ca/about-the-cfia/acts-and-regulations/list-of-acts-and-regulations/eng/1419029096537/1419029097256

CFIA: Food Labelling for Industry
www.inspection.gc.ca/food/labelling/food-labelling-for-industry/eng/1383607266489/1383607344939

CFIA Guidance Document List of Ingredients and Allergens
www.inspection.gc.ca/food/labelling/food-labelling-for-industry/list-of-ingredients-and-allergens/
eng/1383612857522/1383612932341

1220 Enhanced Labelling for Allergen and Gluten Sources and Added Sulphites

Regulations Amending the Food and Drug Regulations (1220-Enhanced Labelling for Food Allergen and Gluten Sources and Added Sulphites). February 16, 2011.
www.gazette.gc.ca/rp-pr/p2/2011/2011-02-16/html/sor-dors28-eng.html

Health Canada Food Allergen Labelling
www.hc-sc.gc.ca/fn-an/label-etiquet/allergen/index-eng.php

Questions and Answers About the New Regulations to Enhance the Labelling of Food Allergens, Gluten and Added Sulphites. August 16, 2012.
www.hc-sc.gc.ca/fn-an/label-etiquet/allergen/project_1220_qa_qr-eng.php

Precautionary Statements

Health Canada: The Use of Food Allergen Precautionary Statements on Prepackaged Foods
www.hc-sc.gc.ca/fn-an/label-etiquet/allergen/precaution_label-etiquette-eng.php

CFIA Guidance Document: Allergen-Free, Gluten-Free and Precautionary Statements
www.inspection.gc.ca/food/labelling/food-labelling-for-industry/allergens-and-gluten/eng/1388152325341/1388152326591

Gluten-Free Labeling

Gluten-Free Regulation B.24.018
www.laws-lois.justice.gc.ca/eng/regulations/c.r.c.,_c._870/index.html

Health Canada's Position on Gluten-Free Claims
www.hc-sc.gc.ca/fn-an/securit/allerg/cel-coe/gluten-position-eng.php

CFIA: Compliance and Enforcement of Gluten-Free Claims
www.inspection.gc.ca/food/labelling/food-labelling-for-industry/allergens-and-gluten/gluten-free-claims/
eng/1340194596012/1340194681961

CFIA Guidance Document Allergen-Free, Gluten-Free and Precautionary Statements (also includes oats, gluten-free beer and fortification of gluten-free foods)
www.inspection.gc.ca/food/labelling/food-labelling-for-industry/allergens-and-gluten/eng/1388152325341/1388152326591

Summary of Comments Received on Health Canada's Proposed Policy Intent for Revising Canada's Gluten-Free Labelling Requirements. July 2012.
www.hc-sc.gc.ca/fn-an/consult/gluten2010/summary-sommaire-eng.php

Health Canada's Proposed Policy Intent for Revising Canada's Gluten-Free Labelling Requirements. May 10, 2010.
www.hc-sc.gc.ca/fn-an/consult/gluten2010/draft-ebauche-eng.php

Oats

Gluten-Free Labelling Claims for Products Containing Specially Produced "Gluten-Free Oats"
www.hc-sc.gc.ca/fn-an/securit/allerg/cel-coe/avoine-gluten-oats-eng.php

Celiac Disease and Gluten-Free Claims on Uncontaminated Oats. May 29, 2015.
www.hc-sc.gc.ca/fn-an/consult/2014-cel-oats-contam-avoine-coel/document-consultation-eng.php

Consultation Summary: Notice of Intent to Issue a Food Marketing Authorization to Allow Gluten-Free Claims for Specially Produced Gluten Free Oats and Products Containing Such Oats. May 29, 2015.
www.hc-sc.gc.ca/fn-an/consult/2015-oats-gluten-avoine-eng.php

Marketing Authorization for Gluten-Free Oats and Foods Containing Gluten-Free Oats. May 19, 2015.
www.gazette.gc.ca/rp-pr/p2/2015/2015-06-03/html/sor-dors114-eng.php

Notice of Intent to Issue a Food Marketing Authorization – Proposed Marketing Authorization to allow gluten-free claims for specially produced "gluten-free oats" and products containing such oats under certain conditions. November 14, 2014.
www.hc-sc.gc.ca/fn-an/consult/2014-oats-gluten-avoine-eng.php

Health Canada's Position on the Introduction of Oats to the Diet of Individuals Diagnosed with Celiac Disease (CD). 2007.
www.hc-sc.gc.ca/fn-an/securit/allerg/cel-coe/oats_cd-avoine-eng.php

CFIA Guidance Document Allergen-Free, Gluten-Free and Precautionary Statements (also includes oats)
www.inspection.gc.ca/food/labelling/food-labelling-for-industry/allergens-and-gluten/eng/1388152325341/1388152326591

Canadian Celiac Association Professional Advisory Council Position Statement on Consumption of Oats by Individuals with Celiac Disease. May 29, 2015.
www.celiac.ca/?page_id=2831

Alcohol

Food and Drug Regulations Division 2: Alcoholic Beverages
www.laws-lois.justice.gc.ca/eng/regulations/c.r.c.,_c._870/index.html

CFIA Guidance Document Allergen-Free, Gluten-Free and Precautionary Statements (also includes gluten-free beer)
www.inspection.gc.ca/food/labelling/food-labelling-for-industry/allergens-and-gluten/eng/1388152325341/1388152326591

Labelling Requirements for Alcoholic Beverages
www.inspection.gc.ca/food/labelling/food-labelling-for-industry/alcohol/eng/1392909001375/1392909133296

List of Ingredients and Allergens: Requirements (Alcohol Ingredient Exemption)
www.inspection.gc.ca/food/labelling/food-labelling-for-industry/list-of-ingredients-and-allergens/eng/1383612857522/1383612932341?chap=1

Product Specific Information for Beer
www.inspection.gc.ca/food/labelling/food-labelling-for-industry/alcohol/eng/1392909001375/1392909133296?chap=9

Gluten-Free Claims (Gluten-Free Beer)
www.inspection.gc.ca/food/labelling/food-labelling-for-industry/allergens-and-gluten/eng/1388152325341/1388152326591?chap=2#s4c2

Vintage Wines and Application of Enhanced Allergen Regulations
www.hc-sc.gc.ca/fn-an/label-etiquet/allergen/vintage-wine-vin-millesimes-eng.php

Information for Consumers

Food Allergies and Allergen Labeling – Information for Consumers
www.inspection.gc.ca/food/information-for-consumers/fact-sheets/food-allergies/eng/1332442914456/1332442980290

How To Read a Food Label
www.healthycanadians.gc.ca/eating-nutrition/label-etiquetage/index-eng.php

Food Allergen and Gluten Declaration on a Food Label
www.inspection.gc.ca/food/labelling/food-labelling-for-industry/list-of-ingredients-and-allergens/eng/1383612857522/1383612932341?chap=2#s7c2

Report a Food Safety or Labelling Concern
www.inspection.gc.ca/food/information-for-consumers/report-a-concern/eng/1364500149016/1364500195684

Celiac Disease
www.hc-sc.gc.ca/fn-an/securit/allerg/cel-coe/index-eng.php

Important Information for Canadians with Wheat Allergies
www.healthycanadians.gc.ca/recall-alert-rappel-avis/hc-sc/2011/13606a-eng.php

Codex Alimentarius Commission

About the Codex Alimentarius
www.codexalimentarius.org/about-codex/en/

Standard for Foods for Special Dietary Use for Persons Intolerant to Gluten CODEX STAN 118-1979 (originally adopted in 1979; amendments 1983 and 2015; revision 2008)
www.codexalimentarius.org/standards/list-of-standards/en

Nutrition and the Gluten-Free Diet

Nutritional Status of Individuals with Celiac Disease

Alzaben A, Turner J, Shirton L, et al. Assessing nutritional quality and adherence to the gluten-free diet in children and adolescents with celiac disease. *Can J Diet Pract Res* 2015; 76:56–63.

Barone M, Della Valle N, Rosania R, et al. A comparison of the nutritional status between adult celiac patients on a long-term, strictly gluten-free diet and healthy subjects. *Eur J Clin Nutr* 2016; 70:23–7.

Botero-López J, Araya M, Parada A, et al. Micronutrient deficiencies in patients with typical and atypical celiac disease. *J Pediatr Gastroenterol Nutr* 2011; 53:265–70.

Cheng J, Brar P, Lee A, et al. Body Mass index in celiac disease: Beneficial effect of a gluten-free diet. *J Clin Gastroenterol* 2010; 44:267–71.

Corazza G, Di Stefano M, Mauriño E, et al. Bones in coeliac disease: Diagnosis and treatment. *Best Pract Res Clin Gastroenterol* 2005; 19:453–65.

Crider K, Bailey L, Berry R. Folic acid food fortification: Its history, effect, concerns, and future directions. *Nutrients* 2011; 3:370–84.

Dahele A, Ghosh S. Vitamin B_{12} deficiency in untreated celiac disease. *Am J Gastroenterol* 2001; 96:745–50.

Dickey W. Low serum vitamin B_{12} is common in coeliac disease and is not due to autoimmune gastritis. *Eur J Gastroenterol Hepatol* 2002; 14:425–7.

Dickey W, Kearney N. Overweight in celiac disease: Prevalence, clinical characteristics, and effect of a gluten-free diet. *Am J Gastroenterol* 2006; 101:2356–9.

Duerksen D, Leslie W. Longitudinal evaluation of bone mineral density and body composition in patients with positive celiac serology. *J Clin Densitom* 2011; 14:478–83.

Garcia-Manzanares A, Tenias J, Lucendo A. Bone mineral density directly correlates with duodenal Marsh stage in newly diagnosed adult celiac patients. *Scand J Gastroenterol* 2012; 47:927–36.

Hallert C, Grant C, Grehn S, et al. Evidence of poor vitamin status in coeliac patients on a gluten-free diet for 10 years. *Aliment Pharmacol Ther* 2002; 16:1333–9.

Heikkilä K, Pearce J, Mäki M, et al. Celiac disease and bone fractures: A systematic review and meta-analysis. *J Clin Endocrinol Metab* 2015; 100:25–34.

Kabbani T, Goldberg A, Kelly C, et al. Body mass index and the risk of obesity in coeliac disease treated with the gluten-free diet. *Aliment Pharmacol Ther* 2012; 35:723–9.

Kinsey L, Burden S, Bannerman E. A dietary survey to determine if patients with coeliac disease are meeting current healthy eating guidelines and how their diet compares to that of the British general population. *Eur J Clin Nutr* 2008; 62:1333–42.

Lerner A, Shapira Y, Agmon-Levin N, et al. The clinical significance of 25OH-Vitamin D status in celiac disease. *Clin Rev Allergy Immunol* 2012; 42:322–30.

Mager D, Qiao J, Turner J. Vitamin D and K status influences bone mineral density and bone accrual in children and adolescents with celiac disease. *Eur J Clin Nutr* 2012; 66:488–95.

Martin J, Geisel T, Maresch C, et al. Inadequate nutrient intake in patients with celiac disease: Results from a German dietary survey. *Digestion* 2013; 87:240–6.

Mora S, Barera G, Beccio S, et al. A prospective, longitudinal study of the long-term effect of treatment on bone density in children with celiac disease. *J Pediatr* 2001; 139:516–21.

Saturni L, Ferretti G, Bacchetti T. The gluten-free diet: Safety and nutritional quality. *Nutrients* 2010; 2:16–34.

Shepherd S, Gibson P. Nutritional inadequacies of the gluten-free diet in both recently-diagnosed and long-term patients with coeliac disease. *J Hum Nutr Diet* 2013; 26:349–58.

Simpson S, Thompson T. Nutrition assessment in celiac disease. *Gastrointest Endoscopy Clin N Am* 2012; 22:787–809.

Theethira T, Dennis M. Celiac disease and the gluten-free diet: Consequences and recommendations for improvement. *Dig Dis* 2015; 33:175–82.

Tucker E, Rostami K, Prabhakaran S, et al. Patients with coeliac disease are increasingly overweight or obese on presentation. *J Gastrointestin Liver Dis* 2012; 21:11–5.

Ukkola A, Mäki M, Kurppa K, et al. Changes in body mass index on a gluten-free diet in coeliac disease: A nationwide study. *Eur J Intern Med* 2012; 23:384–8.

Valletta E, Fornaro M, Cipolli M, et al. Celiac disease and obesity: Need for nutritional follow-up after diagnosis. *Eur J Clin Nutr* 2010; 64:1371–2.

Wierdsma N, van Bokhorst-de van der Schueren M, Berkenpas M, et al. Vitamin and mineral deficiencies are highly prevalent in newly diagnosed celiac disease patients. *Nutrients* 2013; 5:3975–92.

Wild D, Robins G, Burley V, et al. Evidence of high sugar intake, and low fibre and mineral intake, in the gluten-free diet. *Aliment Pharmacol Ther* 2010; 32:573–81.

Zanchetta M, Longobardi V, Bai J. Bone and Celiac Disease. *Curr Osteoporos Rep* 2016; 14:43–8.

Nutritional Quality of Gluten-Free Specialty Products

Kulai T, Rashid M. Assessment of nutritional adequacy of packaged gluten-free food products. *Can J Diet Pract Res* 2014; 75:186–90.

Lee A, Ng D, Dave E, et al. The effect of substituting alternative grains in the diet on the nutritional profile of the gluten-free diet. *J Hum Nutr Diet* 2009; 22:359–63.

Mazzeo T, Cauzzi S, Brighenti F, et al. The development of a composition database of gluten-free products. *Public Health Nutr* 2015; 18:1353–7.

Miranda J, Lasa A, Bustamante M, et al. Nutritional differences between a gluten-free diet and a diet containing equivalent products with gluten. *Plant Foods Hum Nutr* 2014; 69:182–7.

Missbach B, Schwingshackl L, Billman A, et al. Gluten-free food database: The nutritional quality and cost of packaged gluten-free foods. *Peer J* 2015; 3:e1337.

Pellegrini N, Agostoni, C. Nutritional aspects of gluten-free products. *J Sci Food Agric* 2015; 95:2380–5.

Thompson T. Folate, iron and dietary fiber contents of the gluten-free diet. *J Am Diet Assoc* 2000; 100:1389–96.

Thompson T. Thiamin, riboflavin, and niacin contents of the gluten-free diet: Is there cause for concern? *J Am Diet Assoc* 1999; 99:858–62.

Thompson T, Dennis M, Higgins L, et al. Gluten-free diet survey: Are Americans with coeliac disease consuming recommended amounts of fibre, iron, calcium and grain foods? *J Hum Nutr Diet* 2005; 18:163–9.

Wu J, Neal B, Trevena H, et al. Are gluten-free foods healthier than non-gluten-free foods? An evaluation of supermarket products in Australia. *Br J Nutr* 2015; 114:448–54.

Enrichment, Fortification and Labeling

Canadian Food Inspection Agency. Fortification of Gluten-Free Foods. www.inspection.gc.ca/food/labelling/food-labelling-for-industry/allergens-and-gluten/eng/1388152325341/1388152326591?chap=3

Canadian Food Inspection Agency. Foods to Which Vitamins, Mineral Nutrients and Amino Acids May or Must be Added [D.03.002, FDR]. www.inspection.gc.ca/food/labelling/food-labelling-for-industry/nutrient-content/reference-information/eng/1389908857542/1389908896254?chap=1

Health Canada. Food and Drug Regulations: B.13.001 (Enriched Flour), B.13.022 (Enriched Bread), B.13.052(2) (Alimentary Paste), B.13.060 (Folic Acid). www.laws-lois.justice.gc.ca/eng/regulations/c.r.c.,_c._870/index.html

Health Canada. Interim Marketing Authorization to Permit the Optional Addition of Vitamins and Mineral Nutrients to Plant-Based Beverages. www.hc-sc.gc.ca/fn-an/legislation/ima-amp/plant_based_beverages-boissons_vegetales-eng.php

Calvo M, Whiting S. "Vitamin D Fortification in North America: Current Status and Future Considerations." *Handbook of Food Fortification and Health*. New York: Springer, 2013: 259–75.

Health Canada. Vitamin D and Calcium: Updated Dietary Reference Intakes. www.hc-sc.gc.ca/fn-an/nutrition/vitamin/vita-d-eng.php#a10

U.S. Food and Drug Administration. Guidance for Industry: Questions and Answers on FDA's Fortification Policy. www.fda.gov/Food/GuidanceRegulation/GuidanceDocumentsRegulatoryInformation/ucm470756.htm

U.S. Code of Federal Regulations (CFR) Title 21 Food and Drugs: Sec. 137.165 (Enriched Flour), Sec. 172.345 Folic Acid (folacin), Sec. 104.20 (Fortification Policy).
www.ecfr.gov/

Dietary Reference Intakes

Health Canada. Dietary Reference Intakes Tables.
www.hc-sc.gc.ca/fn-an/nutrition/reference/table/index-eng.php

National Academy of Sciences. Dietary Reference Intakes Tables and Application.
Food and Nutrition Board, Institute of Medicine of the National Academies.
www.nationalacademies.org/hmd/Activities/Nutrition/SummaryDRIs/DRI-Tables.aspx

General Nutrient References

National Osteoporosis Foundation. Calcium/Vitamin D.
www.nof.org/calcium

Nelms M, Sucher K, Lacey K, et al. *Nutrition Therapy and Pathophysiology*, 2nd ed.
Belmont, CA: Cengage Learning, 2011.

Office of Dietary Supplements, National Institutes of Health. Vitamin and Mineral Supplement Fact Sheets.
www.ods.od.nih.gov/factsheets/list-VitaminsMinerals/

Osteoporosis Canada. Nutrition: Healthy Eating for Healthy Bones.
www.osteoporosis.ca/osteoporosis-and-you/nutrition/

Whitney E, Rolfes S. *Understanding Nutrition*, 14th ed.
Belmont, CA: Cengage Learning, 2013.

Nutrient Composition

Nutrient composition values can vary considerably depending on factors such as:

- specific variety, growing conditions and processing of the grain, legume, nut or seed;
- coarseness of the grind of the grain and sifting process used to produce the flour; and
- individual laboratory analytical methods and testing equipment used for nutrient analysis.

Most of the nutritional information for the tables and appendices on pages 72–74, 76, 81–84, 86–88, 90, 91, 93–96 and 318–323 was obtained from:

USDA Nutrient Database for Standard Reference Release #28
U.S. Department of Agriculture, Agricultural Research Service, Nutrient Data Laboratory.
USDA National Nutrient Database for Standard Reference (Release 28, released September 2015, slightly revised May 2016).
https://ndb.nal.usda.gov/

Other nutrient information from:

Food/Ingredient	Weight Source	Nutrient Analysis Source
Almond Flour (blanched)	Bob's Red Mill (BRM)	USDA
Almond Meal (natural with skins)	BRM	USDA
Amaranth Flour	BRM	Ardent Mills*
Black Bean Flour (whole)	Canadian International Grains Institute (CIGI)**	Best Cooking Pulses (BCP)
Chestnut Flour	Allen Creek Farm	Calculated from USDA (chestnuts); Allen Creek Farm (fiber content)
Chickpea Flour (whole)	CIGI**	BCP
Garfava™ Flour	Authentic Foods	Authentic Foods
Guar Gum	BRM	USDA

* Ardent Mills www.ardentmills.com
** Canadian International Grains Institute (CIGI) www.cigi.ca

Food/Ingredient	Weight Source	Nutrient Analysis Source
Hazelnut Flour	BRM	USDA
Lentil Flour (whole)	CIGI**	BCP
Mesquite Flour	Peter Felker; Casa de Mesquite	References: see Mesquite section, below
Navy Bean Flour (whole)	CIGI**	BCP
Nutritional Yeast	BRM	BRM (vitamin B_{12})
Oat Flour (gluten free)	Cream Hill Estates	Cream Hill Estates; Avena Foods (magnesium, zinc, folate, vitamin B_6 values)
Oats – Steel-Cut (gluten free, raw)	Avena Foods	Calculated from USDA
Oats – Steel-Cut (gluten free, cooked)	Oats from Avena Foods cooked by S. Case to determine prepared weight	Calculated from USDA
Pea Flour – Yellow (whole)	CIGI**	BCP
Pinto Bean Flour (whole)	CIGI**	BCP
Potato Starch	BRM	BRM
Quinoa Flour	BRM	Ardent Mills*
Rice Flour – Sweet	BRM	BRM
Sorghum Grain – White (refined/pearled, raw)	Wondergrain	Calculated from USDA (using refined sorghum flour)
Sorghum Grain – White (refined/pearled, cooked)	Sorghum from Wondergrain cooked by S. Case to determine prepared weight	Calculated from USDA (using refined sorghum flour)
Sorghum Grain – White (whole grain, cooked)	Sorghum from Wondergrain cooked by S. Case to determine prepared weight	Calculated from USDA
Tapioca Starch/Flour	BRM	BRM
Teff Flour	BRM	Ardent Mills*
Teff Grain (raw)	USDA	USDA Silliker Labs (folate value)
Xanthan Gum	BRM	BRM

* Ardent Mills www.ardentmills.com
** Canadian International Grains Institute (CIGI) www.cigi.ca

Mesquite and Mesquite Flour

Becker R, Grosjean O. A compositional study of pods of two varieties of mesquite (Prosopis glandulosa, P. velutina). *J Agric Food Chem* 1980; 28:22–5.

Felker P, Grados N, Cruz G, et al. Economic assessment of production of flour from Prosopis alba and P. pallida pods for human food applications. *J Arid Environ* 2003; 53:517–28.

Felker P, Takeoka G, Dao L. Pod Mesocarp Flour of North and South American Species of Leguminous Tree Prosopis (Mesquite): Composition and Food Applications. *Food Reviews International* 2013; 29:49–66.

Grados N, Cruz G. New approaches to industrialization of algarrobo (Prosopis pallida) pods in Peru. www.researchgate.net/publication/237729419

Meyer D. Processing, utilization and economics of mesquite pods as a raw material for the food industry. Swiss Federal Institute of Technology. PhD Diss. ETH 7688. 1994.

Prokopuik D. Sucedáneo del café a partir de algarroba de Prosopis alba Griseb (Coffee substitute from the pods of Prosopis alba Griseb). Tesis Doctoral (PhD Thesis). Registro N°2183. Universidad Politécnica deValencia, Espana 2005.

Saunders R, Becker R, Meyer D, et al. Identification of commercial milling techniques to produce high sugar, high fiber, high protein and high galactomannan gum fractions from Prosopis pods. *Forest Ecology Management* 1986; 16:169–80.

Teff Grain – raw (folate value)

Analyzed December 14, 2005, by Silliker Canada Co., 90 Gough Road, Markham, ON, Canada L3R 5V5.

Index

A

Absolutely Gluten Free, 222, 224, 256, 264
Additives, 25–26, 295
Against The Grain, LLC., 287
Agave Nectar/Syrup, 14, 17, 25, 32
Alcohol
    about, 15, 17, 31–34
    Alcohol and Tobacco Tax and Trade Bureau (TTB), 51, 52, 56, 63–64, 308, 311, 328, 333
    beer, 10, 15, 17, 24, 33, 34, 63–64, 262, 311, 328, 333, 335
    distilled, 15, 17, 32, 34, 63–64, 311, 327
    Food and Drug Administration (FDA), 64, 333
    hard cider, 15, 18, 22, 34, 63–64, 333
    Health Canada, 64, 328, 335
    gluten-free status, 15, 17, 22, 24, 32–34
    labeling, 51, 52, 56, 63–64, 308, 311, 333, 335
    liqueurs, 15, 17, 32, 34, 63–64, 311
    specialty premixed, 15, 22, 34, 63–64
    wine, 15, 22, 32–34, 63–64, 311, 327–328, 333, 335
Ale, see Alcohol – Beer
Aleias Gluten Free Foods, 218, 242, 264, 305
All But Gluten (Weston Bakeries, Ltd.), 67, 212, 214, 215, 217, 264
Allen Creek Farm, 231, 238, 264
Allergens, 52, 53
Almonds
    flour, meal, 147, 149, 238
    gluten-free status, 11, 13
    nutrition, 318, 321, 322
Amaranth
    about, 16, 97, 98, 144
    flour, 98,148
    gluten-free status, 11, 12, 16, 98
    nutrition, 318, 319, 322, 323
Amy's Kitchen, Inc., 212, 217, 218, 246, 250, 253, 256, 257, 264, 305
Ancient Harvest Quinoa Corporation, 208, 227, 239, 243, 244, 250, 254, 264, 305
Andean Dream, LLC., 218, 250, 257, 264
Anemia, 1, 2, 7, 66, 79, 84, 89
Anheuser-Busch, Inc., 262, 264, 282
Annie Chun's, Inc., 244, 250, 264
Annie's Homegrown, Inc., 218, 227, 254, 264, 305
Apetito, 246, 265
Appendices, 305–323
Applegate Farms, 247, 249, 265
Arnel's Originals, 231, 265
Arrowroot
    about, 111, 148
    gluten-free status, 11
    starch / flour, 111, 148
    thickening with, 155
Aspartame, 25, 63
Atta, 10, 11, 23
Authentic Foods, 16, 149, 231, 238–24, 265
Autoimmune Diseases/Disorders, 1, 3, 74, 89
Avena Foods, Ltd., 211, 235, 239, 243, 265, 280, 305
Avenin, 9, 28, 312

B

Bagels – Ready-to-Eat, 215
Baguettes – Ready-to-Eat, 213
Bakeries – Cross-Contamination, 132
Bakery On Main, 208, 224, 227, 243, 265, 305
Baking
    gluten-free, 147–156
    gluten-free flour blends, 152
    mixes, 231–237
Baked/Canned Beans, 13, 20
Baking Powder, 15, 22, 153
Balsamic Vinegar, see Vinegars
Banza, 250, 254, 265
Barbara's, 67, 208, 265, 305
Bard's Tale Beer Company, LLC., 262, 265
Barilla (Barilla America, Inc.), 250, 266
Barkat (Gluten Free Foods), 208, 212–214, 216, 218, 221, 222, 224, 227, 231, 242, 250, 254, 260, 266
Barley
    about, 9, 10
    beer, see alcohol–beer
    gluten-free status, 10–12, 57, 98
    grass, 15, 37, 42, 328
    labeling, 49–55, 57, 59–62, 63, 64, 309, 329
    malt, 10–12, 33, 34, 37, 42, 309, 329
    malted barley flour, 10, 39, 42, 62
    malt extract / malt syrup, 10, 38, 42, 309, 329
    malt flavoring, 10, 38, 42, 309, 329
    malt vinegar, see vinegars
Beanfields Snacks, 225, 266
Beanitos, Inc., 225, 266
Beans (Dried), see Legumes
Beetnik Foods, LLC., 247, 254, 266
BeFreeForMe.com, 133
Benedictine Sisters of Perpetual Adoration (BSPA), 19, 224
Best Cooking Pulses, Inc., 238, 266
Beverages
    gluten-free status, 11, 15, 17, 21, 22, 24, 31–34
    non-dairy, 11, 69, 74, 77, 101–103,105, 109
Beyond Celiac, 50, 289, 292, 293, 303, 304
BFree Foods, Ltd., 212–215, 266
Bgreen Foods (Big Green (USA) Inc.), 238–240, 251, 261, 266
Bionaturae, LLC., 251, 266
Biopsy – Small Intestinal, 3–7
Birkett Mills, The, 211, 235, 238, 243, 266, 277, 281, 286
Blended Vinegar, see Vinegars
Blood Tests, 3, 4
Blue Cheese, 11, 16, 328
Blue Diamond Almonds (Blue Diamond Growers), 222, 266, 305
Blue Horizon (Elevation Brands, LLC.), 247, 249, 267
Bob & Ruth's Gluten-Free Dining & Travel Club, 302
Bobo's Oat Bars, 227, 267, 305
Bob's Red Mill Natural Foods, Inc., 208, 209, 232, 237–241, 243, 267, 305
Bold Organics, 256, 267
Bone Disease / Bone Health, 77–78
Books, 294–296, 303–304
Bouillons, Bouillon Cubes
    gluten-free status, 14, 21
    products, 257–260
Boulder Organic Foods, LLC., 257, 267

Bourbon, *see* Alcohol – Distilled
Brandy, *see* Alcohol – Distilled
Bread Crumbs, Breading
    cooking, 133, 148, 149, 151
    products, 241, 242
Bread
    baking mixes, 231–237
    dough, 221
    gluten content, 44
    ready-to-eat, 212–213
    sticks, 222–223
Breads From Anna (Anna's Allergen Free, Inc.), 232, 267
Breton (Dare Foods), 222, 225, 267
Brewer's Yeast, *see* Yeast
Broths
    gluten-free status, 14, 21
    products, 257–260
Brownies
    baking mixes, 231–237
    ready-to-eat, 217
Brown Rice Syrup, *see* Rice Syrup
Buckwheat
    about, 16, 99, 144
    flour, 19, 99, 148
    gluten-free status, 11, 12, 16, 19, 98
    noodles / pasta, 19, 99
    nutrition, 318, 319, 322, 323
Bulgur, 10, 11, 23
BumbleBar, Inc., 227, 267, 275
Buns and Rolls
    baking mixes, 231–237
    ready-to-eat, 214, 215
Burgers
    gluten-free status, 13, 20
    ready-to-eat, 247, 249, 250

C

Caesar's Pasta, LLC., 245, 254, 267
Cakes
    baking mixes, 231–237
    ready-to-eat, 217, 218
Calcium
    about, 70
    deficiency, 77–78
    Dietary Reference Intake, 70
    food sources, 71, 72–74, 318–321
    supplements, 71, 76
Campbell Company of Canada, 247, 257, 267
Campbell Soup Company, 257, 267
Canadian Celiac Association (CCA), 289, 292, 295, 302, 306, 307
Canadian Food Inspection Agency (CFIA), 51, 334
Candy, 24, 226
CanMar Grain Products, Ltd., 238, 268
Canyon Bakehouse, 212, 214, 215, 217, 268
Canyon Oats (GF Harvest, LLC. [GFO, Inc.]), 209, 268, 272, 305
Cappello's, 221, 245, 251, 256, 268
Caramel
    gluten-free status, 25, 38, 42, 329
    labeling, 58, 60, 309
Carbohydrate Content of Foods, 318–323
Carob Chips / Powder, 15
Casa de Mesquite, 239, 268, 339
Cassava, *see* Tapioca
Catelli (Catelli Foods Corporation), 251, 268

Celiac Disease
    about, 1–5, 324–325
    alternative therapies, 5
    centers and programs, 291, 292
    organizations, 289, 290
Celiac Disease Foundation (CDF), 289, 304
Celiac Support Association, Inc. (CSA), 50, 289, 292
CelifibR (Maplegrove Gluten Free Foods, Inc.), 257, 268
Cereals
    gluten-free status, 12
    ready-to-eat, 208–211
Chapatti, 10
Chebe, 221, 232, 268
CheeCha (CadCan Marketing & Sales, Inc.), 225, 268
Cheese
    gluten-free status, 11, 16, 19
    lactose intolerance, 69
Cherrybrook Kitchen (Healthy Brands Collective), 232, 268
Chestnut Flour, 148, 318, 322
Chia, 13, 17, 108, 321, 323
chic-a-peas, LLC., 225, 268
Chickpeas, *see* Legumes
Chicory, *see* Coffee Substitutes
Chips
    gluten-free status, 14, 21, 24
    products, 224–226
Chocolates / Chocolate Bars, 14, 15, 21
Cider/Apple Vinegar, *see* Vinegars
Cloud 9 Specialty Bakery, 232, 238, 239, 268, 305
Club House (McCormick Canada), 240, 241, 260, 269
Coatings and Crumbs, *see* Bread Crumbs, Breading
Coconut Flour, 148
Code of Federal Regulations (CFR), 51, 53, 56, 308–310, 314, 316, 332, 338
Codex Alimentarius Commission,
    about, 55, 317, 336
    Codex Standard: *Foods for Special Dietary Use for Persons Intolerant to Gluten*, 55, 312, 313, 317, 321, 336
Coffee, Coffee Substitutes, 15, 21, 24
Colors / Coloring Agents, 25
Communion Hosts/Wafers
    gluten-free status, 12, 17, 19
    products, 224
Compliance Policy Guide (CPG), 308, 309–311, 332
Condiments, 15, 17, 22, 24, 136
Confectioner's Sugar, 14, 25
Contains Statement, 49, 50, 52, 53, 58–62, 64
Conte's Pasta Co., Inc., 245, 254, 256, 269
Cookies
    baking mixes, 231–237
    dough, 221
    ready-to-eat, 218–220
Cooking
    gluten free, 143–147, 155–156
    resources, 297–300
Cooksimple (The Healthy Pantry, Inc.), 67, 244, 247, 251, 254, 269
Corn
    about, 99–100
    bran, 11, 100, 148
    flour, 100, 148
    gluten, 9
    gluten-free status, 11, 12, 14, 25, 98
    nutrition, 318, 322
    starch, 11, 40, 59, 100, 111, 149
Cornmeal, 11, 12, 99, 149, 318, 322
Corn Thins (Real Foods), 224, 282

Couscous, 10, 11, 23, 244, 245
Crackers
    gluten-free status, 14, 21
    products, 222–223
Cream Hill Estates, 209, 239, 243, 269, 277, 305
Cross-Contamination, 28, 46, 58, 135–142, 331
Croûtons, 241–242
Crunchmaster (TH Foods, Inc.), 222, 225, 269, 305
Cuisine Santé (Haco, Ltd.), 257, 260, 269
Cuisine Soleil, 209, 232, 238, 239–241, 269
Cup4Cup, LLC., 232, 269
Cybele's (Free to Eat, Inc.), 218, 269, 305

D

Dairy
    beverages, 11, 23, 69
    calcium content, 72
    lactose intolerance, 68, 69
    vitamin D content, 76, 77
Daiya Foods, Inc., 218, 254, 256, 270
Dapsone, 6
Dasheen, see Taro
Dates, 14, 20
DeBoles (The Hain Celestial Group, Inc.), 67, 251, 254, 270
Deep Fryers, 139, 140
Deli Meats, 13, 20
Dempster's Bakery (Canada Bread Company, Limited), 212, 270
Dermatitis Herpetiformis, 5–6, 325
Dextrin
    gluten-free status, 10, 41, 42, 329
    labeling, 59, 310
Dextrose, 25
Dietary Fiber, see Fiber
Dietary Reference Intake (DRI), 67, 70, 75, 79, 85, 90, 92, 338
Dinkel, see Spelt
Dinner Rolls, see Buns and Rolls
Distilled Alcoholic Beverages, see Alcohol
Distilled Vinegar, see Vinegars
DNA Tests, see Genetic Tests
Doctor in the Kitchen, LLC., 222, 270
Domata, 232, 242, 270
Doughnuts
    baking mixes, 234
    ready-to-eat, 218
Dowd & Rogers, 233, 238, 239, 270
Dr. Praeger's Sensible Foods, Inc., 244, 249, 250, 270, 305
Drugs, see Medications
Duinkerken Foods, Inc., 67, 233, 240, 241, 270
Durum, 10, 11, 23, 98

E

Eating Away From Home
    resources, 300–303
    restaurants, 136–140
    social events, 141
    traveling, 142,
Edamame, 105, 146, 321, 323
Eddo, see Taro
Eden Foods, 225, 243, 251, 257, 260, 261, 270
Edward & Sons, 222, 258, 271, 277, 281, 282, 286
Eggs, Egg Products, 13, 20, 51, 56
Einkorn, 10, 11, 23, 98

Element Snacks, Inc., 223, 271
ELISA (Enzyme-Linked Immunosorbent Assay) Tests, 46, 58, 331
El Peto Products, 209, 212–218, 221, 233, 238–242, 271
Emmer, 10, 11, 23, 98
Ener-G Foods, Inc., 67, 212–215, 217–219, 221, 222, 224, 225, 227, 233, 239–242, 271
English Muffins – Ready-to-Eat, 215
Enhanced Labelling For Food Allergens and Gluten Sources and Added Sulphites, 53, 316, 334
Enjoy Life Foods, 67, 219, 225, 227, 233, 271
Enrichment and Fortification, 67, 98, 318–323, 337–338
Entrées – Ready-to-eat, 246–249
EnviroKidz (Nature's Path Foods), 209, 227, 271, 305
Enzyme Supplements, 5
Erewhon (Attune Foods, LLC.), 209, 271, 305
Evol Foods (Boulder Brands USA, Inc.), 247, 254, 271
Explore Cuisine, Inc., 251, 258, 271

F

Farina, 10, 11, 23
Farro/Faro, see Spelt
Feel Good Foods, 244, 247, 271
Fiber
    about, 91
    Dietary Reference Intake, 92
    food sources, 92–96, 318–321
    supplements, 92
Fining Agents, 32, 64, 327
Fish
    gluten-free status, 13, 20
    oils, 76
    products, 244, 246, 248, 249
Flatbreads – Ready-to-Eat, 213
Flavors, Flavorings, 25, 37–39, 42, 52, 60–62, 309, 310, 328
Flax
    about, 108–109, 149,
    gluten-free status, 11, 13
    nutrition, 318, 321–323
Flax4Life, 209, 214, 216, 217, 272, 305
Flours
    about, 147–151
    baking, 153–156
    blends, 152
    gluten-free status, 11, 16, 17, 19, 23
    products, 237–240
Focaccia, 213, 232
FODMAP Carbohydrates, 7–8
Folate
    about, 84
    deficiency, 84
    Dietary Reference Intake, 85
    food sources, 85–88, 318–321
    folic acid, 84, 85
Fondation Québécoise de la Maladie Coeliaque (Quebec Celiac Disease Foundation), 289, 302
Food and Drug Administration (FDA)
    about, 51, 56–62, 64, 308–311, 314, 331–333
    Food Allergen Labeling Consumer Protection Act (FALCPA), 52, 332
    gluten-free labeling, 53, 56–64, 308, 314–316, 331–332
Food and Drug Regulations
    Canada, 53–54, 56–58, 64, 308–311, 316, 334, 335
    USA, 52–53, 56–58, 63–64, 308–311, 314–316, 331–333
Food For Life, 212, 213, 215, 272

Food Safety and Inspection Service (FSIS), *see* U.S. Food Safety and Inspection Service (FSIS)
Foods By George, 215–218, 221, 256, 272
Frankfurters/Wieners, 13, 20
Freedom Foods North America, Inc., 209, 227, 233, 272, 305
Free For All Kitchen (Partners Company), 219, 222, 272
Freekeh, 10, 11, 23
French Fries, 14, 20, 139
Fruits, 14, 20, 83, 88, 95, 96
Fu, 10, 13, 24

G

Gabriella's Kitchen, 245, 253, 254, 272
Garbanzo Beans, *see* Legumes
Garden Lites (Classic Cooking, LLC.), 216, 244, 272, 305
Garfava™ Flour, 11, 16, 149, 238, 265, 318, 322
Gelatin, 14, 26, 156
Genetic Tests, 4
GFB: Gluten Free Bar, The, 225, 227, 272, 305
GF Harvest, LLC. (GFO, Inc.), 209, 239, 243, 268, 272, 305
gfJules, 67, 233, 272, 305
G-Free NYC, 287
Gin, *see* Alcohol – Distilled
Gliadin, 3, 9, 28, 330, 331
Glucose Syrup
    gluten-free status, 25, 41, 42, 330
    labeling, 58, 60, 310, 330
Glutelins, 9, 53
Gluten
    challenge, 4, 7, 43
    definition, 1, 9
    testing, 29, 43, 46, 58, 330, 331
    threshold levels, 43–45, 56–58, 315, 330
Glutenberg, 262, 273
Gluten Free
    claims and symbols, 49, 50, 58, 63, 64, 332, 334, 335
    labeling, *see* labeling
    resources, 289–304
    stores and online retailers, 287, 288
Glutenfree Bakehouse (Whole Foods Market), 212, 214–219, 221, 242, 273, 305
Gluten Free Bistro, LLC., The, 221, 256, 273
Gluten Free Café (The Hain Celestial Group, Inc.), 67, 227, 247, 254, 258, 273
Gluten-Free Certification Organization (GFCO), 50, 292
Gluten-Free Certification Program (GFCP), 50, 292
Glutenfreeda Foods, Inc., 209, 210, 213, 218, 243, 248, 273, 305
Gluten-Free Diet
    by food groups, 11–24
    overview, 9
Gluten-Free Food Program (GFFP), 302
Gluten-Free Food Service (GFFS) Training and Accreditation Program, 303
Gluten-Free Mall, Inc., 288
Gluten-Free Naturals, LLC., 233, 273
Gluten Free Palace, LLC., 288
Gluten-Free Prairie, 210, 219, 233, 239, 243, 273, 305
Gluten-Free Products
    certification, 49, 50, 58, 292
    enriched and fortified, 67
    list of, 205–262
    manufacturers of, 263–286
    nutritional quality, 66–67, 336–337
Gluten-Free Resource Education Awareness Training (GREAT) Kitchens, 303

Gluten Free Watchdog, LLC., 293, 300, 328, 329, 331
Glutenin, 9
Gluten Intolerance Group (GIG), 50, 289, 292, 303, 304
Glutino (Boulder Brands USA, Inc.), 67, 212, 215, 218, 219, 222, 225, 227, 234, 242, 256, 273
Glutinous/Sweet Rice, 11, 16, 102, 150
Gnocchi, 245, 246
GoGo Quinoa, 210, 219, 234, 239, 243, 244, 250, 251, 258, 273
Goldbaum's Natural Foods, 222, 225, 227, 242, 244, 251, 274
Golden Platter Foods, Inc., 249, 274
GoMacro, 228, 274, 305
Good Bean, The, 225, 228, 274
Goodbye Gluten, 287
Good Manufacturing Practices (GMPs), 50, 205
Goodness Knows (Mars, Inc.), 228, 274
GoPicnic, 225, 274, 305
Gorilly Goods, 226, 274
Graham Flour, 10, 11
Grain-Free JK Gourmet, Inc., 210, 226, 228, 234, 238, 274
Grainful, 244, 248, 274, 305
Grains
    about, 97–104
    cooking, 143–145
    cross-contamination, 28, 46, 331
    gluten-free status, 10–12, 16, 17, 19, 23, 27–30, 98
    incorporating into meals and snacks, 112, 116, 118–127
    products, 243
Granola, 12, 208–211
Granola Bars, 227–231
Gravy, Gravy Mixes, 155, 260
Guar Gum, 15, 18, 26, 149, 153, 241, 319

H

Habitant (Cambell Company of Canada), 258, 274
Hail Merry, LLC., 218, 219, 274
Hain Celestial Group, *see* De Boles; Gluten Free Café; Imagine Foods; Rudi's Gluten-Free Bakery
Hamburger Buns, *see* Buns and Rolls
Hamburgers, *see* Burgers
Hard Cider, *see* Alcohol – Hard Cider
Hazelnuts,
    flour, 149, 239
    gluten-free status, 11
    nutrition, 318, 321, 322
Health Canada (HC)
    about, 51, 308–311, 334
    allergen labeling, 53, 64, 334
    gluten-free labeling, 51, 53, 54, 56–62, 64, 316, 334
    oats, 27–30, 54, 57, 326, 335
Hemp, 11, 13, 109, 321, 323
Herbalicious, 287
Herbs, 15, 39, 42, 309, 329
Hilary's Eat Well, 242, 244, 250, 274
HLA (Human Leukocyte Antigen), 4
Hodgson Mill, Inc., 210, 234, 238–243, 245, 251, 275, 305
Hol•Grain, 222, 234, 242, 260, 275
Homefree, LLC., 219, 275, 305
Hominy, 12, 16, 99, 149
Honey, Honey Powder, 14, 21, 25
Hordein, 9, 312, 331
Hosts, *see* Communion Hosts/Wafers
Hot Chocolate, 15, 21

Hot Dog Buns, *see* Buns and Rolls
Hydrolyzed Plant/Vegetable Proteins, 10, 39, 42, 61, 309
Hydrolyzed Wheat Protein, 10, 39, 42, 61, 309

I

Ian's (Elevation Brands, LLC.), 216, 242, 245, 248, 249, 256, 275
Ice Cream, 11, 69, 72
Ice Cream Cones/Cups, 14, 227
Icing Sugar, *see* Confectioner's Sugar
IgA
    Deamidated Gliadin Peptide (DGP), 3
    deficiency, 3
    Endomysial (EMA), 3
    Tissue Transglutaminase, (tTG), 3
IgG
    Deamidated Gliadin Peptide (DGP), 3
    Tissue Transglutaminase, (tTG), 3
Imagine Foods (The Hain Celestial Group, Inc.), 258, 260, 275
Imitation Seafood, *see* Surimi
Ingredient List, 49, 50, 52, 58–62, 64
International Celiac Organizations, 290
Iodine and Dermatitis Herpetiformis, 6
Iron
    about, 79
    deficiency, 79
    Dietary Reference Intake, 79
    food sources, 80–84, 318–321
    supplements, 80
Irritable Bowel Syndrome (IBS), 3, 7
Isomalt, 25

J

Jake's Gluten-Free Market & Bakery, 287
Janell's Gluten-Free Market, 287
Jerky, 13
Joe's Gluten-Free Foods, 245, 275
Jovial Foods, Inc., 219, 234, 251, 275
Juno Bar (BumbleBar, Inc.), 227, 267, 275

K

Kamut, 10, 11, 23, 98
Kaniwa, 11, 16, 101, 102, 144, 149
Karaya Gum, 26
Kashi Canada (Kellogg Company), 210, 276
Kashi Company, The (Kellogg Company), 210, 216, 228, 276
Kay's Naturals, 210, 219, 226, 276
Kellogg Canada, Inc. (Kellogg Company), 67, 210, 228, 276
Kellogg Company, 67, 210, 216, 228, 276, 305
Kikkoman, 242, 261, 276
KIND, LLC., 67, 210, 228, 229, 276, 305
King Arthur Flour, 67, 234, 237–239, 241, 243, 276, 305
Kinnikinnick, 67, 212, 214–219, 221, 235, 242, 276
Kitchen Basics (McCormick & Company, Inc.), 258, 276
Kitchen Table Bakers, 222, 276
Koji, 15, 22

L

Labeling
    alcohol, 63–64, 308, 311, 327–328, 335
    Canadian regulations, 53–54, 64, 308–311, 316, 327–328, 334–335
    gluten free, 50–64, 331–336
    how to read a food label, 49–50
    precautionary advisory statements, 50, 58, 334–335
    United States regulations, 53, 63–64, 308–311, 314–316, 331–333
Lactase, *see* Lactose Intolerance
Lactose Intolerance, 68–70
Lager, *see* Alcohol – Beer
Lakefront Brewery, Inc., 262, 277
La Messagère (Les bières de la Nouvelle-France), 262, 277
Lärabar (Small Planet Foods Canada), 229, 277
Lärabar (Small Planet Foods, Inc.), 229, 277
Lara's (Cream Hill Estates), 209, 269, 277, 305
Larrowe's (The Birkett Mills), 235, 266, 277
La Tortilla Factory, 214, 277
Le Asolane (Molino di Ferro), 252, 277
Legumes
    about, 104–108
    cooking, 145–147
    flours, 11, 16, 105, 147–151
    gluten-free status, 11–13, 16
    incorporating into meals and snacks, 113, 116, 118–127
    nutrition, 318, 319, 321–323
Lentils, *see* Legumes
Leo's Gluten Free, 246, 253, 254, 277
Les bières de la Nouvelle-France, 262, 277
Let's Do... (Edward & Sons), 227, 277
Let's Do... Organic (Edward & Sons), 227, 238–241, 277
Le Veneziane (Molino di Ferro), 219, 223, 246, 252, 272
Libre Naturals, Inc., 210, 229, 243, 277, 305
Licorice, 14, 24, 224, 226
Liqueurs, *see* Alcohol – Liqueurs
Little Northern Bakehouse, 213, 214, 278
Lorenzo's Specialty Foods, Ltd., 288
Lotus Foods, Inc., 223, 245, 252, 258, 278
Louise Sans Gluten Free, 288
Lucy's, 217, 219, 278, 305
Luncheon Meats, *see* Deli Meats
Lundberg Family Farms, 223, 245, 252, 254, 278

M

Magazines, 296–297
Magnesium, 318–321
Malabsorption, 1, 66
Malt, *see* Barley – Malt
Malted Barley Flour, *see* Barley – Malted Barley Flour
Malted Milk, 10, 11, 23
Malt Extract/Syrup, *see* Barley – Malt Extract / Malt Syrup
Malt Flavoring, *see* Barley – Malt Flavoring
Maltitol, Maltitol Syrup, 25
Maltodextrin
    gluten-free status, 26, 41, 42, 330
    labeling, 58, 60, 310, 330
Maltol, Ethyl Maltol, 25
Maltose, 25
Manini's, 214, 235, 253, 255, 278
Manioc, *see* Tapioca
Maplegrove Gluten Free Foods, Inc., *see* CelifibR; Pastariso; Pastato
Mary's Gone Crackers, 219, 223, 226, 278
Masa Harina Flour, 16, 99, 149

Matzo/Matzoh/Matzah, 10,12, 17, 23
Meal Ideas
    breakfast, 112–114, 118, 121, 128, 129–130
    lunch, 112–114, 119, 122–124, 129–130
    snacks, 112–114, 120, 126–130
    supper/dinner, 112–114, 119, 124–126, 129–130
Meal Planning, 115–130
Meats and Alternatives
    gluten-free status, 13, 17, 20, 24
    nutrition, 80, 82, 87, 90, 91, 321, 323
Meat Substitutes,
    gluten-free status, 10, 13, 17, 20, 24
    types, 105, 106
Medication Resource, 304
Mesquite
    about, 107–108, 339
    flour, 16, 149, 239
    gluten-free status, 11, 16
    nutrition, 318, 322, 339
Mikey's, LLC., 215, 221, 278
Milk
    calcium, 71, 72
    gluten-free status, 11, 23
    lactose intolerance, 68–70
    vitamin B_{12}, 91
    vitamin D, 76, 77
Millet
    about, 16, 100, 144, 243
    flour, 100, 149
    gluten-free status, 11, 12, 16, 98
    nutrition, 318, 320, 322, 323
Milton's Craft Bakers, 219, 223, 278
Miso, 15, 17, 22, 24, 106
Modern Table, Inc., 252, 255, 278, 305
Modified Food Starch
    gluten-free status, 40, 42
    labeling, 59, 310
Molasses, 14, 25, 84
Monosodium Glutamate (MSG), 15, 25
Mrs. Leeper's (World Finer Foods), 252, 255, 258, 278
Muffins
    baking mixes, 231–237
    ready-to-eat, 215–216
Mustard
    condiment, 15, 17, 22
    flour, 15, 17, 22
    pickles, 15, 22

N

Namaste Foods, 235, 238–242, 255, 258, 279
National Foundation for Celiac Awareness (NFCA),
        see Beyond Celiac
Natural Flavorings, see Flavors, Flavorings
Nature's Path Foods, 210, 211, 216, 229, 271, 279, 305
Neat Foods, LLC., 248, 279, 305
Niacin, see Vitamin B_3
NoGii (SBI Brands), 229, 279
Non-Celiac Gluten Sensitivity (NCGS), 6, 7, 325, 326
NorQuin (Northern Quinoa Corporation), 239, 243, 279
North American Society for the Study of Celiac Disease
        (NASSCD), 289
Nourish Snacks, 226, 279, 305
Nu Life Market, LLC., 235, 240, 243, 279
Nutritional Concerns, 67–96, 336–338
Nutrient Composition of Grains, Flours, Starches, Gums,
        Legumes, Nuts and Seeds, 318–323, 338–339
Nutritional Status, 66, 336–337

Nuts
    flours, 147–150
    gluten-free status, 11, 13, 20, 21
    incorporating into meals and snacks, 114, 116, 118,
        120, 121, 125, 126, 129, 130
    nutrition, 318, 321, 322, 323

O

Oats
    about, 100–101, 326–327
    companies with gluten-free oat products, 305
    flour, 101, 150
    gluten-free status, 10, 11, 12, 16, 19, 27–30, 98,
        306–307, 326, 327, 335
    labeling, 49, 53, 54, 55, 57, 335
    mechanical and optical sorting, 29
    nutrition, 318, 320, 322, 323
    purity protocol, 28
O'Doughs, 213–217, 256, 279
Olivia's Croutons, 242, 279
1-2-3 Gluten-Free, 67, 217, 235, 280
Only Oats (Avena Foods, Ltd.), see Avena Foods, Ltd.
Orgran, 211, 220, 223, 226, 236, 242, 252, 255, 258,
        260, 280
Orzenin, 9
Orzo, 12, 23
Osteomalacia, Osteopenia, Osteoporosis, see Bone
        Disease / Bone Health

P

Pacific Foods, 248, 259, 260, 280
Pamela's Products, Inc., 220, 229, 236, 280, 305
Pancakes, Waffles
    baking mixes, 231–237
    ready-to-eat, 216
Parts Per Million (PPM), 43–46, 330
Pasta
    dry, 250–253
    fresh, 253
    gluten-free status, 12, 19
    pasta meals, 253–255
Pasta Legume, LLC., 252, 280
Pastariso (Maplegrove Gluten Free Foods, Inc.), 252, 255,
        280
Pastato (Maplegrove Gluten Free Foods, Inc.), 67, 252,
        255, 280
PatsyPie, 217, 220, 221, 236, 280
Peas (Dried), see Legumes
Pea Flour, 150, 318, 322, see also Legumes
Peanut Flour, 150, 318, 319, 322
Perfect Bar, 230, 280
Perogies – Products, 245
Pie/Pastry
    baking mixes, 231–237
    crusts, dough, 221
    ready-to-eat, 218
Piping Gourmets, The (Batter Up, LLC.), 217, 280
Pitas – Ready-to-Eat, 213–214
Pizza
    crusts, 221
    dough, 221
    gluten-free status, 12
    mixes, 231–237
    ready-to-eat, 256
Plum-M-Good (Van's Rice Products), 223, 224, 242, 281
Pocono, (The Birkett Mills), 211, 238, 243, 266, 281

Polenta, 19, 100, 102, 144, 149
Potato
    chips, *see* chips
    flour, 150, 239
    gluten-free status, 11
    nutrition, 319, 322
    starch, 11, 59, 111, 150, 155, 241
Poultry, 13, 20, 80, 82, 87, 90
PPM, *see* Parts Per Million
Precautionary Advisory Statements, *see* Labeling
Premier Japan (Edward & Sons), 261, 281
Premium Gold Flax, Inc., 211, 236, 281
President's Choice (Loblaw Companies, Ltd.), 67, 213,
        214, 216, 217, 220, 223, 226, 236, 242, 245,
        248–250, 252, 253, 255, 281
Pretzels–Ready-to-Eat, 224–226
Prolamins, 9, 53, 312
Promax Nutrition Company, 230, 281
Promise Gluten Free (Cuisine Royale Manufacturing, Ltd.),
        213, 215–217, 230, 281
Protein Content of Foods, 318–321
Psyllium, Psyllium Husks,15, 18, 26
Puddings, 14
Pulses, *see* Legumes
Pumpkin Seeds, 13, 20, 110, 321, 323
PureFit, 230, 281, 305
Pure Genius Provisions, 217, 281, 305
Purely Elizabeth, 211, 281, 305
Pure Organic (The Pure Bar Company), 230, 281
Pyridoxine, *see* Vitamin B$_6$

Q

Qrunch Foods, 216, 250, 282
Quaker (PepsiCo Canada), 211, 224, 226, 282, 305
Quaker (PepsiCo, Inc.), 211, 224, 226, 282, 305
Quattrobimbi Imports, Inc., 288
Quickbreads
    baking mixes, 231–237
    ready-to-eat, 215–216
Quinn Foods, LLC., 226, 282
Quinoa
    about, 101–102, 144
    flour, 102, 149, 150
    gluten-free status, 11, 12, 16, 98
    nutrition, 319, 320, 322, 323

R

Real Foods, 224, 269, 282
Really Great Food Company, The, 236, 282
Recipes – Gluten Free
    Breads
        Apple Date Bread, 166
        Banana Seed Bread, 167
        Brown Rice Bread, 158–159
        Cornbread, 161
        Flax & Peanut Focaccia, 165
        Injera (Ethiopian Flatbread), 164
        Oatmeal Bread, 163
        Pumpkin Bread, 168
        Teff Polenta, 162
        Wholesome Flax Bread, 160
    Cake, Cookies & Snack Bars
        Carrot Apple Energy Bars, 176
        Chocolate Banana Rum Cake, 181
        Coconut & Banana Lentil Bites, 178
        Cranberry Pistachio Biscotti, 180
        Fruit n' Nut Bars, 177
        Sorghum Peanut Butter Cookies, 179
        Sweet Sorghum Banana Date Breakfast Cookies,
            175
    Cereals & Trail Mix
        Spiced Apple Cranberry Buckwheat Cereal, 174
        Cajun Lentil Trail Mix with Dark Chocolate, 182
    Entrées & Side Dishes
        Black Bean Chili, 197
        Fresh Rolls with Peanut Dipping Sauce, 189
        Hoisin Lentil Lettuce Wraps, 194
        Lentil Pizza Squares, 202
        Moroccan Millet, 192
        Multi-Grain Pilaf, 191
        Oven-Fried Chicken, 201
        Pepperoni Pizza, 203
        Sahara Stew over Superblend Grains, 198
        Spicy Sweet Potato Bean Burgers, 193
        Tabbouleh with Shrimp on Mixed Greens, 200
        Turkey Meatballs with Lemon Sauce, 199
        Vegetable & Beef Lasagna, 196
        Wild Rice, Chicken & Vegetable Casserole, 195
        Wondergrain Sorghum Stuffing, 190
    Miscellaneous
        Thai Hot-and-Sour Sauce, 204
    Muffins
        Blueberry Almond Muffins, 170
        Mighty Tasty Muffins, 171
        Shelley's Orange Cranberry Muffins, 169
    Pancakes
        Carrot Cake Pancakes, 172
        Teff Banana Pancakes, 173
    Salads
        Brown Rice, Chickpea, Kale Salad, 186
        Moroccan Salad, 185
        Quinoa Salad, 187
        Wild Rice Salad, 188
    Soups
        French Canadian Pea Soup, 184
        Lentil Vegetable Soup, 183
Recognition Seal Program (CSA), 50, 292
Redbridge (Anheuser-Busch), 262, 264, 282
References, 324–339
Resources, 289–304
Restaurants, *see* Eating Away From Home – Restaurants
Riboflavin, *see* Vitamin B$_2$
Rice
    about, 102–103, 144
    bran, 103, 150
    cakes, 223–224
    flour, 103, 150, 156
    gluten-free status, 11, 12, 16, 98
    nutrition, 319, 320, 322, 323
    polish, 16, 103,150
    syrup/malt, 42, 60, 310, 330
    vinegar, *see* vinegars
    wild, *see* wild rice
    wine, *see* alcohol – wine
Rickets, 77
Rise Bar, 230, 282
Rizopia, 252, 282
Road's End Organics (Edward & Sons), 255, 260, 282
Rolls and Buns, *see* Buns and Rolls
Ronzoni, 252, 282
RP's Pasta Company, 253, 282
Rudi's Gluten-Free Bakery (The Hain Celestial Group, Inc.),
        213–215, 230, 283, 305
Rum, *see* Alcohol – Distilled
Rustic Crust, 221, 283

Rye
about, 9
gluten-free status, 10, 11, 12, 98
labeling, 49, 52–55, 57, 59
whiskey, *see* alcohol – distilled

S

Saffron Road (American Halal Co., Inc.), 223, 226, 248, 259, 261, 283
Sago, 11, 16
Sake, *see* Alcohol – Wine
Salad Dressings, 15, 22
Sandwich Tips, 124
San-J International, 223, 259, 261, 283
Sauces
gluten-free status, 15, 17, 18, 22, 24
products, 260–261
thickening, 155–156
Sausages
gluten-free status, 13, 20
products, 247, 248, 250
Savory Choice (Savory Creations International), 259, 261, 283
Schär, Schär USA, 67, 213, 215, 217, 218, 220, 221, 223, 236, 242, 252, 255, 256, 283, 305
Scones/Biscuits
baking mixes, 231–237
ready-to-eat, 215
Scotch Whiskey, *see* Alcohol – Distilled
Sea Fare Pacific (Oregon Seafoods), 248, 259, 283
Seasonings
gluten-free status, 15, 22, 39, 42, 329
labeling, 61, 309, 329
Secalin, 9, 312
Seeds
about, 108–111
gluten-free status, 13, 20
incorporating into meals and snacks, 114, 118–122, 125, 126, 128–130
nutrition, 318, 321 322, 323
Seitan, 10, 13, 24
Semolina, 10, 11, 23
Sesame Seeds, 13, 110, 321, 323
Shopping
list, 134
tips, 131–133
Side Dishes – Products, 244–246
Silver Hills Bakery, 213, 283
Simple Mills, 223, 237, 283
Simply Asia (Simply Asia Foods, Inc.), 261, 284
SimplyProtein (Wellness Foods), 226, 230, 284
Simply Shari's, 220, 284
Smart Flour Foods, 215, 221, 237, 256, 284
Smoke Flavoring
gluten-free status, 39, 42, 328
labeling, 62, 310, 328
Smoothies, 14, 20, 128
Snack Bars – Products, 227–231
Snacks
gluten-free status, 14, 21, 24
ready-to-eat, 224–231
Soba Noodles, *see* Buckwheat – Noodles/Pasta
Sol Cuisine, 249, 250, 284
Sorghum
about, 16, 103, 144, 243
gluten-free status, 11, 12, 16, 98
flour, 103, 151, 156, 240
nutrition, 319, 320, 322, 323

Soups
gluten-free status, 14, 21
products, 257–260
Soy
about, 105–106, 145–146
beans, *see* legumes
flour, 105, 151
gluten-free status, 11, 12, 13, 14, 15, 17, 20, 21, 24
nutrition, 319, 321, 322, 323
sauce, 15, 17, 24, 106, 261
SOYJOY, 230, 284
Specialty Food Shop, 288
Spelt, 10, 11, 23, 98
Spices
gluten-free status, 15, 22, 39, 42, 329
labeling, 61, 309, 329
Starches
about, 40, 42, 111, 148–151
cooking, 155
gluten-free status, 10, 11, 16, 23, 26, 40, 329
labeling, 58, 59, 310
nutrition, 318, 319, 322
products, 240–241
Stocks
gluten-free status, 14, 21
products, 257–260
Stout, *see* Alcohol – Beer
Strictly Gluten Free, 288
Stuffing – Products, 241–242
Suet, 15, 22, 117
Sugar, Sugar Alcohol, Sweeteners, 25
Sunflower Seeds, 13, 20, 110–111, 321, 323
Sunshine Burger and Specialty Food Company, Inc., 250, 284
Surimi / Imitation Seafood, 13, 20, 139
Swanson (Campbell Soup Company), 259, 284
Sweet Potato Flour, 11, 151, 240

T

Tabouli (Tabbouleh), 12, 23
Tahini, 110
Tapioca
about, 111
baking/cooking, 155, 156
gluten-free status, 11, 16
nutrition, 319, 322
starch/flour, 11, 16, 59, 111, 151, 319, 322
Taro, 11, 17
Taste Adventure (Will-Pak Foods, Inc.), 245, 249, 259, 284
Taste of Nature, 231, 284, 305
Tea, 15, 21
Teff
about, 17, 104, 144
flour, 104, 151, 240
gluten-free status, 11, 17, 98
nutrition, 319, 320, 322, 323
Teff Company, The, 240, 243, 284
Tempeh, 13, 20, 106
Tempura, 15, 24
Tequila, *see* Alcohol – Distilled
Teriyaki Sauce, 15, 24, 261
Textured Soy Protein (TSP), 13, 20, 105
Thai Kitchen (Simply Asia Foods, Inc.), 249, 252, 255, 260, 261, 285
Thiamin, *see* Vitamin B_1
Thickeners / Thickening Agents, 155–156

Three Bakers (Gluten Free Food Group, LLC.), 213, 215, 220, 221, 223, 242, 256, 285
Threshold Levels, *see* Gluten –Threshold Levels
Tinkyada, 253, 285
Toaster
  bags, 136, 142
  cross-contamination, 136, 140
Tofu, 13, 17, 20, 106
Tofurky Company, The, 249, 250, 256, 285
Tolerant Foods (MXO Global, Inc.), 253, 285
Tonya's Gluten Free Kitchen, 226, 285
Tortillas, Wraps
  gluten-free status, 12, 19
  ready-to-eat, 213–214
Toufayan Bakeries, Inc., 214, 285
Travel, *see* Eating Away From Home – Traveling
Triticale, 9, 10, 11, 12, 23, 57, 98
TruRoots (The JM Smuckers Company), 243, 245, 253, 285

U

Udi's Gluten Free (Boulder Brands USA, Inc.), 67, 211, 213–218, 220, 221, 226, 231, 243, 249, 255, 256, 285, 305
Udon, 12, 23
U.S. Alcohol and Tobacco and Trade Bureau (TTB)
  about, 51, 52, 308
  labeling, 56, 63–64, 308, 311, 328, 333
U.S. Department of Agriculture (USDA)
  about, 51, 52, 333, 338
  labeling, 56, 59–62, 308–310, 333
U.S. Food Safety and Inspection Service (FSIS), 51, 52, 308–310, 333

V

Vanilla Extract, Flavoring, Imitation, Pure, 15, 18, 25
Van's (Van's International Foods, Inc.), 211, 216, 223, 226, 231, 255, 285, 305
Vegetables, 14, 20, 84, 88, 96
Viki's Foods, 211, 286, 305
Villi, 1, 43, 66, 68, 69
Villous Atrophy, 1, 2, 4, 5, 7, 43
Vinegars
  about, 18, 36, 42, 103, 328
  balsamic, 18, 36, 42
  blended, 18, 36
  distilled white, 18, 36, 42
  gluten-free status, 15, 18, 22, 24, 36, 42, 328
  labeling, 52, 57, 59, 62, 310
  malt, 10, 15, 18, 24, 36, 42, 57, 62, 310
  rice, 22, 36, 42, 103
Vitamin B_1/Thiamin, 318–321
Vitamin B_2/Riboflavin, 318–321
Vitamin B_3/Niacin, 318–321
Vitamin B_6/Pyridoxine, 318–321
Vitamin B_{12}
  about, 89
  deficiency, 89
  Dietary Reference Intake, 90
  food sources, 90–91
Vitamin D
  about, 74–75
  deficiency, 77, 78
  Dietary Reference Intake, 75
  food sources, 76
  fortification, 67, 77
  supplements, 76
Vodka, *see* Alcohol – Distilled

W

Waffles, *see* Pancakes, Waffles
Wasabi Peas, 14, 21
Watusee Foods, 226, 242, 286
Weight Management, 68
Wheat
  about, 9, 10, 98
  bran, 10, 11, 319
  flour, 10, 11, 319
  flour substitutes, 147–151, 155–156
  germ, 10, 11
  gluten, 10, 11, 23, 61
  gluten-free status, 10, 11, 12, 23, 57, 98
  grass, 14, 37, 42, 328
  labeling, 49, 50, 52–55, 57–64, 328, 329
  starch, 10, 11, 23, 26, 40, 42, 329
Whiskey, *see* Alcohol – Distilled
Whole Note Food Company, 237, 286, 305
Wild Rice
  about, 104, 144
  flour, 104
  gluten-free status, 11, 12, 98
  nutrition, 320, 323
Wine, *see* Alcohol – Wine
Wine Vinegar, *see* Vinegars
Wizard's, The (Edward & Sons), 261, 286
Wolff's (The Birkett Mills), 211, 243, 266, 286
Wondergrain (Nature2Kitchen), 237, 240, 243, 286
Woodstock Mini Me's (Blue Marble Brands), 224, 286
Worcestershire Sauce
  gluten-free status, 15, 22
  products, 260–261
WOW Baking Company, 217, 220, 221, 237, 286, 305
Wraps – Ready-to-Eat, *see* Tortillas, Wraps

X

Xanthan Gum, 15, 18, 26, 151, 319
XO Baking Co., 237, 286, 305

Y

Yeast
  autolyzed, 15, 18, 22, 37, 42, 61, 309, 328
  baker's, 15, 18, 26
  brewer's, 10, 15, 24
  extract, 15, 22, 37, 42, 328
  nutritional, 15, 18, 26, 90
  torula, 15, 18, 26
Yeast-Free Breads – Ready-to-Eat, 213
Yogurt
  gluten-free status, 11
  lactose intolerance, 69
Yuca, *see* Tapioca

Z

Zein, 9
Zinc, 318–321
Zing (Northwest Nutritional Foods, LLC.), 231, 286, 305

Gluten Free: The Definitive Resource Guide

Number of copies _____ x $29.95 U.S. = $ _____

Number of copies _____ x $29.95 CDN = $ _____

Shipping and handling (see below) = $ _____

Subtotal = $ _____

In Canada add GST (5%) = $ _____
GST# 867639122

Total enclosed = $ _____

Shipping and Handling

	United States	Canada
1 Book	$8.00	$10.00

More than one book, contact Case Nutrition Consulting, Inc.

✦ Please allow 7–10 days for delivery. Books shipped by USPS or Canada Post.
✦ Payment Methods: Check payable to: **Case Nutrition Consulting, Inc.** (see below)
   Credit Card (Visa or MasterCard)
✦ U.S. orders payable in U.S. funds.

NAME: _____

ORGANIZATION: _____

STREET:_____

CITY:_____ STATE/PROV.:_____

COUNTRY: _____ ZIP/POSTAL CODE:_____

PHONE: _____ FAX: _____

Email: _____

We do not rent, lease or share our mailing list.

Credit Card Orders:

____ Visa ____ MasterCard   Expiry: _____ / _____   Security Code ___ ___ ___

Card Number: _____

Name on Card: _____

Signature: _____

Mail to: **CASE NUTRITION CONSULTING, INC.,**
Suite 1403 | 3520 Hillsdale St.,
Regina, Saskatchewan,
Canada   S4S 5Z5

Online ordering: www.shelleycase.com
Email: info@glutenfreediet.ca
Phone/FAX: 306-751-1000